D1695388

Sports Medicine

Sports Medicine

Finley Edwards

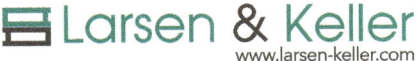
www.larsen-keller.com

Sports Medicine
Finley Edwards
ISBN: 978-1-64172-503-3 (Hardback)

© 2020 Larsen & Keller

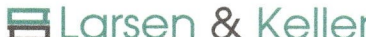

Published by Larsen and Keller Education,
5 Penn Plaza,
19th Floor,
New York, NY 10001, USA

Cataloging-in-Publication Data

Sports medicine / Finley Edwards.
   p. cm.
Includes bibliographical references and index.
ISBN 978-1-64172-503-3
1. Sports medicine. 2. Sports sciences. 3. Medicine. I. Edwards, Finley.
RC1210 .S66 2020
617.102 7--dc23

This book contains information obtained from authentic and highly regarded sources. All chapters are published with permission under the Creative Commons Attribution Share Alike License or equivalent. A wide variety of references are listed. Permissions and sources are indicated; for detailed attributions, please refer to the permissions page. Reasonable efforts have been made to publish reliable data and information, but the authors, editors and publisher cannot assume any responsibility for the validity of all materials or the consequences of their use.

Trademark Notice: All trademarks used herein are the property of their respective owners. The use of any trademark in this text does not vest in the author or publisher any trademark ownership rights in such trademarks, nor does the use of such trademarks imply any affiliation with or endorsement of this book by such owners.

For more information regarding Larsen and Keller Education and its products, please visit the publisher's website www.larsen-keller.com

Table of Contents

Preface .... **VII**

Chapter 1 Introduction to Sports Medicine **1**
    a. Sports Chiropractic 4
    b. Sport Psychology 6
    c. Diagnostic Imaging in Sports Medicine 9

Chapter 2 Orthopedic Sports Medicine **32**
    a. Quality Metrics and Sports Medicine 54
    b. Orthopedic Rehabilitation 56
    c. Orthopedic Physical Therapy 60

Chapter 3 Types of Sports Injuries **71**
    a. Physiology of Sports Injuries 79
    b. Sprains and Strains of Sporting Injuries 108
    c. Sport-related Concussion 109
    d. Knee Injuries 111
    e. Hip Tendonitis 115
    f. Diagnosis of Tendon Injury 116
    g. Sports Hernia 122
    h. Shin Splints 124
    i. Shoulder Injuries 127
    j. Muscle Injuries 136
    k. Tennis Elbow 140
    l. Sports Specific Injuries 147

Chapter 4 Sports Injury: Treatment, Prevention and Rehabilitation **163**
    a. Sport Injury Prevention 164
    b. Price Method 167
    c. Cryotherapy 168
    d. Hydrotherapy 171
    e. Treatment Options for Low Back Pain 173
    f. Non-surgical Treatments 179
    g. Sports Injury Rehabilitation 182
    h. Injury Recovery and Rehabilitation Exercises 190
    i. Recovery Techniques for Athletes 194
    j. Regenerative Therapy 200

Chapter 5 Sports Nutrition and Supplements **205**
    a. Sports Supplements 209

b. Dietary Supplements	216
c. Performance-enhancing Supplements	242
d. Energy Bars	243
e. Sports Drinks	244

Permissions

Index

Preface

The branch of medicine which deals with physical fitness along with the prevention and treatment of sports and exercise injuries is known as sports medicine. Several kinds of ailments and injuries are treated under this field such as ligament, muscle, bone and tendon problems. Chronic illnesses which might deter athletes from performing optimally such as asthma and diabetes are also treated within sports medicine. It helps in making the performance of the athlete more advanced. It also ensures their safety while performing the activity. Common sports injuries include fractures, ankle sprains, knee and shoulder injuries, cartilage injuries, etc. This book provides comprehensive insights into the field of sports medicine. It will also provide interesting topics for research which interested readers can take up. Coherent flow of topics, student-friendly language and extensive use of examples make this book an invaluable source of knowledge.

Given below is the chapter wise description of the book:

Chapter 1- The branch of medicine that is concerned with the prevention and treatment of injuries related to sports and exercise is referred to as sports medicine. It includes sports chiropractic, sport psychology, orthopaedic sports medicine, etc. The topics elaborated in this chapter will help in gaining a better perspective about these branches of sports medicine.

Chapter 2- Orthopedic Sports Medicine focuses on identifying, preserving and restoring musculoskeletal system affected by athletic activity. It includes medical, surgical and rehabilitative methods of treatment. This chapter has been carefully written to provide an easy understanding of orthopedic sports medicine.

Chapter 3- There are some common injuries that are experienced by athletes such as ankle injuries and sprains, fractures and concussions, shoulder injuries, muscle injuries, hip tendonitis, shin splints etc. This chapter discusses these common types of sports injuries in detail.

Chapter 4- Cryotherapy, hydrotherapy, PRICE method, etc. are some methods that are widely used in sports injury preventions. Rehabilitation and physical therapy such as regenerative therapy seek to restore functional ability to those with physical impairments or disabilities. All these aspects related to sports injury treatment, prevention and rehabilitation have been carefully analyzed in this chapter.

Chapter 5- Sports nutrition is defined as the study and practice of implementing appropriate diet and nutrition to improve the athletic performance of a person. It studies the nutrition and quantity of fluids and food taken by an athlete. This chapter closely examines the different dietary supplements under sports nutrition to provide an extensive understanding of the subject.

Indeed, my job was extremely crucial and challenging as I had to ensure that every chapter is informative and structured in a student-friendly manner. I am thankful for the support provided by my family and colleagues during the completion of this book.

Finley Edwards

Introduction to Sports Medicine

The branch of medicine that is concerned with the prevention and treatment of injuries related to sports and exercise is referred to as sports medicine. It includes sports chiropractic, sport psychology, orthopaedic sports medicine, etc. The topics elaborated in this chapter will help in gaining a better perspective about these branches of sports medicine.

Sports medicine is the medical and paramedical supervision, of athletes in training and in competition, with the goal of prevention and treatment of their injuries. Sports medicine entails the application of scientific research and practice to the optimization of health and athletic performance.

Since the revival of the Olympic Games in 1896, increased participation in sport and training for sports have resulted in the need to not only prevent and treat sports injury but also advance the scientific knowledge of the limits of human exercise performance and the causes of fatigue. Moreover, with increased training levels and specialization across the spectrum of recreational sports and with opportunities for sport participants to become professionals, there has been a parallel increase in the careers to support the care and training of athletes and physically active individuals.

Sports Medicine Specialties

Sports medicine is an umbrella term representing a broad array of specialties that bridge the academic disciplines of medicine and physical education as well as the basic sciences (e.g., physiology, chemistry, and physics). Within clinical medicine, physicians in primary care or pediatrics may become team physicians for competitive teams at all levels (interscholastic, intercollegiate, professional, and amateur sports). Other members of a sports medicine team typically include an orthopedic surgeon, a certified athletic trainer, a physical therapist or kinesiotherapist, and a strength-and-conditioning specialist. Other professionals, such as those in the areas of sports nutrition, sports psychology, sports physiology, podiatry, sports vision, sports dentistry, and chiropractic, are valuable consultants.

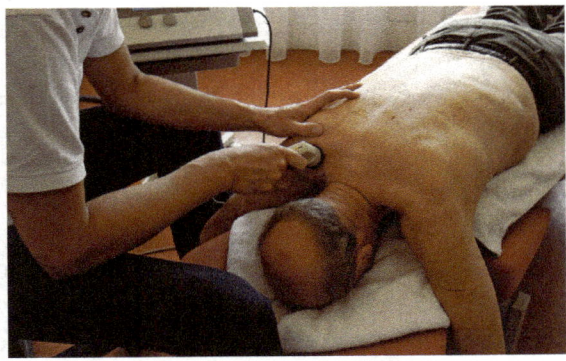

Sports medicine: Physiotherapy A physiotherapist treating the shoulder of a senior patient.

Although sports medicine is more commonly thought to be related specifically to orthopedic medicine, with respect to the treatment and prevention of injuries occurring in a sport, other medical specialties in cardiology, psychiatry, gynecology, and ophthalmology can also play an important role in comprehensive sports medicine. For example, cardiac rehabilitation is an important area in sports medicine that employs not only doctors but also allied health professionals, such as registered clinical exercise physiologists and nurses. These individuals help patients recover and improve their functional capacity following cardiovascular events such as heart attack or cardiac surgery.

A sports medicine team physician can be called upon to treat a wide variety of sports-related injuries or illnesses. One example is an overuse type of injury, such as a stress fracture in the foot or lower leg. An injury such as this can be caused by any of a variety of problems, including muscle imbalance, muscular weakness arising from a lack of proper strength training, improper footwear or abnormal gait, inadequate mineral or other nutrient intake that upsets the caloric balance necessary for training, hormonal deficiency, and overload of exercise training volume, frequency, and intensity. Thus, to effectively treat an overuse injury, a team physician needs expertise and knowledge in a wide range of sports medicine issues.

Sports Medicine and Health

The use of exercise and sport as a therapy to prevent chronic disease is well established. The wide range of health benefits of exercise stem from the several key elements that comprise physical fitness: cardiorespiratory endurance, muscular strength, muscular endurance, flexibility, agility, and body composition.

The relationship between regular physical activity and health has been well established worldwide. Governments of numerous countries have published guidelines that describe the amount of physical activity needed for health, although these guidelines may vary slightly.

In 2008 the U.S. government released *Physical Activity Guidelines for Americans*, the country's first published set of guidelines on the "dose," or amount, of physical activity needed to maintain health for individuals aged six and older. This document was based on a rigorous review by an expert panel of the scientific literature available on exercise and health. The panel found strong evidence indicating that 150 minutes of moderate to vigorous exercise per week for adults helped prevent a wide range of diseases, including cardiovascular disease, stroke, diabetes, hypertension (high blood pressure), certain types of cancer, and depression. This amount of exercise for adults was also associated with a reduced risk of early death, of falls, and of weight gain. There was also moderate evidence indicating that this level of physical activity aids in the prevention of hip fracture, osteoporosis, lung cancer, and endometrial cancer; facilitates weight maintenance after weight loss; and improves sleep quality.

The 2008 U.S. report also indicated that for individuals aged 6 to 17 the baseline dose of exercise needed to obtain health benefits was 60 minutes or more of physical activity every day (physical activity was defined as aerobic or endurance exercise of moderate or vigorous intensity). The greatest health benefits were associated with vigorous activity at least three days per week. Muscle-strengthening and bone-strengthening activities performed at least three days per week for children and at least two days per week for adults were also found to improve health.

In Canada, youths are encouraged to obtain even more minutes of daily activity (60 moderate and 30 vigorous minutes). In general, similar guidelines have been established for all individuals, and they are not considered to be optimal training doses for various sports and athletes. Training for competitive sports generally requires additional sports medicine expertise.

Exercise in therapeutic doses is powerful in preventive medicine. Therefore, in the broadest of terms, sports medicine is applicable to any individual who includes movement as a part of his or her daily life as well as to those who compete on teams or in individual sports—from youth to masters-level events.

Importance of Sports Medicine

Because of the drive and motivation of the people today to push towards a health-conscious world and society, there is an increased interest in participating in recreational sports over the past couple of years. It has given more opportunities for sports medicine. Back in the day, sports medicine was all about treating illnesses and injuries of athletes. Nowadays, with the help of research and technology, sports medicine comes a long way. Sports medicine extends to proper health care, health examination of athletes before they even engage themselves in sports, injury prevention and treatment, rehabilitation, proper exercises, and proper training and nutrition.

The presence of sports medicine is becoming more important these days. If you are an athlete or you engage a lot in different sports, make sure to consult a sports doctor. Just like a family doctor, a sports doctor is more familiar with your activities so it's easier to identify injuries and problems that might be brought about by sports. If you get injured because of sports and you consult other specialists instead of going for someone who is more specialized in sports medicine, there is a risk of having physician negligence.

- Specialized care: Physicians with a specialization in sports medicine are well trained to take good care of sports athletes, sports enthusiasts, fitness professionals, and active individuals. They understand everything about sports including the impact that exercise and sports bring about on an individual's body such as repetitive motion injuries, concussions, etc. They work hand in hand with physical therapists and orthopaedic surgeons to come up with tailored treatment plans that correspond to each patient's specific needs. They can recommend the proper diet and nutrition, training and exercise that are needed by an individual depending on their body's capacity and their activities.

- Enhanced performance: Specialists in sports medicine help athletes and other sports enthusiasts enhance their performance when it comes to sports based on each individual's strengths, weaknesses, and needs. They usually come up with a training plan to help athletes and other enthusiasts maximize their full potential. They are considered experts in sports and they have the knowledge and tools in order to evaluate an individual's strengths and weaknesses, give specific recommendations, and identify areas for improvement.

- Enhanced prevention of injuries: Specialists in sports medicine have a deep knowledge and understanding of how athletes use their bodies in sports practices and actual games. Because of this, they can give expert advice and specific instructions on how to avoid injuries and how to also avoid re-injury of an area that has previously been damaged. They also help athletes decide on whether to return or resume to playing after having an injury which they usually do by running physical exams to make sure that they can already resume to their sporting events and activities.

- Better treatment: Aside from avoiding malpractice, going to a sports medicine specialist for concerns or issues caused by exercise or sports activities guarantees a better treatment. Sports medicine surgeons and physicians use the latest procedures and techniques in helping patients restore function to areas that were injured.

Sports medicine isn't just for athletes. If you are a sports enthusiast who is actively engaged in sports, exercise, and other fitness activities, then it is important to consult sports medicine professional for your sports healthcare needs. Sports medicine is increasingly becoming more important as more and more individuals are becoming health conscious.

Sports Chiropractic

Sports chiropractic (or chiropractic sports medicine) is a relatively new subspecialty in the field of chiropractic healing. As chiropractic care becomes more mainstream, more practitioners are starting to specialize in a variety of healing methods. Sports chiropractors specialize in the care of musculoskeletal injuries, including prevention. This branch of chiropractic expertise is an excellent resource for athletes. Whether you need a little advice on performance issues or treatment for a sport-related injury, any type of athlete will find that a sports chiropractor is an important part of keeping their body in peak condition.

Chiropractic care has been around for thousands of years, but it wasn't until 1980 that the first chiropractor was added to the United States Olympic medical team. Since then, spinal adjustments have become an important part of many sports medical teams. Athletes from every walk of life are starting to realize the long-term benefits of chiropractic care.

Sports chiropractors take a multidisciplinary approach to treat their patients. They also have an extensive knowledge of sports and sports-related injuries. This means that they're uniquely qualified to diagnose and treat an athlete's body without the use of drugs or invasive surgical procedures. Because chiropractic medicine is defined by its "hands on" approach to healing and the belief in caring for the entire body, it's becoming an increasingly popular way to stay in the game without relying on drugs or surgeries.

Sports chiropractic is a highly specialized field that typically focuses on professional or aspiring athletes. If you don't spend a good portion of your life participating in a sport, you probably don't require that level of specialized care. Your local chiropractic team is trained in the same type of spinal manipulation and pain relief techniques as a sports chiropractor, and can perform the same techniques as a specialist. They're also able to offer a more general approach to your overall health.

Every chiropractor treats injuries with the same basic techniques. They use spinal manipulation to align your spine and traction tables to relieve pressure in the discs in your back. A good chiropractor will also be eager to educate you on the proper way to move your body to avoid injury. Chiropractors are strong believers in holistic care. This means that they're concerned with the health of your whole body and can be an excellent resource for the sports-minded individual.

Anyone who plays sports regularly can benefit from chiropractic care. Your chiropractor can help you with aches and pains that come along with an exercise regimen, as well as helping you to stay fit and healthy. If exercise pains are slowing your workout down, get going to your chiropractor for an adjustment. They'll have you back at the gym in no time at all.

Benefits of Chiropractic Care

It helps Relieve the Torture Inflicted by Strenuous Exercises

As you cheer and watch your favorite athletes perform in the arena, what you don't understand is the fact that they subject their bodies to unimaginable torture and endure lots of muscle and body pains. However, thanks to chiropractic care, athletes no longer have to live with these pains. This is because the procedure helps relieve the pains and torture. And yes, athletes also suffer spinal pains due to the stress they subject their bodies to while performing. All this is easily treated with chiropractic care.

It can Treat Various Injuries

As testified by several athletes, chiropractic care helps reduce chances of one getting injured. And yes, the practice also helps the body to heal fast from both minor and major injuries. How is that? Chiropractic care helps the muscles to relax and also helps in enhancing proper blood circulation. All these are paramount if at all an athlete is to perform perfectly. With care focused on spinal manipulation, it also heals headaches, ankle pains, and spinal pains. Therefore, it is crucial for any athlete to visit a chiropractor every now and then in order to stay away from these complications.

It is Non-invasive and Drug-free

Given an option, it is crystal clear that most of us would prefer to not opt for taking medications. This is because drugs are not so good for our bodies. For that reason, this therapeutic procedure is non-invasive and drug-free, making it quite convenient for athletes. This is, in fact, a major benefit since it does not pose side effects to one's body. And yes, being non-invasive implies that one can get into action immediately they come from this procedure as opposed to invasive procedures where one has to give their body some time to recover.

It Prevents Injuries and Enhances Performance

In case you visit an Orange County chiropractor, you will not only get treatment but also get into a program that will ensure that you do not get injuries easily. In fact, your performance will be enhanced using chiropractic care. How is that? Well, studies have shown that chiropractic care greatly helps enhance an athlete's performance.

It Reduces Pain

As pointed out earlier, chiropractic care focuses on spinal manipulation. From science, it is obvious that the spine is basically the nervous system. For that reason, with manipulation of the spine, one could have their pain greatly reduced. All this is achieved thanks to chiropractic care. Therefore, this is a great way to relieve pain.

It Increases Strength

Although initially meant for treatment purposes, studies indicate that chiropractic care also helps in increasing the strength of an athlete. In fact, it has been proven that those athletes who use this practice are stronger than those who don't. And yes, strength and performance are almost synonymous; one can never work without the other. It follows that being strong translates to great performance.

It Causes Relaxation

This is obvious. Given the fact that your body is carefully massaged and every pressure point professionally worked on, there is no doubt that the results will be a unique relaxation. For any athlete who wants to feel relaxed and have pressure relieved from their body, this is the procedure to seek.

Sport Psychology

Sport psychology is an aspect of sport training and preparation; this science is primarily directed at assisting individual athletes and teams maintain an optimal balance between mind and body, both in terms of the physical execution of the technical aspects of the sport and the related functions of emotion and mood. Many athletes who possess superior physical gifts are rarely able to seemingly combine athletic talent and mental control; sport psychology is directed at the building and reinforcement of that connection. Sport psychology is a separate but related study from sports medicine.

Formal psychological training is a combination of intense academic study and practical applications; sport psychology is an accepted subscript of the science. Sport psychologists typically are persons with an interest in and an understanding of the mechanics and the dynamics of both sport and sport coaching. At an elite competitive level, the athlete/coach/psychologist triangle is usually very tightly formed, particularly in support of athletes who compete in individual sports.

Sports psychology was not generally accepted as a formal science until the 1970s, when a body of knowledge began to develop concerning how athletes could be motivated to train harder and to maintain a peak emotional level prior to competition. Modern sport psychology is a multifaceted science, covering a broad and sometimes contradictory range of professional opinions about how to best stimulate the mind of the athlete to assist in the achievement of a desired result.

There is no single sports psychology approach. Team sports and the dynamics of group interaction are entirely different than the pursuits of individual competition. The nature of the sport itself will play a significant role in how the athlete may be assisted; certain sports, by their nature, are likely to attract certain types of personalities. A cross-country skier and the object of the sport are a polar opposite to the goals of a weightlifter or a boxer. While individuals in their sport may require varying psychological approaches, the science of sports psychology is founded on a number of constants. Sport psychology, as a support to the athlete, will invariably include work in three general areas: goal setting, imagery and simulation, and development of better powers of concentration.

Goal setting is a planning process that occurs as a part of an assessment of the overall needs and abilities of an athlete. Goals must ultimately be realistic; to set objectives that are unattainable for an athlete is to guarantee failure. Goal setting involves the determination of such issues as the athlete's ability to self-motivate and the personal measure of self-confidence. The sports psychologist, along with the athlete and the coaches, can play a role in the prioritizing of competitive events within the training year; effective coaches will create a schedule that is often referred to as periodization of training, when the year is divided into the constituent parts of competitive season, off-season and preseason. Sport psychology principles are of particular application in the athlete's development of a feedback loop, where the constant analysis, re-evaluation, and refocusing of training and competitive direction, occurs regarding performance.

Imagery and simulation training and techniques form the second branch of sport psychology. Although commonly treated as a single entity, imagery and simulation are two distinct psychological approaches to sport training and preparation.

The physical training undertaken by any athlete requires the development of the athlete's brain and the pathways of the nervous system, particularly those of the peripheral system that extend to the musculoskeletal structure that is directed and powered to achieve movement. The more specific and focused the nerve impulses initiated by the brain in respect of the intended physical movements of the sport, the more effective the athlete will be in execution of the required movements of the sport.

Imagery is a psychological technique where the athlete is conditioned to prepare for sport through the use of the mind. Imagery includes the development of set thought patterns, composed of often abstract words or images that the athlete finds helpful in reinforcing the focus on the activity. Images are developed between the athlete and the psychologist to trigger certain types of emotions that the athlete may wish to harness at appropriate times. The common emotions that are tied to imagery are those that calm the athlete in a tense environment, ones that motivate the athlete to increase intensity where the athlete may be at a lower level of intensity than is desired, or images to heighten the ability to block out all extraneous activity or distraction.

The images may be personal to the athlete's experience, or they may be created to spur a particular reaction. Once taught, imagery is a self-motivational tool, portable in that the images and their keys are carried in the athlete's mind. An example is the use of the word "wind" and words associated with the performance and the nature of wind in relation to how a distance runner might imagine his or her own performance. The abstract wind is connected to the reality of what the athlete seeks to achieve.

Simulation is a mental training process that is a direct linkage between mental control and the sport. Simple simulations include the mental rehearsal of sport-specific techniques such as the mental review of all aspects of a foul shot in basketball, from the first approach to the foul line to the ball falling through the cylinder. An important component of effective simulation is the appreciation of all of the senses that the athlete would expect to engage at the time of the actual event being simulated. Using the basketball foul shot as an example, the player would be encouraged to think not only of the mechanics of the shot, but how the ball feels in the shooter's hand, the sensation of the player's shoes on the floor, and the sound made by the ball as it swishes through the mesh of the basket on a successful attempt. Simulation seeks to build the entire act and its surrounding physical circumstances in the mind, to better equip the athlete to deal with those related sensations during competition.

Simulation is the mental companion to the physical training involved in sports practice. The live drills used by teams to prepare for competition are the mirror to the mental training and psychological preparation of simulation. The overriding purpose of both imagery and simulation in sport is to assist in the development of confidence in the athlete.

The development of the athlete's powers of concentration is the third general component of sport psychology. In many respects, the maintenance of concentration powers is the most difficult mental effort extended by an athlete, as concentration is influenced by both physical circumstances such as fatigue or injury, as well as the mental aspects of competitive pressure and other distracting variables. Sports psychologists often seek to develop a number of specific attributes to mental performance as a general increase in the powers of concentration in an athlete. The first of these qualities is focus. In both training and competitive situations, an athlete must maintain a relentless attention on the matters at hand. Focus is applicable to both the mechanics of the sport, as well as the maintenance of the required intensity to perform at the desired level.

Mood is the next factor to be controlled in the enhancement of concentration powers. Sport psychology provides for an intensely individualized analysis when determining the ideal mood suitable for the best performance in any given athlete. As a general proposition, the psychologist will seek to assist the athlete in attaining the desired mood. Imagery is sometimes employed, as are external stimuli such as music.

The athlete's activation level is a concept closely related to the mood of the athlete, as every athlete has an emotional point where he or she is sufficiently mentally stimulated to possess the desire and the drive to perform, without being so excited by the prospect of competition that the athlete loses concentration regarding the execution of the required physical aspects of the sport. The phrase "to get psyched up" is a simple example of words that are used to take the athlete to the activation level. Another tool to maintain activation level in an athlete is positive self-talk, where the athlete is encouraged to talk silently for constant self-encouragement throughout an event.

Sports psychologists will also seek to equip the athlete with personal stress management tools; if an athlete succumbs to the stress of competition, he or she will not be able to succeed. The control of stressful factors by the athlete, especially when the athlete is able to direct some of the energy that is created by stress into positive performance, is among the goals of the psychologist.

Pressure is a more generalized emotional factor that is closely related to stress. Pressure is often driven by external circumstances, such as the expectations of a parent, a team, or a coach. It is a factor that tends to undermine the power of concentration. Pressure is often subtle and more diffuse than the stress that is associated with a specific event. Pressure may often be related to insecurity or a poor self-image on the part of the athlete. Sports psychologists often work with athletes to establish reasonable expectations to assist with the ability to deal with the variables of sport performance.

The overall maintenance of mental and emotional balance on the part of the athlete's mental outlook is a powerful weapon against overtraining. The science of psychology has long recognized two general classifications of personalities, labeled type A and type B. Type A persons are those who are intense, perfectionist, and demanding individuals; Type B are relaxed and easy-going people. Type A athletes are the most vulnerable to overtraining syndrome, as these persons will tend to push themselves past healthy physical and emotional limits in their pursuit of excellence.

Diagnostic Imaging in Sports Medicine

Imaging should be considered only after a provisional clinical diagnosis is reached, and only if it will influence management.

Musculoskeletal imaging in sports medicine is a rapidly developing field, being driven by both continuously advancing technology and improved understanding of the disabilities that may result from sporting injuries, many of which can be minimised or avoided by early diagnosis and appropriate treatment.

Paradoxically, as imaging tests become ever more sophisticated and sensitive, the importance of clinical judgement in determining both when to order tests and the relevance of abnormal findings increases. This is because real but incidental anatomical derangements, such as normal developmental variants, and asymptomatic degenerative changes which become more prevalent with age and high-level sporting activity, are frequently detected. Studies have shown that subclinical pathological change is present in a large proportion of asymptomatic or minimally symptomatic athletes. It has long been recognised that even gross pathological derangements, such as osteoarthritic joints, intervertebral disc protrusions and rotator cuff tears, can sometimes be completely asymptomatic. Thus, physicians must always remember to "treat the patient, not the scan".

Indications for Imaging

The common-sense rule of only ordering a test if the result is likely to influence management applies. In sports medicine, a specific anatomical diagnosis is not always required and does not necessarily constitute best practice. For example, mild-to-moderate back pain in young adults without neurological signs may be appropriately managed with physiotherapy alone, irrespective of the actual anatomical diagnosis. A recent interesting study has found that in back pain, early use of computed tomography (CT) or magnetic resonance imaging (MRI) leads to slightly better patient outcomes without changing management. Despite this, the study concluded that whether such imaging was cost effective remained unresolved.

In general, the indications for imaging are as follows:

- When the clinical diagnosis is uncertain and management may be affected by one or more of the particular possibilities being considered;
- When clinical "red flags" are present and sinister or systemic abnormality must be excluded;
- When the clinical diagnosis is obvious, but the extent of injury or presence of complications is unclear and either of these considerations may affect management;
- When treatment has failed and the reasons for this are unclear (was the original diagnosis correct?);

- When objective evidence is required to document the existence, progression or resolution of disease (eg., medicolegal situations);
- When preoperative localisation or planning information is needed.

Imaging Techniques

The selection of the best test or tests will vary, depending on (i) the provisional clinical diagnosis, (ii) the local availability of appropriate radiological equipment and expertise, (iii) patient considerations such as cost, convenience, and compliance, (iv) safety considerations such as patient age, radiation dose and contrast sensitivity, and (v) other costs such as that to the tax payer or insurance company. Radiation safety is an important consideration, as adverse effects are known to occur. In particular, multislice CT, which can readily generate large exposures, should be used judiciously. The United States Food and Drug Administration estimates that an effective dose of 10 mSv may carry a one in 2000 lifetime risk of inducing fatal cancer. A short list of relative radiation doses. The actual dose delivered in any given CT examination can vary greatly, depending on the type of scanner and scan technique used. It has been estimated that over one million CT scans are performed each year and that the collective radiation dose arising from these studies could be inducing as many as 280 fatal cancers per year. Thus, in sports medicine, where disease is not life-threatening, the question of whether CT scans or isotope bone scans are essential to management is important. For younger patients in particular, safer tests such as ultrasound or MRI should be used wherever they will provide equivalent diagnostic efficacy.

It is always important to provide a request form which offers a guiding differential diagnosis or asks specific questions that the radiologist must attempt to answer. This not only allows appropriate optimisation of imaging protocol, but also increases the likelihood of disease detection (because subtle or equivocal findings are easily overlooked if the clinical notes provided do not adequately direct the radiologist's search pattern and analysis). It is worth asking your local radiologist for advice if uncertain about such issues of cost, access, accuracy, safety or the significance of the report findings.

Plain X-ray

This provides a comprehensive anatomical overview at low cost and relatively low radiation dose, and should generally be the first imaging test. Combined with the clinical assessment, plain films alone will often allow a reasonable provisional diagnosis and management plan to be formulated without the need for more sophisticated tests. Even when the clinical features suggest that an injury involves soft tissue structures alone, plain films may be required to detect important features that other tests may miss (eg., soft-tissue calcifications, foreign bodies, bone spurs, accessory centres of ossification, periosteal reactions, joint malalignments, old injuries and other predisposing conditions, clinically unsuspected fractures). X-rays that show no abnormalities are not a waste of time, as they help to exclude or reduce the likelihood of many conditions. Failure to obtain plain films can lead to significant errors in the interpretation of more sophisticated tests, such as MRI, bone scans or ultrasound.

Isotope Bone Scans

Isotope bone scans provide a "functional" image of current skeletal osteoblastic activity which is sensitive but non-specific. They are often used in sports medicine to confirm and localise a bone or joint abnormality before targeted characterisation by another form of imaging, but may also be used to diagnose a few specific conditions including long bone stress fracture, osteonecrosis, osteitis pubis, and reflex sympathetic dystrophy. The clinical context will heavily influence the interpretation of isotope scans, as a number of pathological processes (including degeneration, trauma, infection, tumour, and osteonecrosis) can produce the same appearance. As abnormalities appear on bone scans for many months after clinical resolution, this form of imaging should not be used for monitoring healing of a lesion.

Computed Tomography

CT is the ideal imaging modality whenever the cortical and trabecular architecture of bone or the bony anatomy of complex joints must be further assessed. CT is better than MRI at showing fracture lines, small calcifications, loose bodies, subtle bone erosions, and bone mineral loss or destruction. CT has a role in assessing non-weight bearing joint alignment (eg., patellofemoral tracking disorders, sternoclavicular joint dislocation, or femoral anteversion). CT can be used to assist with guided injections into deep structures that are beyond the resolution of ultrasound (eg., sacroiliac joint, facet joint). CT can also be used to give the surgeon a better preoperative 3D understanding of complex bony derangements or prosthesis complications. While detection of focal lumbar disc protrusions by CT is equivalent to MRI, MRI should be used in most circumstances as it does not expose patients to radiation.

Magnetic Resonance Imaging

MRI provides a comprehensive, panoramic, and multi-planar image of both superficial *and deep* soft-tissue structures. Although MRI resolves bone mineral poorly, it is the ideal modality whenever a detailed characterisation of bone marrow disorder is sought. This gives MRI a special place in evaluating osteochondral injury, osteonecrosis, bone bruising, bone stress, transient osteoporosis of the hip, and tumours. MRI has equivalent sensitivity to isotope bone scanning for the detection of bone stress, but provides considerably more anatomical information without exposing patients to ionising radiation. MRI also provides excellent delineation of both deep and superficial soft tissues in a more panoramic and less operator-dependent format than ultrasound, and is the best non-invasive imaging test for injuries of articular cartilage and fibrocartilage (eg., meniscal tears). Some types of ligament, muscle and tendon injury are also best seen with MRI, especially when these involve deep or inconveniently positioned structures that do not afford ready ultrasound access. In recent years, MRI has been shown to be very useful in helping to provide a prognosis for muscle strain injuries in professional athletes, although the cost makes it inappropriate as a routine test in amateurs (on the basis that management would not be changed). MRI may be contraindicated or complicated by factors such as cardiac pacemakers, cerebral aneurysm clips, claustrophobia, inability to remain still, prostheses and other surgical hardware.

Under the current Australian health system, cost and access are also significant issues because Medicare rebates do not apply to MRI scans ordered by primary care providers (including sports physicians, even if they are consulted on a referral basis). For both CT and MRI examinations of joints where intra-articular abnormality is suspected (particularly for the hip and shoulder), joint surface resolution may be improved by the use of an intra-articular contrast material. The benefits of this must be weighed against the added patient discomfort and risks, such as allergic reaction, chemical synovitis or, rarely, septic arthritis.

Ultrasound

Ultrasound is a safe and powerful, but highly operator-dependent, method of imaging superficial soft tissues, especially tendons (eg., rupture, adhesions, tendonitis) and associated structures such as bursae. Ultrasound is particularly useful for detecting radiolucent foreign bodies, ganglion cysts and other fluid collections, and small soft tissue masses. It is a targeted and interactive test in which the examiner is in the room with the patient, actively interrogating the site of symptoms and correlating clinical features such as localised tenderness directly with the imaging appearances. Ultrasound is cheaper, faster and better tolerated than MRI. It is often the best method of assessing soft tissue pathodynamics such as abnormal tendon glide, soft tissue impingement and hernial protrusion. Doppler techniques give ultrasound a role in some vascular conditions (eg, arterial aneurysm, deep vein thrombosis). It also allows the accurate guidance of percutaneous therapeutic procedures such as injections.

New and impressive medical imaging techniques emerging over the last two decades have greatly expanded our ability to non-invasively interrogate complex anatomical structures in fine detail, and to diagnose a variety of conditions in sports medicine. Nevertheless, the complicated array of available imaging technology now makes the choice of exactly which test to order, and when, challenging. In many situations, there are simply no authoritative guidelines available, and the choice of test may also be influenced by individual patient or local community circumstances.

It must never be forgotten that imaging does not replace or reduce the need for a thorough clinical evaluation. Such evaluation, coupled with knowledge of the relevant anatomy and an understanding of likely pathological conditions, remains the cornerstone of accurate diagnosis. Only when a provisional clinical diagnosis has been reached can a rational decision be made about the need for additional diagnostic tests and the significance of any subsequent results.

Imaging of Muscle Injuries in Sports Medicine

Muscle injuries represent a major challenge for professional athletes, accounting for up to one-third of all sports-related injuries, and they are responsible for a large part of time lost to competition. The main goal of the sports medicine physician is to return the athlete to competition—balanced against the need to prevent the injury from worsening or recurring. Prognosis based on the available clinical and imaging information is crucial. Imaging is crucial to confirm and assess the extent of sports-related muscle injuries and may help to guide management, which directly affects the prognosis. This is especially important when the diagnosis or grade of injury is unclear, when recovery is taking longer than expected, and when interventional or surgical management may be necessary. Several imaging techniques are widely available, with ultrasonography (US) and magnetic resonance (MR) imaging currently the most frequently applied in sports medicine.

Mechanisms of Injury and Clinical Features

The most common mechanism of injury of muscles in elite athletes is related to muscle strain (indirect muscle injury), mainly in the lower limbs. Muscles are at risk for disruption during eccentric contraction, as the force of active contraction is added to the passive stretching force applied to the myotendinous junction (MTJ). Acute muscle injuries in the lower limbs are associated with both sprinting and stretching activities, mainly affecting the hamstring muscle complex. For these MTJ injuries there is more pronounced loss of function initially but with faster recovery for sprinting-related injuries, while for stretching injuries there is less loss of function initially but slower recovery. Factors related to muscles and activities that increase the risk for indirect muscle injury include eccentric contraction, involvement of muscles with high content of fast twitch type 2 fibers, a sudden change in muscle function, muscles crossing multiple joints (biceps femoris, rectus femoris, gastrocnemius muscles), failure to absorb or counteract forces from other muscle groups or ground reaction, and muscle imbalance. Indirect mechanisms may further lead to acute avulsion injuries, usually resulting from extreme, unbalanced, and eccentric forces. With muscle injuries, athletes present with an immediate sudden onset of pain usually localized in a specific muscle compartment during a period of eccentric contraction, which prevents the athlete from continuing the activity. Flexibility and strength measurements are usually used to obtain additional information on injury severity. Clinically, muscle strains may be categorized into grade 1, no appreciable tissue tearing, with no substantial (less than 5%) loss of function or strength; grade 2, tissue damage of the MTJ with reduced strength and some residual function; and grade 3, complete tear of the myotendinous unit with complete loss of function and occasionally a palpable gap.

Blunt trauma is the most common mechanism of direct muscle injury in sports, mainly affecting the lower limbs in sports that may involve collisions as in soccer, football, and rugby. Depending on the dissipation pattern of the blunt force, different degrees of muscle contusion may be observed, usually (but not always) occurring deep in the muscle belly: An intramuscular hematoma may be present. High-grade injury is commonly seen in cases of massive blunt force directed toward the bone, with a massive amount of energy dissipated from the deep muscle to the bone. Penetrating trauma with muscle laceration rarely occurs in elite sports. Clinically, muscle contusions can be categorized as mild (range of motion loss less than one-third with shorter recovery times), moderate (range of motion loss from one-third to two-thirds of normal, with moderate recovery times), and severe contusions (range of motion loss greater than two-thirds with longer recovery times). Muscle contusions tend to show fewer symptoms than muscle strains.

US Assessment of Skeletal Muscle Injuries

Advances in hardware and transducer technology now allow visualization of muscular architecture at in-plane resolution under 200 μm and with a section thickness of 0.5–1.0 mm, which exceeds current MR imaging. Although the evaluation of muscle injuries by using MR imaging has been extensively described, US can have a number of distinct advantages: It offers dynamic muscle assessment, it is fast, relatively inexpensive, easier for patients, and allows serial evaluation to follow healing, and it can be used to perform real-time interventions. In addition, US can demonstrate the muscle structure and other relevant anatomy surrounding an injury that can often be obscured by edema on MR images.

US Technique

Initial assessment commences with a clinical history and pertinent physical examination. This allows the subsequent US examination to be targeted toward the most relevant areas. The majority of skeletal muscles lie superficially within the body and therefore are optimally assessed by using linear transducers. Modern multifrequency transducers (center frequency greater than 10–17 MHz) allow visualization of most muscle groups. Lower-frequency linear (8–10 MHz) probes may be needed in very muscular patients, especially in the gluteal region and proximal thigh. Modern software and transducers now allow trapezoid fields of view (FOVs) or composite image formation for which the latter can extend the transducer's FOV to 60 cm. After obtaining the optimal transducer setting, the examination begins with longitudinal and transverse scanning of the symptomatic area. In the majority of muscle injuries, the symptomatic area accurately locates the muscle lesion, but the examiner must be confident of the anatomy being examined and the exact position of the lesion. After assessing the appearance of the muscle and any lesion at rest, the abnormal area and surrounding tissues should be assessed dynamically with active and passive contraction. This allows the consistency of the abnormality (eg, solid or cystic), alteration in muscle function, and any movement of disrupted fibers (helping differentiate grades of tears) to become more apparent. Additional maneuvers, especially in the case of muscle hernias, may be required since the hernia may only become apparent when the patient is standing.

US Features

Normal muscle fibers are arranged in parallel hypoechoic bundles (fascicles) surrounded by echogenic fibrofatty septa in a "pennate" configuration. The muscle fibers and fascicles are of low echogenicity compared with adjacent fascia and nervous tissue. Because of its thickness, the perimysium, which appears relatively echogenic due to its fibrous (collagen) content, can be seen in pennate muscles at longitudinal scanning as multiple parallel lines forming oblique angles (separated by the hypoechoic fascicles) with the MTJ. The orientation of perimysium to the long axis of muscle is oblique in uni-/bipennate muscles and parallel in fusiform muscles. These linear structures converge to the MTJ with the tendon seen as a discrete fibrillar echogenic structure as it becomes more defined. In the transverse plane, the muscle fibers are hypoechoic with the intervening septae seen as smaller linear areas and echogenic "dots". Finally another thick layer of fascia called the epimysium surrounds the entire muscle and again is echogenic due to its fibrous content.

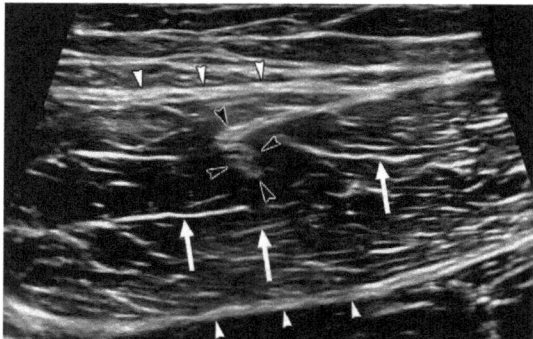

Transverse sonogram of rectus femoris shows normal echogenic epimysium (white arrowheads), perimysium (arrows) with intervening hypoechoic fascicles, and normal echogenic MTJ (black arrowheads).

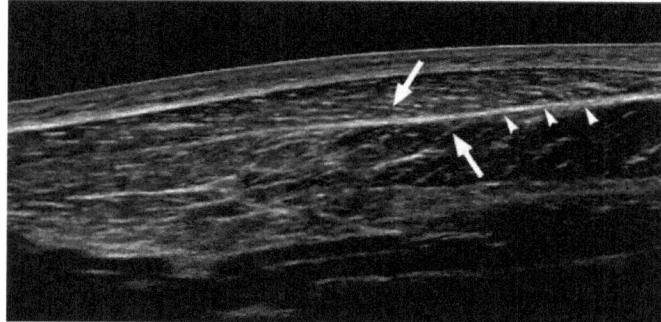

Longitudinal extended FOV sonogram of gastrocnemius shows normal echogenic perimysium (arrows) with intervening hypoechoic fascicles converging in a pennate orientation to the MTJ (arrowheads).

The spectrum of US features of muscle strain was previously described by Peetrons. In clinically grade 1 injuries, US images may be either negative or exhibit focal or diffuse ill-defined areas of increased echogenicity within the muscle at the site of injury. Grade 1 injuries may also include injuries exhibiting minimal focal fiber disruption occupying less than 5% of the cross-sectional area of the muscle, represented by a well-defined focal hypoechoic or anechoic area within the muscle. There is no consensus about this definition, with some authors considering any degree of partial fiber disruption as a grade 2 injury. The presence of areas of partial fiber disruption (less than 100% of the cross-sectional area of the muscle affected) seen at US represents grade 2 injury. Usually, there is discontinuity of the echogenic perimysial striae around either the MTJ or the myofascial junction. An intramuscular hematoma may be depicted as well in grade 2 injuries, and its echogenicity is dependent on the temporal evolution of the injury. Initially (24–48 hours), intramuscular hematomas usually appear as an ill-defined muscle laceration separated by hypoechoic fluid with marked increased reflectivity in the surrounding muscle. During this period, hematomas may solidify and display increased echogenicity in comparison to the surrounding muscle. After 48–72 hours, hematomas will develop into a well-defined hypoechoic fluid collection with an echogenic margin, which gradually enlarges, potentially filling the hematoma in a centripetal fashion.

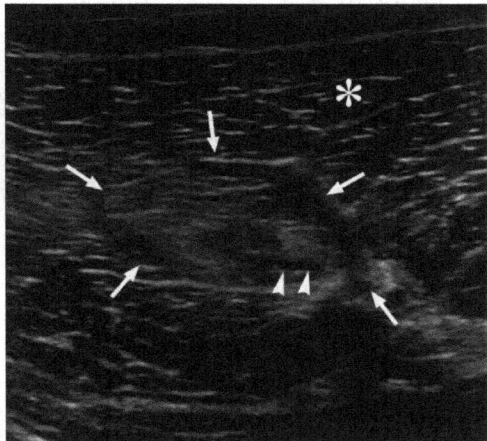

Grade 1 injury of the biceps femoris. Transverse sonogram of left thigh shows normal muscle with a small area of echogenic edematous muscle (arrows) containing a tiny area of hypoechoic disruption (arrowheads).

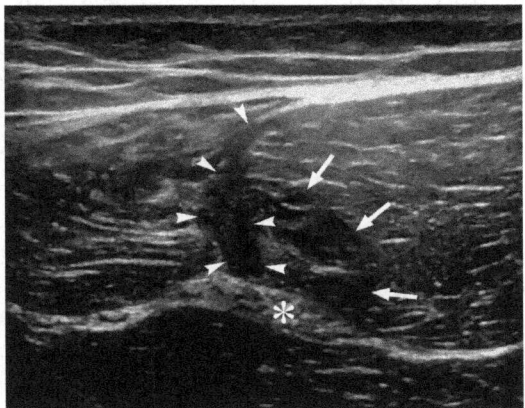

Grade 2 injury of the semitendinosus with diffuse leg pain: Transverse and longitudinal sonograms of left thigh show hypoechoic muscle disruption (arrows) with hematoma (arrowheads) also present extending along the disrupted perimysium and abutting the sciatic nerve.

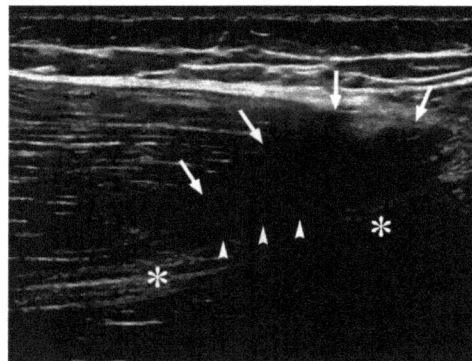

A complete discontinuity or disruption of the MTJ with different degrees of retraction depicted at US represents grade 3 injury. Grade 3 lesions are usually clinically evident with a palpable gap between the retracted ends of the muscle affected. Also, perifascial fluid may be depicted with US, which may have an increased echogenicity due to the presence of extravascular blood but is usually hypoechoic because most examinations occur more than 24 hours after injury. Perifascial fluid detection is not a specific feature as it can occur in any grade of injury.

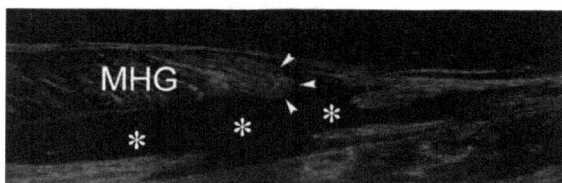

Grade 3 injury of the medial head gastrocnemius (MHG). Longitudinal extended FOV sonogram shows edematous muscle (medial head gastrocnemius) with complete tear causing retraction (arrowheads) and extensive hematoma (*).

Artifacts and Pitfalls in US Evaluation of Muscle Injury

The linear configuration of the septae makes them susceptible to anisotropy artifact leading to decreased echogenicity or absent of conspicuity of septae, which can be mistaken for an injury. Careful probe repositioning is needed to ensure that the apparent absence of septae is due to the artifact rather than an injury. Other potential sources of artifacts are prominent intramuscular vessels, which can mimic tears. Errors due to this artifact can be avoided through the use of Doppler as well as by carefully tracing of the vessels through the septae to their neurovascular bundles and by determining that the surrounding muscle structure is normal right up to the vessel boundary. Occasionally thickened or scarred septae can cause acoustic shadowing that makes the underlying muscle appear hypoechoic. During exercise, blood flow through the muscle and connective tissues can normally increase 20-fold, with resultant muscle swelling and displacement of the overlying fascial planes (a muscle volume increase of 10%–15%).

Routine MR Imaging Assessment of Skeletal Muscle

MR Imaging Technique

MR imaging is considered the reference imaging method to assess the morphology of muscles in athletes owing to its ability to visualize soft tissues with excellent contrast and provide high spatial-resolution and multiplanar assessment, especially in cases in which traumatic lesions are clinically suspected. MR imaging is well suited to confirm and evaluate the extent and severity of muscle injuries. Furthermore, MR imaging may be better suited than US for the assessment of muscle injuries located in deep muscle compartments. MR imaging is usually performed unilaterally (affected limb only) by using a dedicated surface coil, to ensure higher resolution images with thinner sections and smaller FOV. Simultaneous acquisition of images of the contralateral lower limb by using a higher FOV should be ideally performed in selected cases (eg., when bilateral injury is suspected). The coil selection should be based on the desired FOV. A skin marker (capsule filled with fish oil or vegetable oil) should be placed over the area of symptoms according to the athlete's orientation, to correlate imaging and clinical features. To accurately evaluate morphology and extent of muscle injuries, multiplanar acquisitions (axial, coronal, and sagittal) are required in regard to the long and short axes of the involved muscle. Pulse sequences must include fat-suppressed fluid-sensitive techniques, which allow for the detection of edematous changes around the myotendinous and myofascial junctions, as well as for the delineation of intramuscular, or perifascial fluid collections or hematomas. Fluid-sensitive techniques include fat-suppressed (fast or turbo) spin-echo T2-weighted, proton density–weighted, intermediate-weighted sequences, as well as the short tau inversion recovery, or STIR, technique. T1-weighted spin-echo sequences are less sensitive to edematous changes within the muscle in acute injury. However, they may be useful in the assessment of subacute hemorrhage or hematoma, as well as to detect and evaluate the extent of atrophy and fatty infiltration and scar tissue formation in chronic injuries.

MR Imaging Features of Muscle Injury

Most muscle injuries occur around the MTJ. Interstitial edema and hemorrhage around the MTJ may often extend along the adjacent muscle fibers and fascicles, which is detected on fluid-sensitive coronal or sagittal MR images as an ill-defined focal or diffuse high-signal-intensity area along the MTJ seen on images obtained with fluid-sensitive techniques, with a classic feathery appearance. The presence of an edematous pattern only, without substantial disruption of muscle fibers or muscle architecture, is commonly referred to as a grade 1 injury, and loss of muscular function is not usually observed. The tendon at the MTJ usually has normal signal intensity and morphology in a grade 1 injury, with regular contours and marked low signal intensity with all pulse sequences. However, it may also be mildly thickened with abnormal signal intensity, but without disruption or laxity. Mild perifascial fluid may accompany grade 1 injuries. In addition to grade 1 features, the presence of a partial disruption of muscle with hematoma formation around the MTJ is commonly referred to as a grade 2 injury, with local distortion of muscle architecture. Partial disruption is usually depicted as a focal area of well-defined high signal intensity on images obtained with fluid-sensitive MR imaging sequences. The tendon adjacent to the MTJ may be thickened and exhibit features of laxity, and partial disruption of the tendon may be depicted as well. There is usually some function loss associated with grade 2 injuries on MR images, depending on the extent. Moderate to severe perifascial fluid is often present in grade 2 injuries. Finally, grade 3 injuries on MR images are usually represented by a complete disruption of the MTJ with a local hematoma filling the gap created by the tear. Clinical examination is usually sufficient to diagnose grade 3 injuries, with complete loss of function, a palpable gap, and muscle retraction observed. Complete avulsion injuries of the MTJ or tendons from the bony attachment are also considered to represent grade 3 injuries.

The MR imaging appearance of intramuscular hematomas, which may accompany not only grades 2 and 3 injuries but also muscle contusions, may change according to the predictable pattern of blood degradation, which is not always true for intermuscular (or perifascial) hematomas. Injuries may occur within the muscle belly and far from the main MTJ, or at the peripheral myofascial junction (around the epimysial interface). One could argue that muscle belly injuries occur from dissipating forces affecting smaller secondary central myoaponeurotic junctions. In injuries at the peripheral myofascial junction, the edema pattern is depicted at the periphery of muscles. These injuries may or may not be associated with focal fascial disruption, as well as with focal partial disruption of the adjacent muscle fibers. Several imaging classification or grading systems for muscle injuries, especially strains, are available for application in clinical practice and clinical research. The widely used grading 1–3 system for muscle injuries, lacks diagnostic accuracy and provides limited prognostic information to sports medicine physicians, since it does not properly cover the full spectrum of muscle injury features. Potentially clinically relevant imaging features should be included in a grading system, which should be capable of providing prognostic information and a diagnostic framework for enhanced clinical decision making in the management of muscle injuries. A consensus statement on new terminology and classification of muscle injuries in sports was published in 2013, which defined grades based on the cause of injuries. The "functional" classes are grade 1 for fatigue-induced disorders and delayed-onset muscle soreness (DOMS); spine-related and muscle-related neuromuscular disorders are grade 2 injuries. The "structural" classes refer to an indirect injury mechanism and include partial muscle tears as grade 3 and subtotal/complete discontinuity of muscle/tendon as grade 4 injuries. Direct injuries leading to muscle contusion or laceration are considered separately in such consensus.

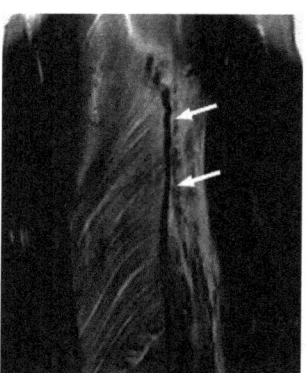

Coronal and axial proton-density fat-suppressed MR images of the thigh (a, repetition time msec/echo time msec, 3900/25; FOV, 23 × 33 cm; section thickness, 4 mm; intersection gap, 1 mm; b, 3900/24; FOV, 28 × 28 cm; section thickness, 5 mm; intersection gap, 1.2 mm). MR grade 1 injury of the semimembranosus muscle is seen, exhibiting the classic feathery pattern of ill-defined muscle edema on the coronal image (a). The edema is mainly distributed around the MTJ, with the central tendon exhibiting normal low signal intensity and thickness (arrows).

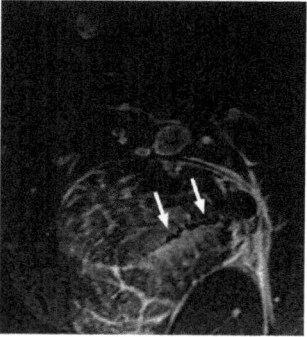

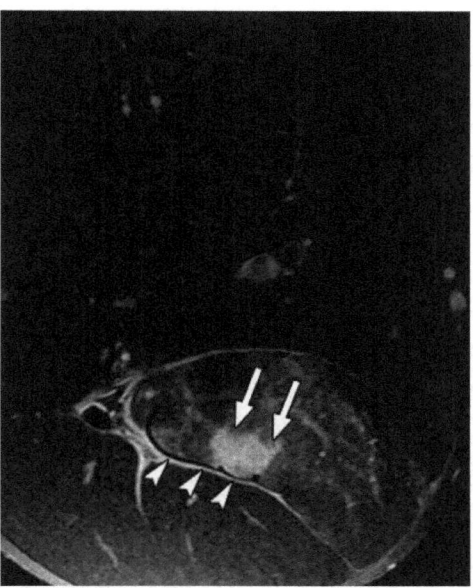

Axial proton-density fat-suppressed MR image of the thigh (3900/24; FOV, 28 × 28 cm; section thickness, 5 mm; intersection gap, 1.2 mm). MR grade 2 injury of the semimembranosus muscle, with a focal partial tear (fiber disruption) represented by a fairly well-defined area of high signal intensity (arrows) adjacent to the MTJ (tendon demonstrated by arrowheads).

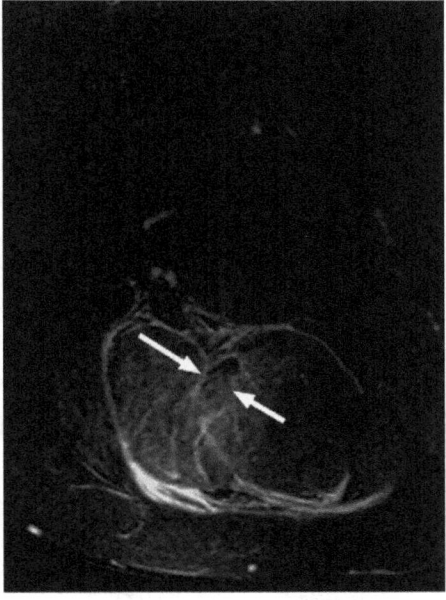

Axial and coronal proton-density fat-suppressed MR images of the thigh (a, 3900/24; FOV, 28 × 28 cm; section thickness, 5 mm; intersection gap, 1.2 mm; b, 3900/25; FOV, 23 × 33 cm; section thickness, 4 mm; intersection gap, 1 mm). Marked thickening and signal intensity changes of the central tendon at the proximal MTJ of the long head of biceps femoris muscle (arrows), with blurring of the tendon contours and foci of partial discontinuity, mainly observed in b (arrows). Discontinuity of the central tendon at the MTJ of the long head of biceps femoris seen with MR imaging was shown to be associated with longer recovery times in athletes.

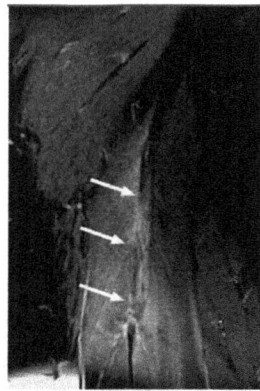

Axial and coronal proton-density fat-suppressed MR images of the thigh (a, 3900/24; FOV, 28 × 28 cm; section thickness, 5 mm; intersection gap, 1.2 mm; b, 3900/25; FOV, 23 × 33 cm; section thickness, 4 mm; intersection gap, 1 mm). Marked thickening and signal intensity changes of the central tendon at the proximal MTJ of the long head of biceps femoris muscle (arrows), with blurring of the tendon contours and foci of partial discontinuity, mainly observed in b (arrows). Discontinuity of the central tendon at the MTJ of the long head of biceps femoris seen with MR imaging was shown to be associated with longer recovery times in athletes.

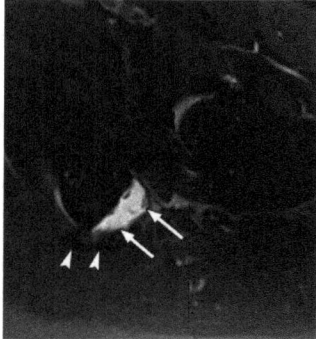

Axial and coronal proton-density fat-suppressed MR images of the thigh. A complete avulsion of the proximal hamstring tendons (grade 3 injury) is depicted at the ischial tuberosity (arrows, a). Note the adjacent sacrotuberous ligament (arrowheads). There is marked distal retraction of the proximal MTJs (arrows, b), with a voluminous hematoma filling the gap (*).

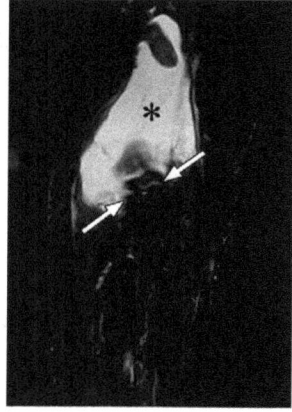

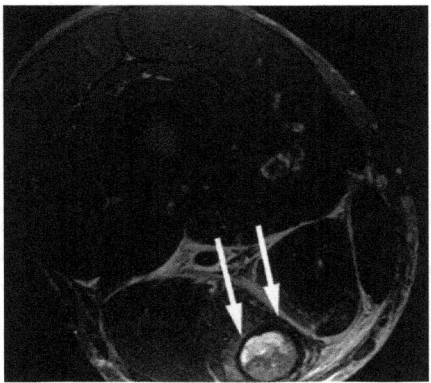

Axial proton-density fat-suppressed image (3900/24; FOV, 28 × 28 cm; section thickness, 5 mm; intersection gap, 1.2 mm) shows an intramuscular hematoma at the semitendinosus muscle after direct trauma (arrows), represented by a well-defined collection with a thick wall and heterogeneous content, with a fluid-fluid level. Note moderate perifascial fluid.

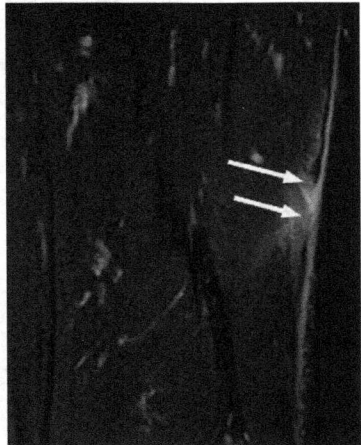

Coronal proton-density fat-suppressed MR image of the thigh (3900/25; FOV, 23 × 33 cm; section thickness, 4 mm; intersection gap, 1 mm) demonstrates injury of the long head of biceps femoris muscle affecting the myofascial junction, with a focal complete tear (disruption) of the adjacent fascia (arrows).

Advanced MR Imaging Techniques

To date, the main advanced MR imaging techniques available for muscle assessment are not applied routinely in clinical practice. These techniques are mainly explored in clinical research and have a great potential to be applied in a sports medicine setting. T2 mapping may be useful from a sports medicine perspective. As T2 values increase in stressed muscles, it is possible to isolate the activated muscles after specific exercises. In some cases even the degree of activation (including muscle activity and muscle strength) can be assessed, as these may be related to the degree of increase in T2 values. Diffusion tensor imaging allows diffusion quantification of anisotropic tissues (eg, muscle) using a series of diffusion-weighted images and subsequent muscle fiber tracking. Diffusion tensor imaging has been shown to be useful for tracking skeletal muscle fiber direction, detecting subclinical changes in muscles after strenuous exercise, detecting muscle injury on a microscopic level, and differentiating injured muscles from normal control muscles. Skeletal muscle MR elastography can be used for studying the physiologic response of normal or diseased and damaged muscles. In fact, it has been found that there is a difference in the stiffness of muscles with and without neuromuscular disease.

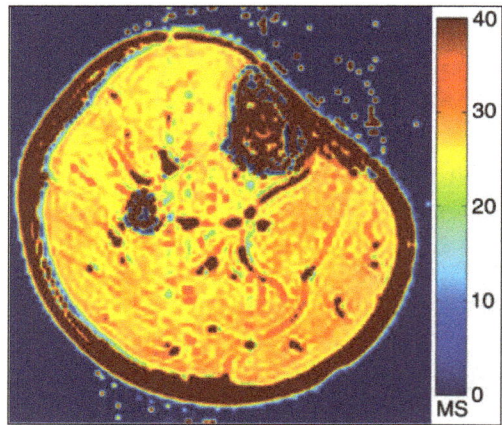

T2 mapping of the right leg of a 31-year-old male volunteer before and 3 minutes after plantar flexion exercise. Parameters of the 3.0-T fat-saturated two-dimensional multi–spin-echo sequence were as follows: matrix size, 128 × 102; FOV, 160 × 130 mm; section thickness, 3 mm; repetition time, 3000 msec; echo times, 10–130 msec (number of echoes = 13); bandwidth, 300 Hz/pixel; refocusing angle, 180°; scan time, 5:15 minutes. Note an increase in T2 values in the gastrocnemius muscles after exercise (arrows) when compared with a.

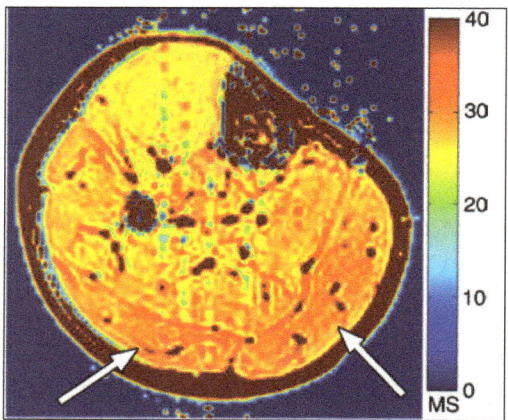

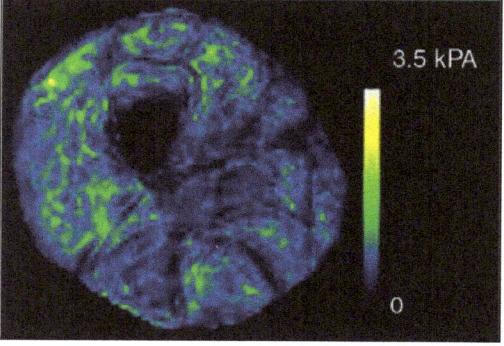

Figure Demonstration of exercise-induced muscle alterations on MR elastograms produced from multifrequency MR elastography data, in a 28-year-old male volunteer. Data were acquired before and 48 hours after an eccentric exercise protocol consisting of 12 sets of eccentric contractions performed on a dynamometer. Increased magnitude shear stiffness is evident on the postexercise elastogram in the rectus femoris and vastus intermedius muscle groups (arrows) when compared with pre-exercise elastogram. Use the color map to compare shear stiffness values between a and b. (MR elastography parameters: 1600/54, section thickness, 2 mm; bandwidth, 1560 Hz/pixel; matrix, 112 × 112; FOV, 224 × 224 mm; resolution; 2 mm isotropic; five sections, two signals acquired, eight phase offsets, one motion encoding gradient cycle at 50 Hz, motion encoding in phase-encoding, section-select, and readout direction. Frequencies acquired = 25, 37.5, 50, and 62.5 Hz).

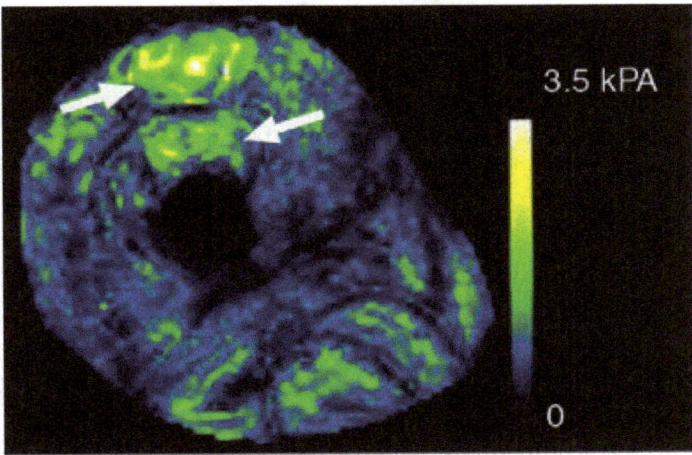

Overuse Muscle Injuries in Sports

In addition to muscle strain, other muscle pathologies related to different sports activities may result in pain and disability. Different from muscle strains, DOMS is an overuse injury related to physical activity, with muscle pain developing hours to days after a specific activity. A decrease of muscle function and strength can be observed. It has been demonstrated that eccentric muscle activity plays a major role in precipitating DOMS. Pain associated with DOMS typically reaches a peak from 24 to 72 hours after physical activity, then decreases slowly. Such clinical presentation is different from muscle strains, with their immediate onset of pain, and represents the main key to diagnosis. The imaging features of DOMS may be similar to muscle strain, making it sometimes difficult to differentiate these two entities based on imaging features alone. Muscle edema is depicted as high signal intensity of the affected muscle belly at fluid-sensitive MR imaging sequences, and perifascial fluid may be present at the early phase of injury. There is no macroscopic fiber disruption or tear associated with DOMS. However, in some cases, DOMS may present with diffuse edema involving the affected muscle belly, not exhibiting the typical "feathery" pattern of strains and without perifascial fluid. There is no linear relationship between the signal intensity on T2-weighted images and clinical symptoms, with a delay between the occurrence of severe symptoms and the maximum intensity of signal abnormalities seen on MR images. The resolution of symptoms and re-establishment of muscle function occur within a period of 10–12 days, whereas abnormal signal intensity on fluid-sensitive MR images may last up to 80 days.

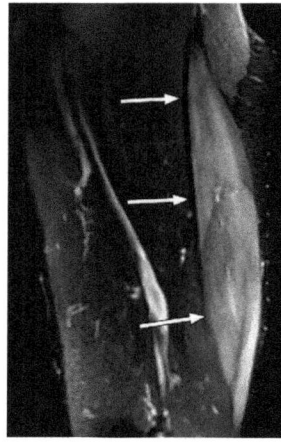

DOMS: Sagittal proton-density fat-suppressed image (3670/25; FOV, 26 × 33 cm; section thickness, 4 mm; intersection gap, 1 mm) shows diffuse edema of the semitendinosus muscle (arrows) in this soccer player complaining of pain that developed 36 hours after intense training. The classic feathery pattern of strain is not observed in this case, and no fiber disruption is depicted. There is no associated perifascial fluid.

Chronic exertional compartment syndrome (CECS) is typically observed in young athletic individuals and is characterized by chronic and recurrent pain induced by physical activity, mainly due to abnormal increase of tissue pressures that lead to reduced perfusion and ischemic pain. The pathophysiology of elevated tissue pressures is not fully understood. Several muscle compartments of the lower and upper limbs may be affected, with—in decreasing frequency—the anterior, deep posterior, lateral, and superficial posterior muscle compartments of the lower limbs the most commonly involved. The typical clinical manifestation of CECS refers to onset of pain in a specific muscle compartment after initiation of a specific physical activity, with increasing pain intensity with continued activity. Pain usually decreases and resolves with rest. Diffuse tenderness over the affected compartment may be documented during clinical examination only after exercise and provocation of symptoms. The reference standard for the diagnosis of CECS is intracompartmental pressure monitoring, with pressures recorded both before and immediately after exercise. This is done by introducing a needle into the affected compartment and monitoring the pressure with a transducer. Postactivity (postexertional) MR imaging may help in the diagnosis of CECS as, unlike asymptomatic subjects, there is usually a greater and mostly delayed increase in T2 signal intensity of the affected compartment after exercise. Subjects not affected by CECS exhibit peak muscle T2 signal intensity during exercise, which tends to normalize 15 minutes after exercise. In contrast, in subjects with CECS the T2 signal peaks in the first recovery phase after exercise, with persistence of abnormal T2 signal intensity after several minutes. A change in T2 values in muscles (before and after exertion) of more than 20% has been suggested as positive for CECS. The specific exercise to be applied in patients or athletes in the radiology facility is often the same one that is responsible for the onset of pain while training or competing, and in most cases it can be accomplished within the facility (ideally the exercise is stopped when pain is produced). Advanced MR imaging techniques such as diffusion tensor imaging also show promise in the evaluation of CECS. As in compartmental syndromes, the increase in compartmental pressure may lead to decreased muscle vascular flow which may be depicted with contrast-enhanced imaging techniques and which can lead to myonecrosis.

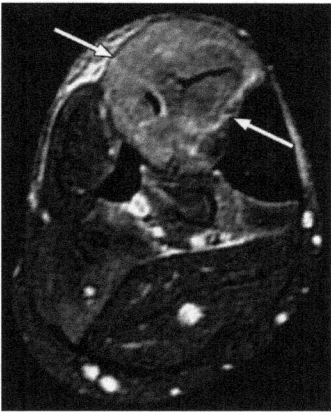

Figure Compartment syndrome affecting the extensor and anterior compartments of the right leg. Axial T2-weighted fat-suppressed MR image (3900/52; FOV, 20 × 20 cm; section thickness, 5 mm; intersection gap, 1.0 mm). T1-weighted fat-suppressed MR image after intravenous gadolinium-based contrast agent injection (824/18; FOV, 20 × 20 cm; section thickness, 5 mm; intersection gap, 1.0 mm). The extensive muscle edema and the extensive lack of enhancement after intravenous contrast agent injection, indicating compromised blood supply.

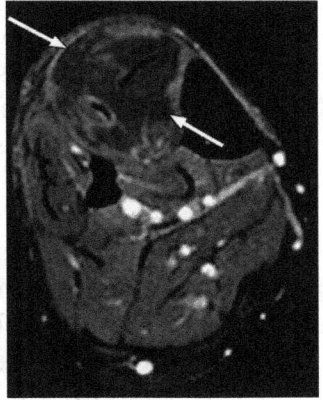

Healing and Complication of Muscle Injuries

Pathophysiology of Muscle Healing

In most types of muscle injuries the repair and healing mechanisms are commonly characterized by three stages. The initial destruction and inflammatory phase, which usually starts immediately after injury, is characterized by rupture and ensuing necrosis of muscle fibers and the formation of hematoma. Since days 2 and 3, the repair phase initiates at the site of injury, consisting of phagocytosis of necrotic tissue, concomitant production of a connective tissue scar accompanied by capillary ingrowth at the injury site, and activation of satellite cells in the regeneration that will differentiate into myoblasts, ultimately responsible of regeneration of the skeletal muscle. Last is the remodeling phase during which maturation of the regenerated fibers, reorganization of scar tissue, and recovery of the functional capacity of the muscle occur. The latter two phases—repair and remodeling—tend to overlap, and their duration depends on the injuries' initial extent. Hemorrhage allows inflammatory cells such as neutrophils and macrophages to enter the site of injury, and an inflammatory response associated with edema at and surrounding the injury site is observed shortly after injury.

Once the destruction phase has subsided, the actual repair of the injured muscle occurs concomitantly with regeneration of disrupted fibers and formation of a connective tissue scar. During phagocytosis, the basal lamina is left intact by macrophages, which acts as scaffolding for reconstitution of the myofibril. Undifferentiated reserve cells called satellite cells below the basal lamina of each individual fiber proliferate, differentiate into myoblasts, fuse to form multinucleated myotubes, and then unite with the remaining portion of injured myofibers. Key events during the remodeling phase include contraction and reorganization of scar tissue, maturation of regenerated myofibrils, gradual resolution of edema, and revascularization of the injured portion of muscle.

Healing and Postinjury Assessment at MR Imaging

While muscle injuries heal there is a decrease in fluidlike signal intensity at the site of injury on MR images. Scar tissue has been observed as early as 6 weeks after initial injury, which can display low signal intensity on T1-weighted and high signal intensity on fluid-sensitive MR images at early stages. At late stages, scar tissue usually displays low signal intensity for all MR imaging pulse sequences. Residual scarring can cause misdiagnosis, leading to both over- and underidentification of new injuries. In the weeks to months after injury during the healing phase, differences in the hydrogen and proton environment due to obtained structural tissue changes including (micro) hemorrhage may contribute to susceptibility artifacts that may be observed during follow-up. Silder and colleagues evaluated MR imaging morphologic changes of musculotendon remodeling following a hamstring strain injury by using quantification of the muscle-tendon scar volumes. They reported that two-thirds of previously injured subjects had residual scarring at the presumed injury site and concluded that the long-term changes in musculotendon structure following injury alter the mechanics of contraction during movement and may raise the risk of reinjury. A recent study found that MR imaging changes may be observed after clinical resolution of symptoms, with 89% of recovered hamstring injuries showing some degree of intramuscular increased signal intensity on fluid-sensitive sequence images. At return to play, one-third of clinically recovered hamstring injuries show low signal intensity suggestive of newly developed fibrous tissues on MR images. The clinical relevance of this finding and its possible association with increased risk of reinjury is uncertain.

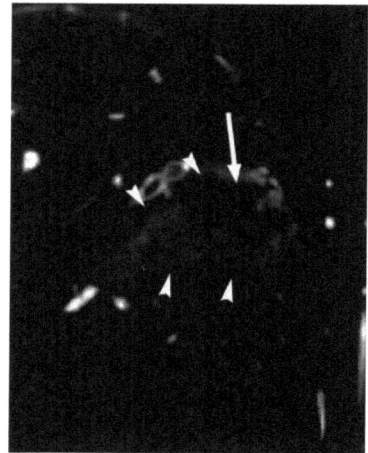

MR findings of chronic muscle injury. Axial T2-weighted fat-suppressed image (640/21; FOV, 350 × 350 mm; 6 mm section thickness with no intersection gap) of the upper thigh of a 23-year-old male soccer player shows diffuse low-grade hyperintensity signal intensity changes in the adductor longus muscle (arrowheads). The signal intensity alterations are subtle and may persist markedly beyond full clinical recovery. Acute grade 1 lesions are commonly more focal involving only specific parts of a given muscle. Note circumscribed hypointensity medially consistent with beginning fibrosis (arrow).

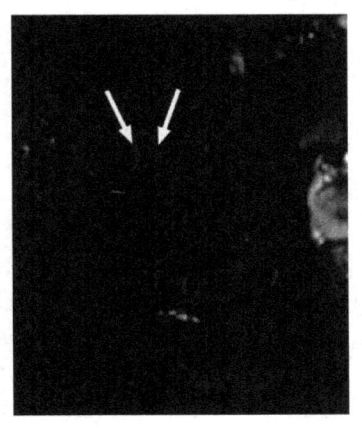

MR imaging findings of chronic muscle injury. Remote injury to the psoas muscle in a 29-year-old male handball player occurred 6 months prior. Axial intermediate-weighted fat-suppressed image (692/23; FOV, 350 × 350 mm; 6 mm section thickness, no intersection gap) of the pelvis shows subtle residual hyperintensity signal intensity changes surrounding the central tendon (arrows). The player had returned to competition 3 months prior and was symptom-free in regard to this lesion at the time of imaging.

Healing and Postinjury Assessment at US

US findings observed during normal healing depend on the nature of the original injury and initial sonographic findings. Minor or grade 1 injuries may appear with increased echogenicity during healing on US studies, which has been documented in up to 50% of cases of grade 1 injuries. In this situation, normal healing is considered a reduction in size or resolution of the region of increased echogenicity. More substantial (grade 2) injuries may present as hypoechoic regions indicative of fluid adjacent muscle fibrils or adjacent to the epimysium. Resolution or substantial decrease in the quantity of fluid is to be expected during the normal healing process. Any hematoma or fluid collection should decrease in size, and macroscopic muscle tears may demonstrate echogenicity of the margins of the tear as healing occurs. Over time small tears may fill with echogenic material, likely representing scar tissue. US is less sensitive than MR imaging to residual morphologic changes after muscle injury, because of the higher soft-tissue contrast and high sensitivity to extracellular fluid offered by MR imaging. Demonstration of scar tissue during follow-up is of significance because it is likely that more extensive scarring results in increased likelihood of recurrent injury. A scar is biomechanically stronger than the native muscle-tendon unit, and it is important to identify these areas of scarring because recurrent injuries may occur nearby. The major advantage of US for the evaluation of healing in muscle injuries is the ability to perform dynamic assessment before and after muscle contraction, which may or may not depict persistence of fiber disruption after clinical management and rehabilitation.

To date, there is no strong evidence in the literature that imaging follow-up should not be routinely performed in athletes sustaining muscle injuries, nor this would relevantly affect management and prognosis. Based on both literature data and clinical experience, we find that follow-up imaging may be useful in two situations: one, for grade 2 injuries (partial fiber disruption) for which clinical symptoms persist after proper management and rehabilitation, being ideally assessed with dynamic US before and after muscle concentric contraction; and two, in cases of clinical suspicion of reinjury, a follow-up US or MR imaging examination may be performed to reassess these injuries. Reinjuries usually display the same imaging features of acute injuries but may occur in a different location within the same muscle or within another muscle of the same muscle group.

Complications of Muscle Injuries

Muscle hernias are a rare complication and are a result of direct trauma to a muscle, which may herniate through a small fascial defect. The lower extremities are most commonly involved, with the tibialis anterior the most frequently affected. Clinically, these patients may present with a chronic mass with or without exertional pain. Imaging is typically not required except where there is clinical uncertainty or the patient needs reassurance. Imaging may not identify any abnormality if there is no herniation at the time of the examination. For this reason US or dynamic MR imaging should be performed also. On US images, normal muscle tissue may be seen extending through a focal fascial defect. The hernia may become more pronounced with contraction. If no abnormality is found, standing with flexion and extension may demonstrate the defect more effectively. Often it is best to ask the patient what produces their lump or what typically produces their pain. On MR images often a subtle contour deformity can be identified with associated edema or a focal outpouching of the muscle through the fascial defect.

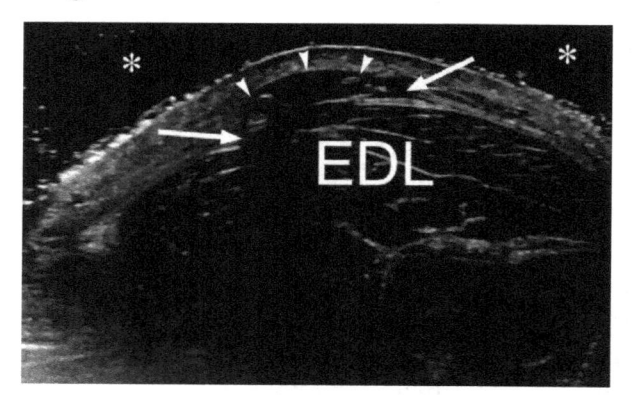

Muscle hernia of extensor digitorum longus. Transverse extended FOV sonogram shows extensor digitorum longus (EDL) with epimyseal defect (arrows) and muscle hernia (arrowheads). A thick layer of coupling gel (*) has been applied so probe pressure does not reduce the hernia.

Myositis ossificans traumatica—Posttraumatic myositis ossificans (PTMO) is a nonneoplastic proliferation of bone and cartilage within the skeletal muscle at the site of previous trauma or repeated injury and hematoma. Being a rare complication, there is little evidence regarding the pathogenesis or the optimal treatment. PTMO most commonly affects the thigh and arm, with anterior muscle groups affected more frequently than the posterior groups. Proximal regions of an extremity are more frequently affected than distal parts. In sports, myositis ossificans is typically associated with prior sports-related muscle injury, the incidence being highest in the contact sports in which the use of protective devices is uncommon, such as rugby. Although it is sometimes possible to detect the first signs of ectopic bone on radiographs as early as 18–21 days after the injury, the formation of ectopic bone usually lags behind the symptoms by weeks, and thus, a definite radiographic diagnosis can only be made substantially later. Although PTMO is a benign self-limiting condition, imaging is an important tool to exclude infection or malignancy. Imaging plays an important role especially in the acute stages, when biopsy or excision should be avoided.

PTMO has a characteristic peripheral calcification pattern, not typically seen in other calcifying soft-tissue lesions. Increased vascularity may be depicted on at Doppler US assessment. US may further help in detecting associated calcifications not visualized on radiographs.

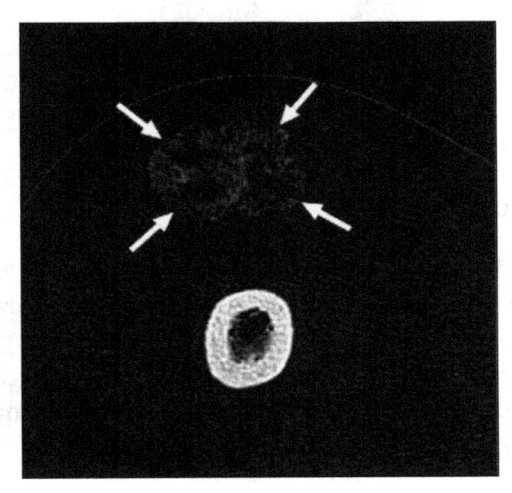

PTMO in a 22-year-old woman who noted, incidentally, a solid mass at the anterior right thigh that was movable beneath the surface. There was previous history of minor direct contact trauma during a hockey game 9 months earlier. Axial nonenhanced computed tomography (CT) image shows a peripherally calcified lesion (arrows) in the rectus femoris muscle (5-mm reconstructed section thickness). On axial T1-weighted nonenhanced MR image (612/18; FOV, 250 × 250 mm; 5 mm section thickness; 1 mm intersection gap), the lesion (arrows) appears hypointense to muscle. No areas of hyperintensity are seen that would reflect lipomatous or hemorrhagic components. Coronal T1-weighted MR image obtained after contrast agent administration (632/24; FOV, 350 × 350 mm; 5 mm section thickness; 1 mm intersection gap) shows marked inhomogeneous enhancement of the lesion (arrows). The peripheral disposition of the calcifications is better depicted with CT than MR imaging.

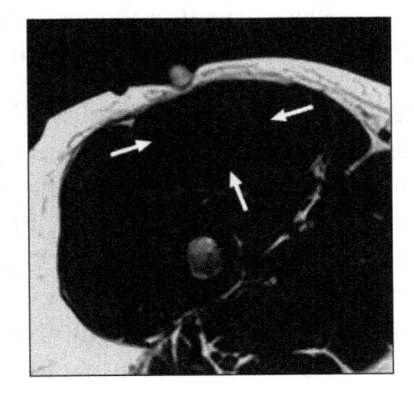

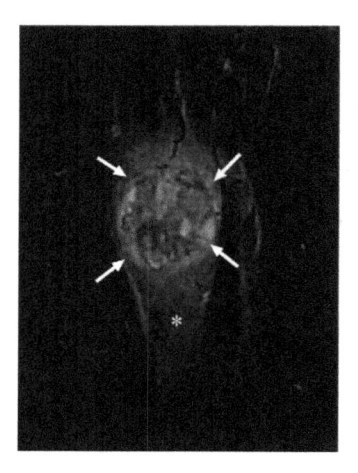

Clinical Relevance of Imaging Findings

Return to Play Prediction

In the elite-athlete setting, MR imaging is considered by some as the modality of choice for predicting time to return to sport after acute muscle injury. Current literature on return to play determination is limited to hamstring-related research applying MR imaging as the imaging modality, since assessment of return to play remains one of the major challenges in dealing with acute hamstring injuries. Previous research has suggested that a number of imaging findings are associated with the time needed to return to play.

However, a recent systematic review found that currently there is no strong evidence that any 1.5-T MR imaging finding is useful for predicting the time to return to sports following hamstring injury. This conclusion was predominantly based on the considerable risk of bias in most studies and the wide variation in time to return, independent of injury severity. The major methodological flaw of the reviewed studies was a lack of blinding of the subjects and clinicians to the MR imaging findings and simple univariate statistical analysis. Also it must be remembered that it is difficult to apply a standard imaging finding to all athletes when they vary greatly in the muscle range and function required to perform specific activities in different sports, which is reflected in the heterogeneity of muscle injuries. Differences and variations in MR imaging protocols used for hamstring injury research are substantial, suggesting that there is no widely accepted reference standard.

Despite these limitations, the review reported limited to moderate evidence for an association of high signal intensity on T2-weighted images affecting the proximal or central tendon, injuries not affecting the MTJ, and complete ruptures with a longer period to return.

Recent studies with a more robust design and using multivariate statistical analysis confirmed that the value of 1.5-T MR imaging or US for predicting return to play was negligible and added little to patient history and clinical examination. Based on the recent literature, routine MR imaging examination therefore cannot be recommended to provide accurate information for prediction of time to return to play after acute hamstring injuries. Nonetheless, this does not imply that MR imaging should be abandoned from daily practice, as it might be of value for confirming the clinical diagnosis, informing the athlete (the images might give the athlete more understanding of the injury), and living up to the expectation of performing imaging in the elite-athlete setting.

Imaging at Return to Play

It is a major challenge to decide whether an athlete can safely return to play, as there are no validated criteria to guide the decision. In clinical practice, MR imaging has been suggested to assist return-to-play decisions. Only three studies have been published and all focused on MR imaging at return to play following hamstring injury. These studies showed persisting increased signal intensity on fluid-sensitive images at return to sport clearance. Normalization of increased signal intensities on MR images is therefore not required for a successful return to play, suggesting that functional recovery precedes structural recovery at imaging.

Risk of Reinjury

High reinjury rates remain a major problem following acute muscle injuries. Reinjuries are often more severe than the initial injury and are associated with a longer absence from sports. Studies have focused on the association of MR imaging parameters and reinjury risk. Especially in hamstring injuries, this association has been studied at two clinically relevant time points: at injury and at return to play. At injury, conflicting results on the predictive value of the MR imaging findings for reinjury have been reported. Studies in Australian rules football revealed only limited evidence that the extent of high-signal-intensity changes seen on T2-weighted images (representing the edemalike changes in muscle injuries), measured by using the longitudinal length and the cross-sectional area, is related to an increased risk of reinjury. Such relationship was not confirmed in a cohort of European professional soccer players, Australian rules footballers, and amateur soccer players. Confirmation of a clinically suspected biceps femoris long head injury with MR imaging might guide the clinician in predicting the reinjury risk, as the reinjury risk is 16% compared with 2% for the medial injured group.

An MR imaging examination at return to play cannot be used to predict which athletes will reinjure and which will not, which is a reflection of the heterogeneity of sports-related muscle injuries. At return to play, persisting T2 high-signal-intensity changes will be present in the majority of cases, and these changes are not associated with an increased reinjury risk. At return to play, an area of abnormal intramuscular low signal intensity on T1-weighted images, suggestive for fibrosis, can be expected in approximately one-fourth of the athletes. These low-signal-intensity abnormalities, however, do not seem to be associated with an increased risk of reinjury.

In summary, with our current 1.5-T protocols, there is no evidence to support the use of MR imaging for identifying athletes at increased risk of reinjury following acute hamstring injury.

References

- Sports-medicine: britannica.com, Retrieved 16 August, 2019
- The-importance-of-sports-medicine: sportsnewsireland.com, Retrieved 05 January, 2019
- Sports-chiropractic-the-athletes-secret-weapon: thejoint.com, Retrieved 23 July, 2019
- 7-benefits-chiropractic-care-athletes: ballerinichiropractic.com, Retrieved 14 June, 2019
- Sport-psychology: sports-fitness-recreation-and-leisure-magazines: encyclopedia.com, Retrieved 26 February, 2019
- 2-use-diagnostic-imaging-sports-medicine: mja.com.au, Retrieved 25 January, 2019

Orthopedic Sports Medicine

Orthopedic Sports Medicine focuses on identifying, preserving and restoring musculoskeletal system affected by athletic activity. It includes medical, surgical and rehabilitative methods of treatment. This chapter has been carefully written to provide an easy understanding of orthopedic sports medicine.

Orthopedic sports medicine is a subspecialty of Orthopedics that focuses on managing pathological conditions of the musculoskeletal system arising from sports practice. When dealing with athletes, timing is the most difficult issue to face. Typically, athletes aim to return to play as soon as possible and at the pre-injury level. This means that management should be optimized to combine the need for prompt return to sport and to the biologic healing time of the musculo-skeletal. This poses a great challenge to sport medicine surgeons, who need to follow with attention to the latest scientific evidence to offer their patients the best available treatment options.

Lower Limb

Knee-meniscal Injuries

Although meniscal injuries are mainly encountered in athletes involved in pivoting maneuvers, even low-impact sports such as swimming have been plagued by meniscal lesions. Meniscal injuries are one of the most common musculo-skeletal issues and one of the most common orthopedic surgeries performed worldwide. Vertical peripheral longitudinal tears as well as root tears should be repaired, leading to superior outcomes in terms of symptoms, function, and return to play, and cartilage preservation compared to meniscectomy. In more recent years, there is an increasing body of evidence in favor of repairing horizontal tears, especially in the young patient. Return to sports after meniscus repair for high-level athletes (basketball, American football, baseball) varies between 80 and 90%. However, studies on meniscal repair in athletes have found that up to one third of the patients underwent reoperation for pain. Concerning the surgical technique of a meniscal repair, there is general agreement to start the procedure performing a debridement and abrasion of the meniscal lesion walls to favor local bleeding, and with regard to the suture technique, vertical or horizontal sutures are recommended, performed either with all-inside, inside-out or outside-in techniques, since no superiority have been demonstrated of one technique over the others.

However, it has been demonstrated that vertical suturing configuration has superior load to failure values compared to a horizontal configuration. Usually, all-inside sutures are used on the far posterior segments, and inside-out for the middle and anterior meniscal segments. Alvarez-Diaz, in a case-series on 29 competitive football players, reported that 26 (89.6%) were able to return to play at the same level of competition at a mean of 4.3 months after surgery.

Anterior Cruciate Ligament Injury

Anterior cruciate ligament (ACL) tears, accounting for about 200,000 injuries per year in the USA, may compromise knee stability and affect negatively sports activity. Although most of the ACL tears result from a non-contact injury, lesions during contrasts in sports such as American football, rugby, or hockey are frequent as well.

Many risk factors have been identified for ACL tear. Some depend on bone morphology (narrower intercondylar notch widths, smaller notch width index, and increased tibial slopes), some others on hormones and gender. Recently, biomechanical factors such as limited hip internal rotation have been associated to ACL tear injury. Conservative management of ACL tears can produce acceptable results, but in athletes, surgical reconstruction is usually preferred. The main advantage of ACL reconstruction (ACLR) is to restore knee stability what will eventually help to prevent secondary injury to menisci and articular cartilage. Different techniques are used to perform ACLR. Transtibial independent drilling (through the antero-medial portal) and the outside-in techniques are the most commonly used ones. A systematic review showed that independent drilling is more likely to lead to better biomechanical and functional outcomes compared to transtibial technique, although no clear clinical evidences support its superiority. Outside-in drilling has the advantages of unconstrained tunnels placement, but it needs two incisions. Single- or double-bundle graft reconstructions have been proposed. Biomechanical studies favored double-bundle graft in terms of rotational stability.

Concerning the graft, it is possible to identify three main categories: autograft, allograft, and synthetic graft. Synthetic graft showed high failure rate, although newer synthetic grafts seem, in the short term, more promising than the older ones.

Allografts are expensive; there is a risk for infections transmission, delayed incorporation, and late failure. Therefore, especially for young athletic individuals, the choice falls on autografts: bone patellar tendon bone (BPTB), hamstrings, and less commonly quadriceps tendon. There is a huge debate on what is better between patellar tendon and hamstring, and no definitive superiority has been shown. BPTB grafts ensure greater post-operative knee stability but exhibit a higher complication rate. On the contrary, hamstring autographs, for which revision surgery is most frequently required, is often associated with post-operative antero-posterior knee laxity, particularly in females. However, despite all the great efforts trying to improve ACL reconstruction, the rate of patients who return to sports ranges between 63 and 92%. This trend confirms the importance of psychological factor and neuromuscular focused rehabilitation as essential elements in determining the return to play rate.

Posterior Cruciate Ligament Injury

Isolate posterior cruciate ligament (PCL) injury has an incidence that ranges between 3 and 44% after acute trauma to the knee. A PCL injury is often part of complex knee injuries, associated respectively in 46, 31, and 62% of cases, to ACL tears, medial collateral ligament (MCL) injury, and posterolateral corner injuries. Isolated PCL injuries in the knees with reduced joint laxity and absence of other peripheral lesion are generally managed conservatively even in athletes, with satisfactory subjective results, and return to sport at the same level in about 50% of cases. In patients with PCL injuries managed conservatively, 41% of the subjects at 14-year follow-up develop early osteoarthritis, with progressive reduction of joint function. Surgical treatment can be performed to optimize joint function. After surgery, competitive sports are practiced again by 67% of the subjects and high functional demand sports by 26%. Clinical outcomes show no differences between single- and double-bundle reconstruction techniques at approximately 30 months of follow-up. However, double-bundle PCL reconstruction mainly improves objective measurement of knee stability.

Hip

Femoroacetabular Impingement

Femoroacetabular impingement (FAI) is a common cause of hip and groin pain in young active people and athletes. FAI initially causes chondral lesions and labral tears and, subsequently, early arthritis. Arthroscopic surgery is undertaken in subjects refractory to conservative management, involving targeted physiotherapy and oral anti-inflammatory drugs. Few studies reported data about surgical procedures, such as femoroplasty, acetabuloplasty, and labral reconstruction, in athletes, and they showed that arthroscopic surgery is effective in terms of both clinical and functional improvement and return to sport (87% of patients). Moreover, timing for arthroscopic treatment is essential; the length of athletic career was significantly affected by symptom duration before arthroscopic treatment in professional hockey players.

Achilles Tendon

Achilles tendinopathy is common in athletes, accounting for 6–17% of all injuries in running athletes. The etiology of tendinopaty is still not well understood, but multiple factors play a role in its pathophysiology. Pharmacological interventions currently lack for scientific evidences supporting their use, while conservative management of chronic midportion Achilles tendinopathy by eccentric exercises and extracorporeal shock waves therapy (ESWT) is strongly supported by several level I studies. Patients resistant to those conservative measures can undergo to high-volume image-guided injection, effective in relieving patients' symptoms and restore tendon function both in the short and long term. In non-insertional Achilles tendinopathy, minimally invasive multiple percutaneous longitudinal tenotomies are valid alternatives to more invasive procedures, at least in patients without evidence of paratendinopathy, unresponsive to 6 months of conservative management. This method leads to satisfactory outcomes in the long term and restores ankle function. Given the renowned complications in terms of infections and difficult wound healing, in most recent years, tendoscopy has been proposed, with satisfactory outcomes, as an alternative method to open surgery, including debridement alone or debridement associated to flexor halluces longus tendon transfer.

Eccentric exercises for insertional Achilles tendinopaty did not show excellent outcomes, while ESWT did better. For those patients not responding to conservative measures, surgery is indicated in order to debride the tendinopathic tissue and to excise the calcaneal bony prominence, with or without tendon detachment and subsequent fixation to calcaneus tuberosity. Surgical management of insertional Achilles tendinopathy is indicated after failure of 3- to 6-month period of nonsurgical management. Thorough debridement is necessary, and this leads often to a near to complete detachment of the tendon's insertion. Therefore, repair with two anchors is recommended; indeed, it is associated with good to excellent results. Outcomes from surgery can be satisfactory, but prolonged rehabilitation is necessary.

Ankle

Lateral Ankle Ligaments

Ankle sprains are common, especially in team sports. They account for up to 40% of all athletic injuries, and 29% of American football injuries can be attributed to ankle injuries. The most common pattern of injury is forefoot adduction, hindfoot inversion, with the tibia externally rotated and the ankle in plantar flexion. This mechanism leads to tears to one or more of the lateral ligaments of the ankle. Up to 70% of the sprains involve the anterior talo-fibular ligament (ATFL) alone. More than 50% of the ankle sprains do not come to medical attention. Patients with ankle sprain grade I and II, accounting for greatest part, will benefit from the use of RICE (rest, ice cryotherapy, compression, and elevation). Grade III has a less standardized management. Some authors have proposed surgical repair for the acute grade III lesion, but many others have reported discouraging outcomes following acute repair in favor of functional treatment.

Chronic ankle instability is defined as the condition of symptomatic ankle instability following an acute ankle sprain managed with conservative measure.

Surgical management of the lateral ligaments of the ankle can be performed with an anatomic reconstruction (the Brostrom-Gould technique) or by several techniques in which a tendon graft, either autograft or allograft, reinforces the local tissue. A recent comparison of lateral anatomic ankle repair (Brostrom-Gould) to allograft reconstruction showed that no revision was needed in patients from both groups, and no significant differences between groups in terms of function and patients' satisfaction were found.

Allografts showed good to excellent results in up to 85% of cases, and they should be considered when multiple ligaments are involved, such as calcaneofibular ligament (CFL) other than ATFL.

At the time of surgical repair of ankle lateral ligaments, it is highly recommended to perform an ankle arthroscopy, since this will allow looking for intrarticular lesions.

Recently, different minimally invasive techniques have been proposed for chronic ankle instability (arthroscopic repair, non-arthroscopic minimally invasive repair, arthroscopic reconstruction, and non-arthroscopic minimally invasive reconstruction). However, there is still a lack for high-level evidences to support their use in daily clinical practice.

Ankle Osteochondral Lesions

About 50% of acute ankle sprain leads to chondral lesions of the talus (OCL), causing persisting pain despite conservative or surgical treatment. Most of the OCL are central-lateral (49%) and follow an inversion ankle sprain. Those kinds of lesions respond poorly to conservative measures. In the acute setting, arthroscopic debridement with excision of the loose OCL is usually indicated for lesions smaller than 1 cm^2. Fragment fixation using bioabsorbable screws is advised for wider lesions.

Chronic OCLs are classified in five types according to Loomer. Type I and II lesions can be addressed by retrograde drilling, a technique that aims to bone marrow stimulation. Type III and IV lesions can be addressed with satisfactory outcomes either by excision or curettage. Finally, type V, a cystic lesion, is usually bone grafted or filled using osteochondral plugs (mosaicplasty).

Spine

Disc Herniation and Disc Degeneration Disease

Injuries of the cervical spine frequently affect athletes who practice contact sports and represent 44.7% of all American football-related spinal injuries. In patients with diagnosis of cervical disc herniations, surgical indications are persistent symptoms, evidence of spinal cord compression on MRI and cervical myelopathy. However, drug (such as anti-inflammatory medications) and physical therapy (strengthening exercises) remains the first-line treatment and produces a higher rate of return to sport if compared with surgical treatment. Furthermore, contact sports are contraindicated in patients who underwent multilevel anterior cervical discectomy and fusion (ACDF) or with cervical myelopathy, residual pain, or muscle weakness.

Low back pain, reported by 75% of elite athletes, is frequent in athletes of all levels. In addition to genetic and anatomic factors, the incidence of lumbar disc degeneration is justified by an abnormal and increased load on the lumbar spine arising from sports activity practiced over the years, which, in the long term, leads to early disc degeneration. Similar to the upper spine levels, in lumbar pathology, the first approach is rehabilitation focused on restoring range of motion and muscular strengthening. Surgery is reserved to symptomatic patients non-responsive to non-operative treatment with imaging evidence of spinal cord compression. Lumbar disc herniation successfully receives non-operative treatment in 90% of patients. Professional athletes who underwent surgery, both total disc replacement or discectomy and fusion, experience significant improvement of symptoms in a high percentage of cases and about 95% of patients return to sport without significant differences with previous sports performances. Lumbar discectomy offers variable results according to the type of sport practiced by professional athletes. Satisfactory outcomes and high rates of return to sport can be found in American football players. On the contrary, baseball players who underwent surgery had a shorter career compared to colleagues with the same diagnosis but treated conservatively. This heterogeneity highlights the importance of load forces as causes of lumbar hernia and possible post-surgical recurrence. Treatment should be guided by surgeon experience and set on athlete's functional requirements.

Upper Limb

Shoulder

In athletes, shoulder injuries commonly involve rotator cuff tendons and the labrum.

Superior Labrum Anterior to Posterior (SLAP) Lesions

Snyder reported an incidence of SLAP lesions ranging from 4.8 to 6.9%. The injury mechanism is usually overhead activity that determines a contact between the articular side of the supraspinatus tendon and the postero-superior glenoid labrum.

The first line of treatment can be conservative, mainly aiming to scapula stabilization, rotator cuff strengthening, and stretching of the postero-inferior capsule. Indeed, an excessive loss of glenohumeral internal rotation (GIRD) is common in overhead athletes.

Surgical indication depends on several factors, such as the kind of lesion, the patient's age, level of activity, and the previous non-operative management. Type II SLAPs are the most common. They present complete detachment of the superior labrum and the biceps anchor from the superior glenoid tubercle. Repairing the lesion in older patients (> 40 years old) showed higher rate of unsatisfactory outcomes and surgical revision. In this instance, the tendon of the long head of the biceps can undergo either a tenodesis or a tenotomy. In young active athletes, the lesion should be repaired. However, this is the most challenging type of lesion: its repair can result in a stiff shoulder, and return to play at the pre-injury level cannot be guaranteed. When choosing the treatment method, in type II lesion, it is of paramount to take into account the patient's type and level of activity. Recent evidences showed that biceps suprapectoral or subpectoral tenodesis is preferable over SLAP repair in young patients practicing overhead activity. Type I lesions are characterized by frying of the labrum, and therefore, the proposed surgical treatment is arthroscopic debridement. Type III lesions show a bucket handle tear of the labrum, while the biceps tendon is normal. For these lesions, resection of the unstable bucket handle tear is indicated. Type IV is a type III lesion with a longitudinal lesion of the biceps tendon, which may dislocate into the joint. When less than 30% of the tendon is torn, the lesion can be abraded together with the degenerated area of the labrum. If the lesion involves more than 30% of the biceps tendon, it will be repaired in young patients or excised in older ones.

Bankart Lesion

Anterior shoulder dislocation is common especially in contact athletes such as American football, ice hockey, and rugby players. The most common injury mechanism in athletes is abduction and external rotation of the arm by an externally rotating force. This injury mechanism generates a Bankart lesion where the antero-inferior capsule-labral complex is detached from the glenoid rim either alone or with a bony fragment (bony Bankart). In athletes, even after the first dislocation, non-operative treatment leads to a high recurrence rate.

Arthroscopic repair of the Bankart lesion has become more popular than open surgery, with similar reoperation and recurrence rate. Return to sport after arthroscopic Bankart repair is variable, going up to 95%. In bony Bankart lesions, following the new concept of glenoid track introduced by Itoi in 2007, there has been much debate on which is the best treatment to address both the humeral (Hill-Sachs) and the glenoid bony lesions. It is suggested to perform arthroscopic Bankart repair for patients with glenoid bone loss < 25% and on-track Hill-Sachs (HS). If the HS is off-track, a remplissage procedure is necessary to restore shoulder stability. When facing a glenoid bone loss > 25%, whether it is on-track or off-track HS, the Latarjet procedure is recommended.

Rotator Cuff Tears

Throwing athletes are at higher risk not only for labrum injuries but also for rotator cuff tears. In addition to the common cuff lesions, the throwing athletes show a higher incidence of partial-thickness articular-sided tears of the postero-superior portion of the cuff compared to the general population. This is secondary to the internal impingement syndrome, a phenomenon described by Jobe and Walch.

That syndrome is due to a conflict between the posterior glenoid rim and the postero-superior rotator cuff insertion on the greater tuberosity. Factors associated with this condition are recurring microtrauma, scapular diskynesis, and posterior capsule contracture with consequent loss of internal rotation.

Surgical options are taken into consideration when conservative measures have failed. In general, partial tears are repaired when the tear involves more than 50% of the tendon thickness; otherwise, the debridement alone is enough. However, it is controversial whether to repair partial lesions of the rotator cuff in a throwing athlete because of the difficulties of returning to play after a rotator cuff repair.

Ankle Ligament Reconstruction

What is an Ankle Sprain?

A sprain is the stretching or tearing of a ligament. Ligaments connect adjacent bones in a joint and provide stability to the joint.

An ankle sprain is a common injury and occurs when you fall or suddenly twist the ankle joint or when you land your foot in an awkward position after a jump. It most commonly occurs when you participate in sports or when you jump or run on a surface that is irregular.

Ankle sprains can cause pain, swelling, tenderness, bruising, and stiffness, numbness in the toes, and inability to walk or bear weight on the ankle accompanied by persistent discomfort.

Inadequate healing of a sprained ligament or incomplete rehabilitation of the affected ligament can result in instability of the ankle.

A complete medical history, including a history of any previous ankle injuries, and a physical examination is essential for an accurate diagnosis of the condition. An X-ray may be ordered to confirm the diagnosis.

Indications for Ankle Ligament Reconstruction

Surgical intervention to reconstruct the injured ligament may be considered in patients with a high degree of instability and in those who have failed to respond to non-surgical treatments.

How is an Ankle Ligament Reconstruction Procedure Performed?

Ankle ligament reconstruction may be performed arthroscopically under general anaesthesia. Your surgeon will make small incisions in your ankle. A tiny camera and a few special instruments are inserted through the incisions to repair and strengthen the ligaments. Stretched or torn ligaments will be shortened and stitched as needed. Sometimes, a weakened ligament is reconstructed with a section of tendon derived from the foot and around the ankle.

The recovery time after ankle ligament reconstruction depends on the extent of injury and the procedure performed. For the first few weeks after surgery, you will be instructed to use crutches or a wheelchair and avoid bearing any weight on the reconstructed ankle joint.

What are the Risks and Complications of Ankle Ligament Reconstruction?

Specific complications of ankle ligament reconstruction include infection, nerve damage, ankle joint stiffness, and recurrent instability.

Bunion Correction

What is a Bunion?

A bunion, also known as hallux valgus, is bony prominence at the base of the big toe, which often results in pain, redness and rubbing in footwear. The 1st metatarsal bone abnormally angles outward towards the other foot from its joint in the midfoot. A bunion can change the shape of your foot, make it difficult for you to find shoes that fit correctly and worsen the symptoms if left untreated.

What are the Causes of a Bunion?

Although it is not clearly understood why bunions occur, possible causes include:

- Family history and genetics.
- Arthritis (inflammation of the joints) including rheumatoid arthritis, psoriatic arthritis and gout.
- Neuromuscular conditions such as cerebral palsy (affects movement and co-ordination).
- Connective tissue disorders such as Marfansyndrome (affects the connective tissues).
- Tight fitting shoes that are too tight, narrow or high heeled.

What are the Symptoms of a Bunion?

The main indication of a bunion is the pointing of the big toe towards the other toes of the foot. Other signs and symptoms include:

- Pain and swelling over the big toe that increases while wearing shoes.
- Swelling with red, sore and calloused skin at the base of the big toe.
- Inward turning of the big toe pushes the second toe out of place.
- Bony bump at the base of the big toe.
- Sore skin over the bony bump.
- Difficulty walking and wearing shoes.

How is a Bunion Diagnosed?

The diagnosis of a bunion by an orthopedic surgeon includes taking a medical history, and performing a physical examination to assess the extent of misalignment and damage to the soft tissues. Your surgeon will usually order weight bearing X-rays (i.e. taken while standing) to access the severity of the bunion and deformity of the toe joints.

What are the Conservative Treatment Options for Bunions?

Your doctor may have already initially recommended conservative treatment measures with the goal of reducing or eliminating your foot pain. Such measures can include:

- Medications for relieving pain and inflammation.

- Wearing surgical shoes with a wide and high toe box, avoiding tight, pointed or high-heeled shoes.
- Use of orthotics to realign the bones of your foot and ease pain.
- Padding the bunions.
- Ice applications several times a day.

Conservative treatment measures can help relieve the discomfort of a bunion, however these measures will not prevent the bunion from becoming worse. Surgery is the only means of correcting a bunion. Surgery is also recommended when conservative measures fail to treat the symptoms of bunion.

What are the Surgical Options for a Bunion?

There are many surgical options to treat a bunion. The common goal is to realign the bones in the foot, correct the deformity, and relieve pain and discomfort. The surgery is performed as a day procedure, under the effect of a light general anesthetic and a regional nerve block. When you wake up, you will not be in pain and will be able to walk on your foot right away.

Osteotomy is a common type of bunion surgery that involves the surgical cutting and realignment of the bones around your big toe. Your surgeon selects the appropriate surgical procedure based on the type of bunion and its severity.

There are 3 main types of osteotomies used by foot and ankle surgeons; namely Akin osteotomy, Chevron osteotomy, and Scarf osteotomy.

- Akin osteotomy: Akin osteotomy corrects the sideways deviation of the big toe. In this procedure, your surgeon makes a small cut in the proximal phalanx (base of the big toe) and removes a wedge of bone to straighten the big toe. The bony fragments are then stabilized using a screw or staples. This procedure is often used in conjunction.
- Chevron osteotomy: A chevron osteotomy is usually recommended for mild to moderate bunion deformities. During this procedure, your surgeon will make an incision over your big toe. The joint capsule is opened, and the bunion is removed using a surgical saw. A V-shaped cut is made on your big toe and the metatarsal bones are shifted to bring your toe into its normal anatomical position. The bunion is then shaved, and the soft tissues are re-aligned to correct the position. Akin osteotomy may be performed if necessary. The mobility of your big toe is examined, and the capsule and wound are re-approximated with sutures. Screws or pins are used to hold the bones in their new position until healing takes place. This procedure can also be performed minimally invasively with keyhole style incisions.
- Scarf osteotomy: Scarf osteotomy is usually recommended for moderate to severe bunion deformities. Your surgeon will make an incision along your big toe and open the joint capsule to expose the bump. The bump on your big toe is then removed using a bone saw. Your first metatarsal bone is then cut in a Z shape and realigned to correct the deformity. Your surgeon will fix the cut bone with pins or screws. The joint capsule and surgical wounds are then re-approximated using dissolvable sutures keeping your toe in a straight position. This is a very powerful corrective procedure with excellent long-term results.

Arthrodesis: This surgery involves fusing the two bones that form the big toe joint. This procedure is used for severe bunions and when arthritis is present. The movement of your big toe is reduced following this procedure, but pain and deformity are very well controlled.

What are the Risks and Complications of Bunion Surgery?

As with any surgery, bunion surgeries involves certain risks and complications and include:
- Infection.
- Recurrence of the bunion.
- Nerve damage.
- Unresolved pain and swelling.
- Joint stiffness or restricted movement.
- Delayed healing or healing in the wrong position.

In rare cases, a second surgery may be necessary to correct the problems.

What is the Postoperative Care for Bunion Surgery?

Patients should follow all instructions given by the surgeon following the surgery. These include:
- Keep your dressings dry and leave them in place until your next outpatient appointment.
- Minimize walking where possible.
- Elevate the foot to minimize swelling as much as possible for the first 6 weeks.
- You will have to wear specially designed Postoperative shoes to protect the wounds and assist in walking.
- You may not be able to wear regular shoes for 6 weeks.

Ankle Arthroscopy

Ankle arthroscopy is a minimally invasive surgical procedure in which an arthroscope, a small, soft, flexible tube with a light and video camera at the end, is inserted into the ankle joint to evaluate and treat a variety of conditions.

An arthroscope is a small, fiber-optic instrument consisting of a lens, light source, and video camera. The camera projects an image of the inside of the joint onto a large screen monitor allowing the surgeon to look for any damage, assess the type of injury, and repair the problem.

What are the Indications for Ankle Arthroscopy?

Ankle Arthroscopy, also referred to as keyhole surgery or minimally invasive surgery, has proven to be highly effective in managing various ankle disorders including ankle arthritis, ankle instability, ankle fracture, osteochondral defects of the talus, infection, and undiagnosed ankle pain.

What are the Benefits of Ankle Arthroscopy?

The benefits of arthroscopy compared to the alternative, open ankle surgery, include:

- Smaller incisions.
- Minimal soft tissue trauma.
- Less pain.
- Faster healing time.
- Lower infection rate.
- Less scarring.
- Earlier mobilization.
- Shorter hospital stay.

How is an Ankle Arthroscopy Procedure Performed?

Your surgeon will make 2 or 3 small incisions around the ankle joint. Through one of the incisions an arthroscope is inserted. Along with it, a sterile solution is pumped into the joint to expand the joint area and create room for the surgeon to work.

The larger image displayed on the television monitor allows the surgeon to visualize the joint directly to determine the extent of damage so that it can be surgically treated. Surgical instruments will be inserted through the other tiny incisions to treat the problem.

After the surgery, the instruments are removed, and the incisions are closed and covered with a bandage.

What is the Post-surgical care for Ankle Arthroscopy?

After the procedure, you will be taken to a recovery room. The ankle joint will be immobilized with a splint or cast. The nature and duration of immobilization will depend on the type of repair performed and the preference of the surgeon. The surgical site should be kept clean and dry during the healing process. Patients may be prescribed pain medication for the management of pain. Elevation of the ankle and ice application helps to reduce pain and swelling. Follow your postoperative instructions for the best outcome.

What are the Risks and complications of Ankle Arthroscopy?

Ankle arthroscopy is a safe procedure and the incidence of complications is low. However, as with any surgery, risks and complications can occur. Some associated risks with ankle surgery can include infection, damage to blood vessels or nerves, bleeding, and compartment syndrome.

Tendon Reconstruction

What is an Ankle Sprain?

A sprain is the stretching or tearing of ligaments, which connect adjacent bones and provide stability to a joint. An ankle sprain is a common injury that occurs when you suddenly fall or twist the ankle joint or when you land your foot in an awkward position after a jump. Most commonly it occurs when you participate in sports or when you jump or run on a surface that is irregular.

Indications for Tendon Reconstruction?

Surgery is recommended in patients with a high degree of ankle instability and in those who have failed to respond to non-surgical treatments.

Tendon Reconstruction Procedure

Tendon reconstruction is a tendon transfer procedure that uses your own tendon or a cadaver tendon as a graft to replace the damaged tendon. The surgery is performed under epidural anesthesia. Your surgeon makes an incision on your ankle. Drill holes are created where the damaged ligament normally attaches to the lower end of the fibula (calf bone) on one side and the talus (anklebone) on the other end. Your surgeon then harvests the peroneus brevis muscle tendon, found on the outer edge of the small toe, and weaves it through the drill holes to form a ligament complex. Range of motion is evaluated; the incision is closed, and a sterile bandage is applied.

Postoperative Care for Tendon Reconstruction

After surgery, your foot will be immobilized with a cast or splint. You will be provided crutches to avoid bearing weight on the operated ankle. Your doctor will remove the splint and provide a removable boot to be worn for 2 to 4 weeks. Physical therapy will be initiated to strengthen your joint and improve range of motion. Complete recovery may take 10 to 12 weeks.

Advantages and Disadvantages of Tendon Reconstruction

The advantages of tendon reconstruction include:
- Provides increased strength.
- Can be used when host tissues are severely damaged.
- Provides additional stability in obese patients.

The disadvantages of tendon reconstruction include:
- Decreased rear foot motion.
- Does not preserve the peroneus brevis, an important structure for the ankle's dynamic stability.

Risks and Complications of Tendon Reconstruction

As with all surgical procedures, tendon reconstruction may be associated with certain complications including:
- Injury to the superficial nerves.
- Chronic pain.

- Stiffness.
- Need for second surgery (rare).

Tendon Transfers

Foot Anatomy and Movement

The foot and ankle is a complex joint involved in movement and providing stability and balance to the body. The foot and ankle consist of 26 bones, 33 joints, and many muscles, tendons and ligaments. Damage to the soft tissues such as nerves and muscles of the foot can cause weakness, decreased movement and difficulty in standing, walking and even wearing shoes.

What is a Tendon Transfer?

In a tendon transfer procedure, a healthy tendon is transferred to replace the damaged tendon and restore the normal movement of the foot.

Indications of Tendon Transfer

Tendon transfer surgery is indicated for the following conditions:
- Flexible flatfoot: The arch of the foot collapses because of the stretching or rupture of the posterior tibial tendon (attaches the calf muscle to the bones on the inside of the foot), leading to pain and discomfort. You tend to walk on the inside of the foot as your foot rolls outward.
- Neurological problem: Charcot-Marie-Tooth disease, nerve damage after an accident or surgery or weakness following a stroke can weaken the muscles of the foot causing pain and fractures. You tend to walk on the outside of the foot as your foot rolls inward.

There are three prerequisites for the surgery to be successful:
- The muscle attached to the tendon should be functional.
- The soft tissue that will receive the tendon should be functional. Scarring or skin damage makes the process of transfer difficult.
- The joints through which the tendon will pass should be mobile and stable.

Tendon Transfer Procedure

Tendon transfer surgery is usually performed under general anesthesia. An incision is made along the foot and the damaged tendon is exposed and removed. A healthy tendon is identified, cut at its normal insertion, rerouted through the soft tissues and bones, and then sutured to another bone in the foot. A tunnel may be drilled to allow the tendon to pass through and then sewn on itself, fastened with a metal or plastic screw, or attached with anchor sutures. The soft tissues and incision are closed, and your foot will be placed in a splint.

What to Expect after Tendon Transfer Care

You will be non-weight bearing for 6 weeks after surgery to allow the tendon to heal. Your splint will remain for 10 to 14 days. Once it is removed, a cast or surgical boot will be placed, and removed 12 weeks after surgery. You will be introduced to physical therapy shortly to strengthen your muscles and help you ambulate.

Complications of Tendon Transfer

As with all surgeries, tendon transfer surgery may be associated with certain complications such as:

- Infection.
- Anesthesia-related risks.
- Bleeding.
- Clot formation.
- Damage to adjacent blood vessels and nerves.
- Non-healing, rupture or loosening of the tendon.
- Progression of the primary neurological condition.
- Need for further surgery.

Osteochondral Allograft Transplantation System (OATS) of the Ankle

OATS of the ankle is a surgical procedure to treat Osteochondral Lesions of the Talus (OCL) or Osteochondritis Dissecans (OCD). It involves the transfer of healthy cartilage to replace the damaged cartilage and restore the normal function of the foot. The cartilage can be taken from your ankle joint (autograft) for smaller defects. An allograft (graft from a donor) is considered for large defects. During an OATS procedure, multiple, tiny plugs of healthy bone and cartilage are transferred and laid in a mosaic pattern, hence, the procedure is also known as mosaicplasty.

What are Osteochondral Lesions (OCL)/Osteochondritis Dissecans (OCD)?

The tibia and the fibula bones of the lower leg join with the talus bone to form the ankle joint. The talus bone is an important bone located between the tibia and fibula and the heel bone (calcaneus). OCL or OCD is the damage to the cartilage and the talus bone of the ankle joint. Usually, the inner or the medial portion of the ankle is affected. OCL may be genetic or may be caused due to trauma, stress fractures in sports, severe sprain, local osteonecrosis, etc. OCL lesions are sometimes asymptomatic. Large lesions are associated with symptoms such as localized ankle pain and discomfort which worsens while walking or running, a clicking or popping sound, swelling, tenderness, weakness of the foot, etc.

Indications for OATS Procedure

The OATS procedure is indicated for large ankle lesions that do not respond to non-surgical treatment methods involving the use of a cast, physical therapy, pain medications, strengthening exercises, etc. Lesions unresponsive to arthroscopic debridement and microfracture also may need the OATS procedure.

Preparation Before Surgery

Before surgery, your doctor will perform a complete physical examination of your ankle. An X-ray, CT-scan, or MRI of your ankle will be ordered. Discuss with your doctor any allergies that you might have and medications you are taking to see which ones you should stop taking before surgery.

OATS Procedure

The surgery is performed under general anesthesia. It involves the following steps:

- An incision is made at the ankle joint. A few ligaments may be incised to expose the joint.
- Your surgeon performs debridement of the chondral surface to remove damaged cartilage. Some damaged bone may also be removed. Care is taken to prevent damage to healthy cartilage.
- An allograft is inserted at the damaged site. Fixation is performed with pins or screws. Your surgeon ensures proper fitting of the allograft.
- Intraoperative fluoroscopy is performed by your surgeon to confirm proper placement of the graft.
- The incision is closed and covered with a bandage.

Rehabilitation after OATS Procedure

- Your leg will be placed in a splint or short leg cast and you will be encouraged to keep weight off your leg for about 6-8 weeks.
- Physical therapy exercises will be taught to improve your flexibility, range of motion and strength of your foot.
- Regularly follow-up with your doctor. Imaging techniques such as X-ray, CT-scan or MRI may be ordered to ensure union of the allograft with the bone.

Outcome of OATS Procedure

Patients typically experience reduced pain with improvement in the movement and functioning of the foot. Complications are rare.

Ankle OCD

The ankle joint is an articulation of the end of the tibia and fibula (shinbones) with the talus (heel bone). Osteochondral injuries, also called osteochondritis dissecans (OCD), are injuries to the talus bone, characterized by damage to the bone as well as the cartilage covering it. Sometimes, the lower end of the tibia or shinbone may also be affected.

Causes of Ankle OCD

Osteochondral injuries are most often caused by trauma to the ankle joint, such as with ankle sprains. Some cases may not have any previous history of ankle injury, and may be caused by local osteonecrosis or a metabolic defect.

Symptoms of Ankle OCD

The predominant symptom of osteochondral injury is pain, which may be localized to the ankle joint. Other symptoms may include tenderness and swelling of the ankle joint with difficulty in weight- bearing, locking of the ankle or instability.

Diagnosis of Ankle OCD

Osteochondral injuries are diagnosed by a physical examination, X-ray and CT and MRI scans. Plain X-ray images can reveal other fractures, bone spurs and narrowing of the joint. A CT scan helps identify any bony fragments and cysts, but is not very helpful to visualize bone edema or cartilage defects. MRI is the best imaging modality, which helps to visualize the cartilage and bone lesions as well as bone edema.

Treatment of Ankle OCD

Non-surgical or surgical treatment may be recommended for the management of osteochondral injuries of the ankle joint. Non-surgical treatment with immobilization, restricted weight-bearing and physical therapy may be ordered to help the bone and cartilage to heal, and improve muscle strength, mobility and coordination. Surgical treatment is recommended for more severe injuries and comprises of debridement (removing) of the damaged cartilage and removal of any loose bodies. Some of the most commonly used surgical techniques include microfracture or drilling of the lesion, grafting of cartilage and bone, or fixation of the fragments with the help of screws.

Osteochondral Lesions

Osteochondral Lesions (OCL) of the Ankle

The tibia and the fibula bones of the lower leg join with the talus bone to form the ankle joint. The talus bone is an important bone located between the tibia and fibula and the heel bone (calcaneus). OCL or OCD is the damage to the cartilage and the talus bone of the ankle joint. Usually, the inner or the medial portion of the ankle is affected.

Causes of OCL of the Ankle

OCL may be genetic or may be caused due to trauma, stress fractures in sports, severe sprain, local osteonecrosis, etc.

Symptoms of OCL of the Ankle

OCL lesions are sometimes asymptomatic. Large lesions are associated with symptoms such as localized ankle pain and discomfort which worsens while walking or running, a clicking or popping sound, swelling, tenderness, weakness of the foot, etc.

Diagnosis of OCL of the Ankle

Osteochondral lesions are diagnosed by a physical examination, X-ray, and CT and MRI scans. Plain X-ray images can reveal other fractures, bone spurs, and narrowing of the joint. A CT scan helps identify any bony fragments, but is not very helpful to visualize bone edema or cartilage defects. MRI is the best imaging modality, which helps to visualize the cartilage and bone lesions as well as bone edema.

Treatment of OCL of the Ankle

Non-surgical Method

Small lesions can be treated non-surgically involving the use of a cast, physical therapy, pain medications, strengthening exercises, etc.

Arthroscopy

An arthroscope is a narrow tube with a tiny video camera on one end. The structures inside the ankle are visible to your surgeon on a monitor in the operating room. Your doctor treats OCL by removing the damaged tissue followed by microfracture, which enables natural healing of the damaged bone and cartilage.

OATS Procedure

Large lesions are treated by the OATS procedure. OATS of the ankle is a surgical procedure to treat Osteochondral Lesions of the Talus (OCL) or Osteochondritis Dissecans (OCD). It involves the transfer of healthy cartilage to replace the damaged cartilage and restore the normal function of the foot. The cartilage can be taken from your ankle joint (autograft) for smaller defects. An allograft (graft from donor) is considered for large defects. During an OATS procedure, multiple, tiny plugs of healthy bone and cartilage is transferred in a pattern that resembles a mosaic, hence, the procedure is also known as mosaicplasty.

Prevention of OCL of the Ankle

OCL of the ankle can be prevented by:

- Learning proper techniques in sports.
- Minimizing overuse activities.
- Practicing strength training exercises.

Cavus Foot Reconstruction

A cavus foot or a high-arched foot refers to a condition that can vary from a slightly high arch to a severe deformity. Cavus foot can lead to symptoms such as pain and instability. The condition may be inherited or associated with neurological disorders or other conditions.

What is Cavus Foot Reconstruction?

Cavus foot reconstruction is performed to reduce pain and increase stability in the foot. It is indicated when conservative treatment including orthotic appliances, shoe modifications, and bracing does not resolve the symptoms.

Cavus foot reconstruction involves various surgical techniques:
- Soft tissue surgery:
  - Tendon release in case of over pull from the muscles.
  - Tendon transfer to correct a deformity in the ankle joint.
  - Achilles tendon lengthening to reduce the tension from the calf muscle, and.
  - Release of a tight plantar fascia, a fibrous band that runs along the bottom of the foot.
- Removal of bone (osteotomy) from the heel, toes or other parts of the foot.
- Joint fusion in case of severe joint deformity and pain.

Recovery Following Cavus Foot Reconstruction

Recovery following cavus foot reconstruction takes approximately 6 weeks for the bone to heal and total recovery may last 8-12 weeks. The postsurgical protocol varies amongst patients, and may be strict non-weightbearing for 6 weeks after the surgery. The decision to initiate an early weight-bearing program depends on the stability of the fixation used to correct the problem. In any case, do not put weight on the foot until instructed by your surgeon.

Risks and Complications Associated with Cavus Foot Reconstruction

As with any surgical procedure, complications can occur and include the risk associated with anesthesia, bleeding, blood clots, infection, damage to surrounding blood vessels and nerves.

Flatfoot Reconstruction

Flatfoot refers to the condition characterized by low foot arches. It can cause foot pain and may interfere with walking. Flatfoot occurs due to a variety of conditions including arthritis, injury, posterior tibial tendon dysfunction, and diabetes.

Procedures for Flatfoot Reconstruction

Flat foot deformity may be surgically treated by correcting any bone deformities and repairing the supporting tendons and ligaments. There are various procedures performed under local or general anesthesia. These include:

- Medializing calcaneal osteotomy: Excision of a portion of the heel bone which is then shifted to the normal anatomic position under the leg and fixed in place with a metal plate and screws.

- Lateral column lengthening: A bone wedge fixed within the outer portion of the heel bone to increase its length and prevent or correct outward rotation of the foot.

- First metatarsal fusion or medial cuneiform dorsal opening wedge osteotomy: An incision is made on the top of the foot and the bones are fused or a portion of bone is removed, and a bony wedge is placed to prevent the big toe portion from raising off the ground.

- Tendon and ligament repair or replacement: This may involve repair or removal of a damaged posterior tibial tendon or lengthening of a tight Achilles tendon. Tendons may be transferred to support the arch. Supporting ligaments are also repaired.
- Double or Triple arthrodesis: Fusion of two or three bones in the hind foot. This is usually performed in the later stages of the disease characterized by arthritis and stiff deformity.

Recovery Following Flatfoot Reconstruction

Depending on the type of surgery, you may be allowed to go home the same day or hospitalized for an overnight stay. Your leg will be immobilized in a splint or a cast and kept elevated for two weeks following which the sutures are removed. Another cast or removable boot may be placed depending on your condition. You will have to avoid weight-bearing on the operated foot for approximately 2 months and then gradually bear weight as tolerated. Your doctor may recommend physical therapy or the use of orthotics or ankle braces.

Risks and Complications Associated with Flatfoot Reconstruction

As with any surgical procedure, complications can occur and include the risk associated with anesthesia, infection, bleeding, and nerve damage. Risks specific to flatfoot reconstruction include non-union of bone, incomplete healing and break down of hardware. However, these complications are rare, and the overall success rate of flatfoot surgery is very high.

Foot Fusion Procedure

Foot Anatomy

The foot has 26 bones, and can be divided into the hindfoot, midfoot and forefoot.

Arthritis of the Foot

Osteoarthritis, rheumatoid arthritis or other conditions may damage these joints that these bones form. The joints may wear out, collapse, cause severe foot deformity and affect the function of the foot.

Foot Fusion

Foot fusion procedures are surgical procedures that fuse the bones of the foot to overcome the painful movement and correct deformities in the region.

Indications for Foot Fusion

Foot fusion is indicated when conservative approaches, such as medications, steroid injections, activity modifications, custom orthotics and modified footwear, fail to provide pain relief. The fusion can treat foot deformity and arthritic joints.

Foot Fusion Procedure

Foot fusion is performed under the effect of general or regional anesthesia. Your surgeon will make 3-4 cm long cuts on the upper or inner surface of the foot, and will open the joints, remove the joint surface, reshape it and correct the deformity. The joints are then fixed and kept in place using screws, plates and staples. During the fusion, your surgeon may add bone grafts to fill the gaps between the joints, if necessary. This procedure stabilizes the joints, prevents movement and provides pain relief.

Postoperative Care for Foot Fusion

After the surgery, keep the operated foot elevated to decrease swelling. After the swelling has reduced, the foot will be put in a plaster cast from knee to toes for about 8 to 12 weeks until the bones have fused. You may have to use crutches for a few weeks. Your physical therapist will guide you to walk without putting pressure on the operated foot. Avoid driving and vigorous exercises for a few weeks after surgery. Follow-up X-ray images will be taken to check for bone fusion.

Risks and Complications of Foot Fusion

As with any procedure, midfoot tarsometatarsal joint fusion may involve certain risks and complications such as:

- Infection and swelling.
- Non-union of bones.
- Nerve injury.
- Malpositioning of the fused bones.
- Loosened pins and screws.
- Rarely, deep vein thrombosis or pulmonary embolism.

Knee Arthroscopy

Knee Anatomy

The knee joint is one of the most complex joints of the body. The lower end of the thighbone (femur) meets the upper end of the shinbone (tibia) at the knee joint. A small bone called the patella (kneecap) rests on a groove on the front side of the femoral end. A bone of the lower leg (fibula) forms a joint with the shinbone.

To allow smooth and painless motion of the knee joint, articular surfaces of these bones are covered with a shiny white slippery articular cartilage. Two C-shaped cartilaginous menisci are present in between the femoral end and the tibial end.

Menisci act as shock absorbers providing cushion to the joints. Menisci also play an important role in providing stability and load bearing to the knee joint.

Bands of tissue, including the cruciate and collateral ligaments, keep the different bones of the knee joint together and provide stabilization to the joint. Surrounding muscles are connected to the knee bones by tendons. The bones work together with the muscles and tendons to provide mobility to the knee joint. The whole knee joint is covered by a ligamentous capsule, which further stabilizes the joint. This ligamentous capsule is also lined with a synovial membrane that secretes synovial fluid for lubrication.

What is Knee Arthroscopy?

Knee Arthroscopy is a common surgical procedure performed using an arthroscope, a viewing instrument, to consider the knee joint to diagnose or treat a knee problem. It is a relatively safe procedure and most the patient's discharge from the hospital on the same day of surgery.

Indications for Knee Arthroscopy

The knee joint is vulnerable to a variety of injuries. The most common knee problems where knee arthroscopy may be recommended for diagnosis and treatment are:

- Torn meniscus.
- Torn or damaged cruciate ligament.
- Torn pieces of articular cartilage.
- Inflamed synovial tissue.
- Misalignment of patella.
- Baker's cyst: A fluid filled cyst that develops at the back of the knee due to the accumulation of synovial fluid. It commonly occurs with knee conditions such as meniscal tear, knee arthritis and rheumatoid arthritis.
- Certain fractures of the knee bones.

Knee Arthroscopy Procedure

Knee arthroscopy is performed under local, spinal, or general anesthesia. Your anesthesiologist will decide the best method for you depending on your age and health condition.

- The surgeon makes two or three small incisions around the knee.
- Next, a sterile saline solution is injected into the knee to push apart the various internal structures. This provides a clear view and more room for the surgeon to work.
- An arthroscope, a narrow tube with a tiny video camera on the end, is inserted through one of the incisions to view the knee joint. The structures inside the knee are visible to the surgeon on a video monitor in the operating room.
- The surgeon first examines the structures inside the knee joint to assess the cause of the problem.
- Once a diagnosis is made, surgical instruments such as scissors, motorized shavers, or lasers are inserted through another small incision, and the repair is performed based on the diagnosis.

The repair procedure may include any of the following:
- Removal or repair of a torn meniscus.
- Reconstruction or repair of a torn cruciate ligament.
- Removal of small torn pieces of articular cartilage.
- Removal of loose fragments of bones.
- Removal of inflamed synovial tissue.
- Removal of baker's cyst.
- Realignment of the patella.
- Making small holes or microfractures near the damaged cartilage to stimulate cartilage growth.
- After the repair, the knee joint is carefully examined for bleeding or any other damage.
- The saline is then drained from the knee joint.
- Finally, the incisions are closed with sutures or steri-strips, and the knee is covered with a sterile dressing.

Postoperative Care Following Knee Arthroscopy

Most patients are discharged the same day after knee arthroscopy. Recovery after the surgery depends on the type of repair procedure performed. Recovery from simple procedures is often fast. However, recovery from complicated procedures takes a little longer. Recovery from knee arthroscopy is much faster than that from an open knee surgery.

Pain medicines are prescribed to manage pain. Crutches or a knee brace may be recommended for several weeks. A rehabilitation program may also be advised for a successful recovery. Therapeutic exercises aim to restore motion and strengthen the muscles of the leg and knee.

Risks and Complications of Knee Arthroscopy

Knee arthroscopy is a safe procedure and complications are very rare. Complications specific to knee arthroscopy include bleeding into the knee joint, infection, knee stiffness, blood clots or continuing knee problems.

Partial Menisectomy

Partial meniscectomy is a surgical procedure to remove the torn portion of the meniscus from the knee joint. Meniscus is the C-shaped cartilage located in the knee that lubricates the knee joint, acts as shock-absorber, and controls the flexion and extension of joint. Meniscal tears can occur at any age, but are more common in athletes playing contact sports. These tears are usually caused by twisting motion or over flexing of the knee joint. Athletes who play sports, such as football, tennis and basketball are at a higher risk of developing meniscal tears.

You may have pain over inner and outer side of the knee, swelling, stiffness of knee, restricted movement of the knee, and difficulty in straightening your knee. If the conservative treatment such as pain medications, rest, physical therapy, and use of knee immobilizers fails to relieve pain, then surgery may be recommended. Surgical treatment options depend on the location, length, and pattern of the tear.

Types of Meniscectomy

There are two surgical procedures for meniscal tears which includes total and partial menisectomy. In total meniscectomy the entire meniscus is removed, but in partial meniscectomy your surgeon will only remove the torn meniscus. Total meniscectomy will help in relieving symptoms, but because the entire meniscus is removed; the cushioning and stability between the joints will be lost. Hence partial meniscectomy is considered.

Procedure of Partial Menisectomy

Partial meniscectomy is performed with arthroscopy, where several small incisions are made around the knee. Through one of the small incision, a miniature camera is inserted to see inside of the knee. Tiny surgical instruments are inserted through other small incisions to repair the tear. During the procedure the torn meniscus is removed, and the remaining edges of the meniscus are smoothened so that there are no sharp ends. Any unstable fragments which are causing locking and catching sensation will also be removed.

Post-operative Care Following Partial Menisectomy

Partial meniscectomy helps in restoring or maintaining knee stability and offers faster and complete recovery. After surgery rehabilitation exercises may help to restore knee mobility, strength and to improve range of motion.

Risks and Complications of Partial Menisectomy

Possible risks and complications of partial meniscectomy include infection, bleeding, and injury to blood vessels or nerves.

Quality Metrics and Sports Medicine

Quality metrics should be followed and measured closely by physicians of all backgrounds and expertise, including sports medicine physicians. While there are certain quality metrics that can be commonly applied to all physicians, such as rate of infections, quality metrics for specifically sports medicine should also be closely measured.

- Measure patients' rate of return to sports: One quality metric He says is hugely underutilized in the field of sports medicine is the patient's return to his or her respective sport. This metric is important, as it allows sports medicine physicians to study and measure the success rate at which they are able to help their patients get back to their sports at the same or higher level previous to the injury.

    "With the [return to sports] quality metric, sports physicians not only want to measure the rate at which patients get back to that sport or activity at the same or higher level but also how long it takes to help patients get there," He says. "Those are two huge metrics and are the basis for why sports medicine physicians get into this field of medicine and why patients go see a sports medicine physician".

- Carefully consider how to follow patients post-surgery: Adequate quality measuring means physicians need to follow their patients post-surgery to measure a wide array of outcomes, including infections, complications and return to sports. long sports medicine physicians choose to follow their patients for and the method of following them should depend on the sport, nature of the injury, the procedure and the patient.

"Typically, what most sports medicine physicians do with surgical injuries is they follow their patients until they are cleared to play [their sports] and then the patients are responsible for calling their physician if they have any problems," "There are some instances that require physicians to follow patients longer, such as kids who may not be done growing".

Sports medicine physicians can also rely on various tools to test how a patient's condition has improved or not improved over a certain period of time. "[For patients playing in team sports], there are muscle strength testing and functional drills sports medicine physicians can use, but that is entirely up to individual physicians," He says.

- Outcomes scores should be stratified: Similarly to how sports medicine physicians should post-surgically follow patients on an individual basis, outcomes scores, as it relates to quality measures, should also be stratified based on the sport, nature of the injury and the surgery and the patient.

"The differences in outcomes may not even be related to individual patients," He says. "Some surgeries have quicker turnarounds, and some surgeries don't do as well as others. For example, meniscal repairs are one of those procedures that are very difficult and the outcomes are not necessarily linked to poor quality. It's simply the nature of the injury".

- Failure rates are not necessarily indicative of quality: Failure rates are defined by the rate at which patients fail to return to play due to a failed procedure. He says failure rates occur at a certain percentage for many procedures, including joint replacement procedures. While these rates should be closely followed and measured, He says failure rates are often out of the hands of sports medicine physicians and can be difficult to bring down to zero.

"Some of these sports medicine injuries, even with the best technique, rehabilitation and most compliant patient, can still fail," He says. "Yes, a complication can occur during or after a surgery, but that does not inherently imply that it was due to the surgeon's technique or quality of care".

In the same example meniscal repairs' failure rate could be associated with a large body of medical literature indicating poor blood supply in the meniscus. However, it is largely out of the sports medicine physicians' control to reverse the poor blood supply in efforts to maximize the outcomes of the surgery.

Orthopedic Rehabilitation

Orthopaedic rehabilitation is a form of therapy that treats a wide variety of conditions affecting the musculoskeletal system and is a cornerstone of the programs and services we provide throughout the country.

Joints and Arthroplasty

Osteoarthritis

Intra-articular administration of hyaluronic acid is a pharmacological approach to the management of knee osteoarthritis. Several formulations of hyaluronic acid are commercially available. Altman performed a meta-analysis of trials assessing the efficacy of hyaluronic acid formulations according to molecular weight. Hyaluronic acid products with a molecular weight of ≥3,000 kDa had a pooled effect size of −0.52 (95% confidence interval [CI], −0.56 to −0.48) when pain reduction was the outcome. These were more efficacious than products that were <3,000 and >1,500 kDa and those that were ≤1,500 kDa in molecular weight.

Whole-body vibration mediates the activation of alpha (α) motor neurons, which cause muscle contractions, thereby leading to increased muscle strength. A recent meta-analysis of 5 studies showed preliminary data for improved pain and function with whole-body vibration training among patients with knee osteoarthritis compared with controls.

Total Knee Arthroplasty

With increasing emphasis on cost-containment and bundled payment, telerehabilitation has become an attractive strategy for delivering rehabilitation services. A randomized controlled trial found that telerehabilitation via videoconferencing was not inferior to face-to-face home visits after primary total knee arthroplasty when the Western Ontario and McMaster Universities Osteoarthritis Index (WOMAC) was used as the primary outcome measure. Another randomized controlled trial showed better pain and functional outcomes for total knee arthroplasty and 12 weeks of rehabilitation compared with only 12 weeks of rehabilitation (without surgery) for patients with knee osteoarthritis.

Hand

A randomized controlled trial compared surgery with physical therapy (manual therapies including desensitization) in females ≤65 years of age with clinical and electrodiagnostic evidence of carpal tunnel syndrome. Patients were classified as having minimal, moderate, or severe median neuropathy on the basis of electrodiagnostic criteria. There were no significant differences in pain and functional outcomes at 6 and 12 months between the 2 treatment groups.

Spine

Back pain accounts for 2% to 5% of all physician visits. While most acute episodes of back pain resolve, many individuals continue to have substantial pain and disability. Early management strategies remain controversial, as increased use of imaging, spinal injections, and prescription medications contributes to rising expenditures. Jarvik performed a prospective cohort study to evaluate early imaging (within 6 weeks of the index visit) including plain radiographs, computed tomography (CT), or magnetic resonance imaging (MRI) for patients ≥65 years of age with a new episode of care for back pain. patients with early imaging had significantly higher resource use and expenditures compared with matched controls. No significant differences were noted between those who underwent early imaging and those who did not in terms of patient-reported pain and disability up to 1 year after the index visit. This suggests that the value of early imaging is uncertain, and early imaging should not be performed routinely for older adults with acute back pain.

Prescription medications, including opioids, are commonly used to help manage acute back pain. Friedman conducted a randomized clinical trial to compare a 10-day course of muscle relaxants or opioids combined with nonsteroidal anti-inflammatory drugs (NSAIDs) and NSAID monotherapy among patients with nonradicular low back pain. All patients received 20 tablets (500 mg) of naproxen to take every 12 hours. Patients also received 60 tablets (1 to 2 tablets every 8 hours) of either placebo (n = 107), cyclobenzaprine (5 mg, n = 108) or oxycodone/acetaminophen (5 mg/325 mg, n = 108). No significant differences were noted across the groups for pain, functional impairment, and the use of health-care resources at 7 days and at the 3-month follow-up. These results did not support providing oxycodone/acetaminophen in addition to naproxen for patients with acute low back pain. Furthermore, this study suggests that combination therapy is not better than monotherapy.

Goldberg performed a randomized clinical trial to determine whether a 15-day tapering course of oral prednisone was effective in improving function and reducing pain among patients with acute radiculopathy associated with a herniated lumbar disc. This study found a small, significant improvement in Oswestry Disability Index (ODI) scores at 3 weeks and 52 weeks in the prednisone group compared with the placebo group. No difference was found for lower-extremity pain scores and the likelihood of undergoing surgery. This suggests that a short course of prednisone (20-mg capsules, 3 daily for 5 days, then 2 capsules daily for 5 days, and then 1 capsule daily for 5 days) may be beneficial for improving patient-reported function among patients with acute radiculopathy.

There is observational evidence to suggest that early referral to physical therapy is associated with lower costs for patients with acute low back pain. Fritz conducted a parallel-group randomized clinical trial to examine whether early physical therapy (manipulation and exercise) is more effective than usual care in improving disability in patients with acute low back pain who had no symptoms below the knee. Both groups were advised that the prognosis of low back pain is favorable and that they should remain active, and a book on back pain was provided to the participants. The usual care group did not receive any further treatment, whereas the early physical therapy group worked with a physical therapist on an exercise program. Early physical therapy (4 sessions over 3 weeks) resulted in significant improvement in ODI scores relative to usual care, but differences were modest and not clinically meaningful. Health-care resource utilization did not differ between the groups. These results support guidelines that advise delaying referral to physical therapy to allow for spontaneous recovery.

Sports Medicine and Shoulder

Anterior Cruciate Ligament (ACL) Rehabilitation

Chmielewski compared high-intensity and low-intensity plyometric exercises during rehabilitation after ACL reconstruction. They found no significant differences between the 2 groups in functional outcomes and biomarkers of articular cartilage degeneration or metabolism.

Rotator Cuff Symptomatology

The relationship between symptoms and the presence of a rotator cuff tear is not clear, as many people with rotator cuff tears are asymptomatic, patient-reported outcome scores for those with failed repairs are similar to those of patients with intact repairs, and nonoperative approaches to treatment have been successful for many patients with a degenerative, full-thickness rotator cuff tear. Two recent studies lend support to the concept that abnormal scapular and glenohumeral kinematics may be responsible for the presence of symptoms. Kolk evaluated shoulder kinematics using 3-dimensional electromagnetic tracking for the humerus and the scapula in 26 patients before and 1 year after rotator cuff repair with a standard postoperative rehabilitation program. Using the uninvolved shoulder as a control, they found that scapular kinematics normalized after rotator cuff repair with postoperative rehabilitation, with lessening of abnormal scapular internal rotation and upward rotation during arm abduction. Miller used dynamic stereoradiography to measure glenohumeral joint translations and subacromial space during coronal plane abduction in 5 patients with full-thickness supraspinatus tears before and after a 12-week exercise program. Abnormal glenohumeral translations decreased and the acromiohumeral interval increased after the exercise program. Patients showed significant improvements in patient-reported outcomes scores, and none of the patients failed the rehabilitation program. These studies suggest that abnormal shoulder kinematics are often seen in patients with symptomatic rotator cuff tears and that both symptoms and kinematics can improve with exercise or surgery followed by rehabilitation.

Postoperative Rehabilitation of Rotator Cuff Repair

In a meta-analysis, Kluczynski compared early rehabilitation (<6 weeks after surgical rotator cuff repair) and delayed rehabilitation (≥6 weeks after surgical repair). Thirty-seven studies met the inclusion criteria of full-thickness tears undergoing primary repair. The outcome of interest was retearing of the repaired tendon, assessed at 1 year with MRI, ultrasound, or arthrogram. The authors concluded that early active range of motion was associated with a higher risk of retearing of the repaired tendon for small and large tears.

Nonoperative Treatment of Labral Tears

The treatment of superior labral tears has evolved away from surgery and toward nonoperative treatment for many patients, as there are data to suggest that nonoperative treatment can be successful in many patients and those surgical outcomes are not always better. In a retrospective cohort comparison, Jang identified a number of features that are associated with the failure of nonoperative treatment of superior labral tears. These included a history of trauma (odds ratio [OR], 9.8; 95% CI, 2.0 to 48.1), participation in overhead activities (OR, 19.1; 95% CI, 3.0 to 119.2), and a positive compression rotation test result (OR, 8.8; 95% CI, 1.5 to 51.9). While patients with these features may be successfully treated nonoperatively, they are less likely to have a successful outcome from nonoperative treatment and are more likely to be headed toward surgery.

Pain Medicine

Ultrasound-guided Injections

Huang performed a systematic review and meta-analysis of double-blinded, randomized controlled trials to evaluate the effectiveness of ultrasound-guided versus landmark-guided intra-articular and peri-articular injections for the knee, hand, shoulder, and hip. This analysis demonstrated that ultrasound-guided injections were significantly more effective in decreasing pain in the short term (2 to 6 weeks); however, no difference was seen at 12 weeks and beyond.

Glucocorticosteroid Injections

Bodick performed a multicenter trial with 228 patients to compare the intra-articular administration of single-dose, immediate-release triamcinolone acetonide (40 mg) and extended-release triamcinolone acetonide (FX006) (10 mg, 40 mg, or 60 mg) in patients with Kellgren-Lawrence grade-2 or 3 osteoarthritis. Primary outcomes were assessed with a numerical pain scale at baseline and 8, 10, and 12 weeks. The 10-mg dose of FX006 proved to be equivalent to immediate-release corticosteroid at 2 to 12 weeks; the 40-mg dose of FX006 was superior at 5 to 10 weeks. The 60-mg dosage did not show any improvement over the 40-mg dosage. Despite a significant difference in outcome using 40 mg of FX006 at 5 to 10 weeks, this difference may not translate to a clinically notable difference from the use of immediate-release corticosteroids.

In a randomized controlled trial, Ranalletta compared the use of unguided, single-dose betamethasone injection and oral NSAIDs prior to physical therapy among 74 patients with adhesive capsulitis of the shoulder. Outcome measures included a visual analog scale (VAS) for pain, the abbreviated Disabilities of the Arm, Shoulder and Hand score for function, the ASES Shoulder Score, passive range of motion, and the abbreviated Constant-Murley score at 2, 4, 8, and 12 weeks. Pain and most functional improvement measures were superior from baseline to 8 weeks in the injection group; however, there was no difference seen at the time of final follow-up.

Cannabinoid use for Chronic Pain and Spasticity

Whiting performed a meta-analysis of 79 trials (6,462 participants) investigating the use of cannabinoids in the management of chronic pain and spasticity as well as for other indications. When compared with placebo, the average reduction in the numerical pain rating and in the Ashworth spasticity scale was greater with cannabinoids. Moderate-quality evidence from studies reviewed in this meta-analysis suggested that cannabinoids can reduce chronic pain and spasticity. However, this may come with increased risks of short-term adverse events, such as dizziness, dry mouth, nausea, fatigue, somnolence, euphoria, vomiting, disorientation, drowsiness, confusion, loss of balance, and hallucination.

Amputation, Prosthetics and Orthotics

Karol assessed the impact of compliance counseling regarding brace use for adolescents with idiopathic scoliosis. Females <1 year post-menarche and with a spine curvature of 25° to 45° were randomized to either the counseled group (sensors embedded in the brace to provide data on compliance, with counseling from the surgeon and orthotist regarding hours of wear) or the non-counseled group (only encouragement to wear the brace provided, without data on compliance). Patients in the counseled group wore the brace a significantly higher number of hours per day compared with the noncounseled group and also had a significantly lower rate of curvature progression.

Physical Modalities

Transcutaneous Electrical Nerve Stimulation (TENS)

The evidence for the use of TENS in pain management is conflicting. Chen performed a systematic review and meta-analysis to determine whether TENS was effective in the management of knee osteoarthritis.

Other types of electrical stimulation include neuromuscular electrical stimulation (NMES), used for muscle strengthening, muscle retraining, and edema control, and functional electrical stimulation (FES), used in the neurorehabilitation of patients with stroke. Morf performed a randomized, single-blinded, crossover study to compare maximal evoked torque, discomfort, and fatigue-related outcomes between multipath NMES and conventional NMES of the quadriceps muscle in patients after total knee arthroplasty. Twenty participants were included in this study. Both groups received two 45-minute sessions (7 days apart). The parameters for multipath and conventional NMES included biphasic symmetrical square pulses of 400 μs with a frequency of 50 Hz and an on:off ratio of 5:10 seconds. Ramp-up and ramp-down times were 1 second each. Multipath NMES generated stronger contractions and induced lower discomfort and muscle fatigue than conventional NMES in patients after total knee arthroplasty.

Kinesiology Taping

Previous systematic reviews that have included low-quality studies have suggested that the use of kinesiology tape may have limited potential in reducing pain in individuals with musculoskeletal injury. Since the effects are unclear with respect to pain caused by knee osteoarthritis, Cho conducted a randomized controlled trial to test whether kinesiology taping (n = 23) improves pain, range of motion, and proprioception compared with sham application (n = 23). They found that the kinesiology taping group had significant improvements in pain during walking, pain-free active range of motion, and proprioception post-treatment, while the sham application group had no significant change in outcomes.

Orthopedic Physical Therapy

Orthopedic physical therapy includes treatment of the musculoskeletal system (which is made up of the muscles and bones of the body) that has been subject to injury or trauma. This includes sprains, strains, post fracture, post surgery and repetitive injuries. The areas of the body include the neck and back as well the extremities.

Orthopedic physical therapy practice, it takes the through a sequential thought process of diagnosis, patient history, physical examination, and, ultimately, treatment.

Orthopedic Physical Therapy Rehabilitation

- Pre and Post Surgical Care of all Orthopedic Conditions.
- Balance/Vertigo Rehabilitation.
- Postural Training.
- Arthritis Management.
- Back/Neck Rehabilitation.
- Joint Pain Management.
- Headache Management.
- Manual Therapy/McKenzie Treatment.
- Spinal Stabilization.
- Muscle and Ligament Strains and Sprains.
- Myofascial Release.
- Auto Accident Injuries.
- Work Injuries.

Basic Orthopedic Physical Therapy Assessment

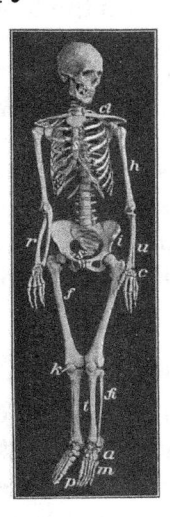

- Patient history.
- Observation.
- Examination of movement.
- Special tests.

- Reflexes and cutaneous distribution.
- Joint play movements.
- Palpation.
- Diagnostic imaging.

In Orthopedic Physical Therapy examining of the musculoskeletal system it is important to keep the concept of function in mind. Note any gross abnormalities of mechanical function beginning with the initial introduction to the patient. Continue to observe for such problems throughout the interview and the examination.

On Orthopedic Physical Therapy examination of a patient who has no musculoskeletal complaints and in whom no gross abnormalities have been noted in the interview and general physical examination, it is adequate to inspect the extremities and trunk for observable abnormalities and to ask the patient to perform a complete active range of motion with each joint or set of joints.

If the patient presents complaints in the musculoskeletal system or if any abnormality has been observed, it is important to do a thorough Orthopedic Physical Therapy examination, not only to delineate the extent of gross abnormalities but also to look closely for subtle anomalies.

To perform an Orthopedic Physical Therapy examination of the muscles, bones, and joints, use the classic techniques of inspection, palpation, and manipulation. Start by dividing the musculoskeletal system into functional parts. With practice the examiner will establish an order of approach, but for the beginner it is perhaps better to begin distally with the upper extremity, working proximally through the shoulder. Then, beginning with the temporomandibular joint, pass on to the cervical spine, the thoracic spine, the lumbar and sacral spine, and the sacroiliac joints. Finally, in the lower extremity, again begin distally with the foot and proceed proximally through the hip.

Use the opposite side for comparisons: It is easier to spot subtle differences as well as identify symmetrical problems. If there is any question, use your own anatomy as a control.

Glean the maximum information from observation. Concentrating on one area at a time, inspect the area for discoloration (e.g., ecchymoses, redness), soft tissue swelling, bony enlargement, wasting, and deformity (abnormal angulation, subluxation). While noting these changes, attempt to determine whether they are limited to the joint or whether they involve the surrounding structures (e.g., tendons, muscles, bursae).

Observe the patient's eyes while palpating the joints and the surrounding structures in Orthopedic Physical Therapy examination. A patient's expression of pain depends on many factors. For this reason the verbalization of pain often does not correlate directly with the magnitude of the pain. The most objective indicator of the magnitude of tenderness produced by presence on palpation is involuntary muscle movements about the eyes. Therefore, the examiner should observe the patient's eyes while palpating the joints and surrounding structures. With practice the examiner will become skilled in evaluating the magnitude of pain produced by the examination and will be able to do a skillful evaluation without producing excessive discomfort to the patient. Note areas of tenderness to pressure, and if possible identify the anatomic structures over which the tenderness is localized.

On Orthopedic Physical Therapy examination should also note areas of enlargement while palpating the joints and surrounding structures. By noting carefully the consistency of the enlargement and its boundaries, one can decide whether this is due to bony widening, thickening of the synovial lining of the joint, soft tissue swelling of the structure surrounding the joint, an effusion into the joint capsule, or nodule formation, which might be located in a tendon sheath, subcutaneous tissue, or other structures about the joint.

While palpating the joints, note areas of increased warmth (heat). A method for doing this that will help even the most inexperienced to perceive subtle increases in heat is to choose the most heat-sensitive portion of the hand (usually the dorsum of the fingers) and, beginning proximally, lightly pass this part of your hand over all portions of the patient's extremity several times. As you proceed from proximal to distal, the skin temperature gradually cools. If you find an area becoming slightly warmer, this represents increased heat.

Have the patient perform active movements through an entire range of motion for each joint in Orthopedic Physical Therapy examination. Defects in function can be most rapidly perceived by having the patient perform active functions with each region of the musculoskeletal system. This reduces Orthopedic Physical Therapy examination time and helps the examiner to identify areas in which there is poor function for more careful evaluation.

Manipulate the joint through a passive range of motion only if the patient is unable actively to perform a full range of motion, or if there is obvious pain on active motion. In passively manipulating a joint, note whether there is a reduction in the range of motion, whether there is a pain on motion, and whether crepitus is produced when the joint is moved. Note also whether the joint is stable or whether abnormal movements may be produced in Orthopedic Physical Therapy examination.

Orthopedic Physical Therapy Examination of the Neck

- Observe the patient as a whole.
- Observe the neck and shoulders from in front and behind.
- Palpate the front and back of the neck with the patient seated and the examiner behind.
- Assess neck flexion by asking the patient to touch their chest with their chin.
- Assess extension by asking the patient to look up and as far back as possible.
- Assess lateral flexion to both sides by asking the patient to touch their shoulder with their ear.
- Assess rotation by asking the patient to look over their shoulder, to the left and right.
- Begin the neurological assessment of the upper limb by examining the motor system. This involves asking the patient to assume a certain position and not let you overcome it. Begin with shoulder abduction.
- Shoulder adduction.
- Elbow extension.
- Elbow flexion.

- Wrist extension.
- Wrist flexion.
- Finger extension.
- Finger flexion.
- Thumb abduction.
- Finger abduction
- Elicit the reflexes of the upper limb beginning with the biceps jerk.
- Triceps jerk.
- Brachioradialis jerk.
- Assess co-ordination of the upper limb.
- Test sensation of the upper limb and determine the distribution of any loss.

Orthopedic Physical Therapy Examination of the Shoulder

- Observe the whole patient, front and back.
- Observe the shoulder.
- Observe the axilla.
- Palpate for tenderness over the sterno-clavicular joint, clavicle, acromioclavicular joint, acromion process, supraspinatus tendon and the tendon of the long head of biceps.
- Observe shoulder abduction from in front and behind, through the entire range of movement. Note the presence of difficulty in initiation or a painful arc.
- Secure the scapula to assess gleno-humeral movement.
- Assess flexion and extension.
- Assess external rotation with elbows in to the sides and flexed to 90°.
- Assess internal rotation by asking the patient to place both hands behind the head.
- Assess internal rotation by asking the patient to reach over their opposite shoulder, behind the neck and behind the back.
- Test biceps function by asking the patient to flex the elbow against resistance.
- Test serratus anterior function by asking the patient to push against a wall, looking for winging of the scapula.
- Test for pain with palpation of subacromial Bursa - indicates impingement of the rotator cuff.
- The apprehension test standing. Abduct, externally rotate and extend the patient's shoulder while pushing on the head of the humerus with the opposite hand to test for anterior

subluxation or dislocation.

- Apprehension test lying down.
- Assess any marked instability in the shoulder. Anterior - instability (moves too far forward); Posterior - instability (moves too far back).

Orthopedic Physical Therapy Examination of the Elbow

- Observe the whole patient, front and back, looking especially for deformity.
- Feel for tenderness.
- Accentuate the pain of tennis elbow.
- Tennis elbow: point tenderness.
- Tennis elbow: pain on resisted extension.
- Tennis elbow: pain on passive stretch.
- Examine extension.
- Examine flexion.
- Examine supination.
- Examine pronation.
- Pivot shift of elbow (instability).
- Provocative test for Cubital Tunnel Syndrome (puts tension on ulnar nerve at elbow).
- Palpate the ulnar nerve.

Orthopedic Physical Therapy Examination of the Wrist and Hand

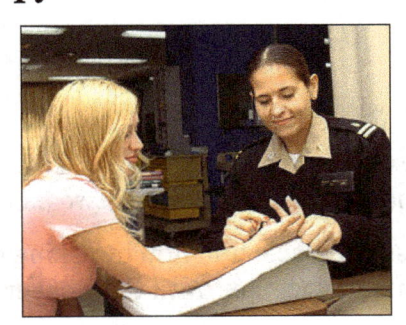

- Observe the hand positioned on a pillow or a table. Ensure you have adequate exposure.
- Observe the palm of the hand.
- Observe the dorsum of the hand.
- Review the anatomy of the hand noting the tip of the styloid process, the anatomical snuffbox bordered by extensor pollicis brevis and extensor pollicis longus tendons and the abductor pollicis longus.

- Feel for tenderness.
- Test active movements of the wrist.
- A useful method for screening of flexion and extension of the wrists.
- Test passive movements of the wrist beginning with extension.
- Flexion.
- Radial deviation.
- Ulnar deviation.
- Pronation.
- Supination.
- Test thumb extension.
- Test thumb abduction.
- Test thumb adduction.
- Test opposition.
- Observe movement of fingers from extension to flexion.
- Test flexor digitorum profundus function by holding the proximal interphalangeal joint extended and asking the patient to flex the finger. Successful finger flexion indicates the tendon is intact.
- Test flexor digitorum superficialis function by holding the other fingers extended while asking the patient to flex the finger being tested. Successful flexion indicates the tendon is intact.
- Assess joint hyperextension.
- Axial compression test.
- Asses ulnar nerve function with Froment's test.
- Asses ulnar nerve/interosseus muscle function by asking the patient to abduct their fingers while slowly pushing the hands together until the weaker one collapses.
- Asses ulnar nerve/interosseus muscle function by asking the patient to abduct their fingers while slowly pushing the hands together until the weaker one collapses.
- Assess median nerve function.
- Assess the function of the hand with the fine pinch grip (paperclip).
- Flat pinch grip (key).
- Tripod grip (pen).
- Wide grip (mug).
- Power grip.

Orthopedic Physical Therapy Examination of the Back

- Observe the patient as a whole, front and back.
- Ask the patient to walk on their toes.
- Ask the patient to walk on their heels.
- Back extension.
- Back flexion.
- Bony Excursion: measure the distance between two bony points when standing.
- Ask the patient to flex forward, the bony points should move at least 5 cm.
- Lateral flexion.
- Rotation (make sure to anchor pelvis).
- FABER test in Orthopedic Physical Therapy Examination: Flexion Abduction External Rotation. Press firmly on the knee. Pain in the groin suggests a hip problem and pain in the back refers to the sacroiliac joint.
- Straight leg raising, dorsiflexion increases the sciatic stretch. Watch for pain and limitation.
- Femoral stretch test: Hip extension and passive flexion of the knee. Watch for pain and limitation.

A Neurological examination including:

- Knee extension.
- Knee flexion.
- Knee jerk reflex
- Ankle jerk reflex.
- Sensation.
- Pain on compression of the head can often be attributed to non-organic pathology.

Orthopedic Physical Therapy Examination of the Hip

- Observe the whole patient.
- Trendelenburg test (normal).
- Positive Trendelenburg Test.
- Ask the patient to walk and observe their gait.
- Test iliopsoas function by asking the patient to lift their thigh off the seat against resistance.
- Ensure the Anterior Superior Iliac Spines are horizontal.
- Check the position of the medial malleoli.

- Measure from the ASIS to the medial malleoli.
- Measure the distance from the xiphisternum to the medial malleoli.
- Feel for the femoral head. It is deep to the femoral pulse.
- Thomas Test in Orthopedic Physical Therapy Examination:

  Flex both hips to eliminate the lumbar lordosis. Extend the hip you are examining and if it is normal it should return to the bed. A fixed flexion deformity of the hip will not allow it to extend to the neutral position.
- Check the patient is not compensating with a lumbar lordosis.
- Check the ASIS are horizontal again. Anchor leg over the edge of the bed and abduct the other hip.
- Assess adduction.
- Internal rotation.

Orthopedic Physical Therapy Examination of the Knee

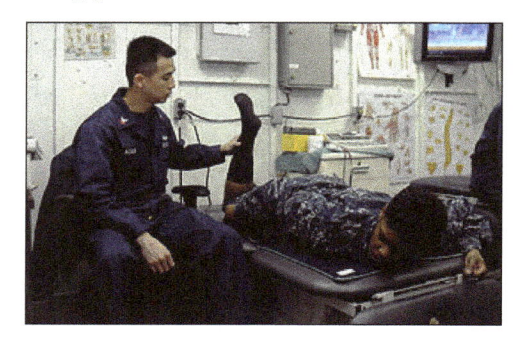

- Observe the patient as a whole.
- Observe the knee joint front and back. Note any genu valgum (a slight degree of which is normal) or genu varum.
- Observe knee from side. Note any genu recurvatum.
- Ask the patient to squat.
- Assess patellae tracking from extension to flexion. Note quadriceps action.
- Patellar apprehension test. Apply lateral pressure to patellar as the patient flexes the knee. Observe facial expressions for fear of impending dislocation.
- Observe the knee with the patient lying on the bed.
- Pick a bony landmark on the knee and measure a fixed distance from it to the approximate centre of the quadriceps.
- Measure the circumference of the knee and leg.
- Feel the temperature of the knee and leg.

- Soloman's test. Lift the patella away from the femur. In synovial thickening it will be hard to grasp.
- Effusion: Tap Test. Push sharply on the patella and with an effusion it will strike the femur and bounce back.
- Effusion: Feel for fluid fluctuance.
- Effusion: Bulge Test. Empty the suprapatellar pouch with pressure above the patella. Wipe hand along the medial side to displace fluid laterally. Compress the lateral side and watch for a bulge medially.
- Feel the superficial and posterior surface of the patella by pushing it medially.
- To test for patello-femoral tenderness press patella against the femur and ask the patient to tighten their thigh muscles.
- Palpate for tenderness with the knee flexed to 90°. Feel along the joint line, the ligaments and the tibial tubercle.
- Assess extension of the knee.
- Flexion.
- Internal and external rotation of the knee is limited.
- Test collateral ligaments by applying medial and lateral pressure to the lower leg which is tucked away under the examiners arm.
- Look for posterior sag of the femur signifying posterior cruciate dysfunction.
- Anterior drawer test. Femur should not move forward significantly unless the anterior cruciate ligament is torn.
- Posterior drawer test. (Posterior cruciate).
- Lachmans test.
- MC test: Lift leg off the bed and if tibia drops there is cruciate dysfunction.
- MacMurrays test: Place the thumb and finger on the joint line. Watching the patients face for pain, flex the leg, externally rotate the foot, abduct and extend leg to test for medial meniscal "clicks". Flex the leg, internally rotate and adduct for lateral meniscal "clicks".
- Ask the patient to lie prone and examine the back of the knee.

Orthopedic Physical Therapy Examination of the Ankle and Foot

Observe patient as a whole from front and back.
- From behind check hind-foot alignment and "too many toes" sign (tib. post dysfunction).
- Check for inversion (tibialis function) and eversion (peroneal function).
- Single stance heel raise test.

- Windlass test.
- Coin test.
- Dorsi flexion.
- Plantar flexion.
- Mid foot abduction/adduction.
- Extension fore foot.
- Flexion fore foot.
- Tibialis anterior test.
- Tibialis posterior test.
- Peroneal tendons test.
- Ankle instability - Inversion test.
- Ankle instability - Anterior draw test.
- Ankle instability - Posterior draw test.
- Simmond's test for TA.
- Examine the sole.
- Check pulses, sensation, reflexes.

Types of Sports Injuries

There are some common injuries that are experienced by athletes such as ankle injuries and sprains, fractures and concussions, shoulder injuries, muscle injuries, hip tendonitis, shin splints etc. This chapter discusses these common types of sports injuries in detail.

Sport injuries are diverse in terms of the mechanism of injury, how they present in individuals, and how the injury should be managed. Defining exactly what a sports injury is can be problematic and definitions are not consistent. Highlighted that definitions of sport injury can be discussed in both theoretical and operational terms.

According to the IOC manual of sports injuries, a sports injury may be defined as "damage to the tissues of the body that occurs as a result of sport or exercise".

The International Classification of Functioning, Disability and Health (ICF) is one of the most well know mechanisms and considered the gold standard for classification of medical conditions but is currently rarely used in the field of sports medicine. For researchers in sport defining simple, pragmatic, consistent, operational criteria which describe an injury that can be applied across a range of sports is vital, particularly when developing injury surveillance systems. Many comprehensive systems have been developed to classify injury in order to assist with development of injury surveillance which can be used across sports. There are many ways to classify sports injuries based on:

- The time taken for the tissues to become injured.
- Tissue type affected.
- Severity of the injury.
- Which injury the individual presents.

Injury Classification

Classification of sporting injuries (adapted from Brukner and Khan's Clinical Sports Medicine).

Site	Acute Injuries	Overuse Injuries
Bone	Fracture Periosteal contusion	Stress fracture Bone strain Stress reaction Osteitis Periostitis Apophysitis

Articular cartilage	Osteochondral/chondral fracture	Chondropathy (e.g. chondromalacia)
	Minor osteochondral injury/lesion	
Joint	Dislocation	Synovitis
	Subluxation	Osteoarthritis
Ligament	Sprain/tear (grades I - III)	Inflammation
Muscle	Strain/tear (grades I - III)	Compartment syndrome (chronic)
	Contusion	Delayed onset muscle soreness (DOMS)
	Cramp	Focal tissue thickening/fibrosis
	Compartment syndrome (acute)	
Tendon	Tear (complete or partial)	Tendinopathy
Bursa	Traumatic bursitis	Bursitis
Nerve	Neuropraxia	Nerve entrapment
		Minor nerve injury/irritation
		Adverse neural tension
Skin	Laceration	Blister
	Abrasion	Callus
	Puncture wound	

Mechanism

According to Brukner & Kahn this is one of the most common methods of classifying sports injuries, and relies on the sports physiotherapist knowing and understanding both the the mechanism of injury and the onset of the symptoms.

Acute

Injury occurs suddenly to previously normal tissue. Acute injuries occur due to sudden trauma to the tissue, with the symptoms of acute injuries presenting themselves almost immediately. The principle in this instance is that the force exerted at the time of injury on the tissue (i.e. muscle, tendon, ligament, and bone) exceeds the strength of that tissue. Forces commonly involved in acute injury are either a direct or indirect. Acute injuries can be classified according to the site of the injury (e.g. bone, cartilage, ligament, muscle, bursa, tendon, joint, nerve or skin) and the type of injury (e.g. fracture, dislocation, sprain or strain).

Direct/Contact Injury

A direct injury is caused by an external blow or force:
- A collision with another person e.g. during a tackle in rugby or football.
- Being struck with an object e.g. a basketball or hockey stick.

Indirect/Non-contact Injury

An indirect injury can occur in two ways:
- The actual injury can occur some distance from the impact site e.g. falling on an outstretched hand can result in a dislocated shoulder.

- The injury does not result from physical contact with an object or person, but from internal forces built up by the actions of the performer, such as may be caused by over-stretching, poor technique, fatigue and lack of fitness.

Common Acute Injuries include:

- Ankle Sprain.
- Quadriceps Strain.
- Clavicular Fracture.
- Shoulder Dislocation.

Overuse Injuries

Any repetitive activity can lead to an overuse injury. Overuse injuries occur over a period of time, usually due to excessive and repetitive loading of the tissue, with symptoms presenting gradually. Little or no pain might be experienced in the early stages of these injuries and the athlete might continue to place pressure on the injured site. This prevents the site being given the necessary time to heal. In contrast to acute injuries, the cause of overuse injuries is often much less obvious. The principle in overuse injury is that repetitive microtrauma overloads the capacity of the tissue to repair itself.

To better understand overuse injury it helps to think in terms of what is happening at the microscopic level to the tissue that has been "stressed" during the repetitive workouts. During exercise the tissues (muscles, tendons, bones, ligaments, etc.) experience excessive physiological stress. When the activity is over the tissues undergo adaptation so as to be stronger to be able to withstand a similar stress in the future if required. Overuse injury occurs when the adaptive capability of the tissue is exceeded and tissue injury then develops. That is, in the over-zealous athlete there is not enough time for adaptation to occur before the next work out and the cumulative tissue damage eventually exceeds a threshold for that tissue causing pain and tissue dysfunction. The adaptive capability of the tissue may be exceeded secondary to excessive repetitive forces attributable to one or more commonly a combination of risk factors including:

Intrinsic	Extrinsic
Age	Training Errors
• Child	• Increased/Excessive Volume
• Adolescent	• Increased/Excessive Frequency
• Adult	• Increased/Excessive Intensity
• Masters	• Excessive fatigue
Physiology	• Inadequate recovery
• Lack of Flexibility	Equipment
• Generalised muscle tightness	• Damaged
• Focal areas of muscle thickening	• Inappropriate
• Restricted joint range of movement	• Worn Out shoes
• Muscle Imbalance	Environmental Conditions
• Muscle Weakness	• Hot
• Fatigue	• Cold
	• Humid

Anatomical	Playing Surfaces
<ul><li>Size</li><li>Body Composition</li><li>Poor Biomechanics<ul><li>Pes Planus</li><li>Pes Cavus</li><li>Rearfoot Varus</li><li>Tibia Vara</li><li>Genu Valgum</li><li>Genu Varum</li><li>Femoral neck anteversion</li><li>Tibial torsion</li></ul></li></ul>Leg length discrepancy Other<ul><li>Genetic factors</li><li>Endocrine factors</li><li>Metabolic conditions</li></ul>	<ul><li>Uneven v Even</li><li>Grass v Concrete</li><li>Cambered</li></ul>Psychological factors Inadequate Nutrition

According to Clarensen overuse injuries is a problem in many sports with athletes exposed to high training loads, tight competition schedules and insufficient recovery thought to be particularly at risk; especially when participating in sports involving repetitive movements or impacts. For example, approximately two-thirds of athletes, who trained between 20 and 35 hours per week, sustained a performance-limiting overuse injury in athletics over a one year period. Similarly between 29% and 44% of elite volleyball players, who often perform over 500 jumps per week, report symptoms of jumper's knee. While it is recognised that overuse injuries are common in elite sport they also occur among recreational athletes, young athletes, and even among sedentary individuals after transient increases in activity.

Table: Common types of overuse injuries in sport.

Site	Type of overuse injury	Common examples in sport
Bone	Bone strain/stress reaction/stress fracture Osteitis, periostitis Apophysitis.	Metatarsal stress fracture in running Medial tibial stress syndrome in running and dancing Osgood-Scl-darter lesion Lumbar stress fracture in gymnastics, cricket fast bowling Pubic ramus in distance running.
Tendon	Tendinopathy (includes paratenonitis, tenosynovitis, tendinosis, tendinitis).	Achilles tendinopathy in footballers Patellar tendinosis in volleyball ("jumper's knee").
Joint	Svnovitis Labrum injuries Chondropathy.	SLAP lesions in throwing athletes Functional acetabalar impingement of the hip in football.
Ligament	Chronic degeneration/micro-tears.	Ulnar collateral ligament injury in baseball.
Muscle/Fascia	Chronic compartment syndrome Delayed-onset muscle soreness (DOMS)Fasciitis/las ciosis.	Illiotibial band syndrome in running (runner's knee").
Bursa	Bursitis.	Greater trochanteric pain syndrome.
Nerve	Altered neuromechanical sensitivity Entrapment.	UInar neuropathy in cycling ("handlebar palsy").

Common overuse injuries:
- Achilles Tendinopathy.
- Tennis Elbow.
- Iliotibial Band Syndrome.

Tissue Type

Sports injuries can also be classified according to which tissue have become damaged. This allows sports physiotherapists to identify soft, hard, and special tissue injuries. In more complex sport injuries damage may occur to more than one tissue type.

Soft Tissue Injuries

Ligament

Joint stability is provided by the presence of a joint capsule of connective tissue, thickened at points of stress to form ligaments, which attach at the ends to bone. There are a number of different grading systems used for the classification of ligament sprains, each have their own strengths and weaknesses. One important consideration is that each therapist will employ different systems so it is important to be aware of a wide variety for continuity of care. This is evident when reading research regarding sprains and authors not disclosing which system they used, reducing rigour and quality of the write up of research. The traditional grading system for ligament injuries focuses on a single ligament.

Grade I Sprain

- Represents a microscopic injury without stretching of the ligament on a macroscopic level.
- Mild - Little Swelling & Tenderness with little impact on function.

Grade II Sprain

- Macroscopic stretching, but the ligament remains intact. Involves a considerable proportion of the fibers and, therefore, stretching of the joint and stressing the ligament show increased laxity but a definite end point.
- Moderate - Moderate Swelling, Pain and Impact on Function, Reduced Proprioception, ROM and Instability.

Grade III Sprain

- Complete tear or rupture of the ligament with excessive joint laxity and no firm end point. Although they are often painful conditions, Grade III Sprains can also be pain-free as sensory fibers are completely torn in the injury.
- Severe - Complete Rupture, Large Swelling, Tenderness+++, Loss of Function and Marked Instability.

Common Injuries:
- MCL Injury Knee.
- LCL Injury Knee.
- ACL Injury Knee.
- PCL Injury Knee.
- Lateral Ligament Injury Ankle.
- Elbow Ligamentous Injuries.

Tendon

Tendons are situated between bone and muscles and are bright white in colour, their fibro-elastic composition gives them the strength required to transmit large mechanical forces. Each muscle has two tendons, one proximally and one distally. The point at which the tendon forms attachment to the muscle is also known as the musculotendinous junction (MTJ) and the point at which it attaches to the bone is known as the osteotendinous junction (OTJ). The purpose of the tendon is to transmit forces generated from the muscle to the bone to elicit movement. The proximal attachment of the tendon is also known as the origin and the distal tendon is called the insertion.

Tendons have different shapes and sizes depending on the role of the muscle. Muscles that generate a lot of power and force tend to have shorter and wider tendons than those that perform more fine delicate movements. These tend to be long and thin.

Tendon Rupture

Acute injuries to tendons usually occur at the point of least blood supply, for example with the Achilles tendon it is usually 2cm above the tendon insertion or at the musculotendinous junction. A complete tendon rupture generally occurs without warning. Also this type of injury usually occurs in older athletes without a history of injury in that particular tendon. The most common tendons to rupture are the Achilles tendon and the Supraspinatus tendon.

Tendinopathy

Tendinopathy refers to the chronic tendon injury with no implication about the etiology (cause) and is the term that the leading researchers in the field of tendon science have been using in recent years. Overuse injuries are commonly seen in tendons. As a tendon is loaded and the strain increases, there is tissue deformation and some fibers begin to fail. Ultimately macroscopic tendon failure occurs. Tendon overuse can not be explained as inflammation as research has shown that the histological findings in athletes with overuse tendon injuries do not show signs of inflammation - (there are no inflammatory cell present in surgical specimens). However, the following are seen with overuse tendon injuries:

- Degenerative changes.
- Changed fibril organisation.

- Reduced cell count.
- Vascular in-growth.
- Occasionally, local necrosis.

Athletes with overuse tendon pain may present with the following clinical features:

- Pain sometime after exercise or the following morning upon rising.
- Can be painful at rest and initially becomes less painful with use.
- Athletes can "run through the pain" or pain disappears when they warm up.
- Pain returns after exercise when they cool down.
- Athlete is able to train fully in the early stages of the condition - this may interfere with the healing process.
- Localised tenderness and thickening upon examination.
- Swelling and crepitus may be present (although crepitus is usually a sign of associated tenosynovitis or due to the water attracting nature of the collage disarray).

Tendinitis

This refers to inflammation of the tendon itself. There is little evidence to support this diagnostic label, though. Tendinitis may occur in association with paratendinitis.

Paratenonitis

This refers to inflammation of the paratenon, either alligned by the synovium or not. A common example is De Quervain's tenosynovitis at the wrist.

Muscle

Skeletal muscle injuries represent great part of all traumas in sports medicine, with an incidence from 10% to 55% of all sustained injuries. They should be treated with necessary precaution since a failed treatment can postpone an athlete's return to the field with weeks or even months and cause re-occurrence of the injury.

Common Injuries:

- Calf Strain.
- Rotator Cuff Tears.
- Rupture Long Head Biceps.

Skin

Skin injuries are common particularly in athletes playing contact sports. Underlying structures such as tendons, ligaments, blood vessels and nerves are always at risk of injury and should also be considered with any skin injury. Open wounds may include abrasions, lacerations or puncture wounds.

Hard Tissue Injuries

Articular Cartilage

The ends of long bones are lined with articular cartilage which provides a low friction gliding surface that acts as a shock absorber and reduces peak pressures on the underlying bone. These are common injuries and there is an increased risk of long term, premature osteoarthritis if not well managed. Articular cartilage can be damaged through shear injuries such as dislocations, and subluxation. Osteochondral injuries may be associated with soft tissue conditions such as injuries to ligaments e.g. ACL. There are three classes of articular cartilage injuries:

- Disruption of the deep layers with or without subchondral bone damage.
- Disruption of the articular surface only.
- Disruption of both the articular cartilage and subchondral bone.

Bone

A bone is a rigid organ that constitutes part of the vertebral skeleton. Bones support and protect the various organs of the body, produce red and white blood cells, store minerals and also enable mobility as well as support for the body. Bone tissue is a type of dense connective tissue.

Fractures

A fracture can result from a direct force, an indirect force or repetitive smaller impacts (as occurs in a stress fracture) and can be classified as transverse, oblique, spiral or comminuted. Fracture complications include:

- Infection.
- Acute compartment syndrome.
- Associated injury (e.g. nerve, vessel).
- Deep venous thrombosis/pulmonary embolism.
- Delayed union/non-union and mal-union.

The signs and symptoms of a fracture include:

- Pain & Tenderness.
- Swelling and Discoloration.
- Restriction of Movement.
- Unnatural Movement.
- Deformity.

Joint

Dislocation

Dislocations are injuries to joints where one bone is displaced from another or complete dissociation of the articulating surfaces of the joint. A dislocation is often accompanied by considerable damage to the surrounding connective tissue. Complications of dislocation can include nerve and vascular damage. Dislocations occur as a result of the joint being pushed past its normal range of movement. Common sites of the body where dislocations occur are the finger, shoulder and patella.

Subluxation

Subluxation is injuries to the joint where one bone is partially displaced from another or partial dissociation of the articulating surfaces of the joint.

Signs and symptoms of dislocation and subluxation include:
- Loss of Movement at the Joint.
- Obvious Deformity.
- Swelling and Tenderness.
- Pain.

Physiology of Sports Injuries

Physiologic processes after injuries are often neglected while much more attention is being paid to the management of symptoms. However, comprehension of these processes is becoming more and more important as therapies are getting increasingly focused on specific molecular and cellular processes. In recent decades, extensive research of tissue regeneration after injury and degeneration, including molecular pathways in healing, helped towards better understanding of this process and led to discoveries of new potential therapeutic targets.

Physiology of Tendon and Ligament Injury and Repair

For skeletal muscles to act properly they must be attached to the bone. Tendons serve as mediators of force transmission that results in joint motion, but they also enable that the muscle belly remains at an optimal distance from the joint on which it acts. Tendons act as springs, which allows them to store and recover energy very effectively. Ligaments on the other hand attach bone to bone and therefore provide mechanical stability of the joint, guide joint motion through their normal range of motion when a tensile load is applied and prevent excessive joint displacement. Although tendons and ligaments differ in function, they share similar physiological features with a similar hierarchical structure and mechanical behavior.

Histoanatomical Features of Tendons and Ligaments

Tendons are made up predominantly of collagen fibers embedded in proteoglycan matrix that attracts water and elastin molecules with a relatively small number of fibroblasts.

Fibroblasts are the predominant cell type in tendons. They are spindle shaped and arranged in fascicles with surrounding loose areolar tissue called peritenon. Cells are orientated in the direction of muscle loading. In mature tendon tissue they are arranged in parallel rows along the force transmitting axis of the tendon. Long cytoplasmic processes extend between the intratendinous fibroblasts, enabling cell-to-cell contact by gap-junctions.

Fibroblasts are connected to the extra cellular matrix (ECM) via integrins that permit the cells to sense and respond to mechanical stimuli which appears vital for their function because this way the mechanical continuum is established along which forces can be transmitted from the outside to the inside of the cell and vice versa. Integrin are also likely candidates for sensing tensile stress at the cell surface. It is also speculated that integrin-associated proteins are involved in signaling adaptive cellular responses upon mechanical loading of the tissue.

Type I collagen is the major constituent of tendons, accounting for about 95% of the dry tendon weight. Collagen type III accounts for about 5% of the dry tendon weight, but smaller quantities of other collagens are also present, including types V, VI, XII and type II collagen. The latter is primarily found in regions that are under compression.

Fibroblasts secrete a precursor of collagen, called procollagen, which is cleaved extracelullarly to form type I collagen. The synthesis of collagen fibrils occurs in two stages: intracellular and extracellular. The pro α-chains are initially synthesized with an additional signal peptide at the aminoterminal end with the function to direct movement of the polypeptides into the rough endoplasmic reticulum where it is cleaved off. Triple helix with three polypeptide chains wound together to form a stiff helical structure is formed intracellularly. Then the procollagen is secreted into the extracellular matrix where it is converted to collagen. Finally, collagen molecules aggregate and the cross-links responsible for its stable structure are formed.

The parallel arrangement of the collagen fibers in tendons enables them to sustain high tensile loads. Collagen molecules group together to form microfibrils, which are defined as 5 collagen molecules stacked in a quarter-stagger array. Microfibrils combine to form subfibrils, and those combine further to form fibrils (50-200 nm in diameter). Fibrils combine together to form fibers (3-7 μm in diameter) which further combine to form fascicles, and this group together to form a tendon. Fascicles are separated by endotenon and surrounded by epitenon. At the level of fascicles, the characteristic "crimp" pattern can be seen histologically.

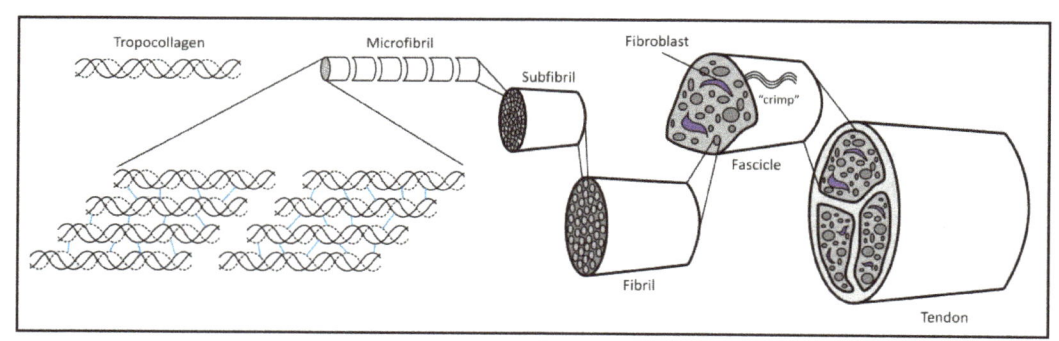

Structure of a tendon.

Proteoglycans (PGs) account for 1-5% of the dry weight of the tendon. PGs are highly hydrophilic they attract water molecules. The predominant proteoglycans in the tendon are decorin and lumican. Biglycan and decorin (and collagen type V) regulate collagen fiber diameter in fibrillogenesis. Because decorin molecules form cross-links between collagen fibers they may increase the stiffness of the fibrils. Proteoglycans are also responsible for lubricating collagen fibers and thus allowing them to glide over each other. Aggreko a normal structure of articular cartilage, in found in tendons that are under compression.

Although tendons and ligaments are very similar in structure, there are some differences between them. (1) Ligaments consist of lower percentage of collagen molecules, but a higher percentage of the proteoglycans and water. (2) Collagen fibers are more variable and have higher elastin content and (3) fibroblasts appear rounder. (4) Furthermore, ligaments receive blood supply from insertion sites.

Table: Differences between tendon and ligament structure.

Content/Feature	Ligaments	Tendons
Fibroblasts	20%	20%
Ground substance	20-30%	lower
Collagen	70-80%	Slightly higher
Collagen type I	90%	95-99%
Collagen type III	10%	1-5%
Elastin	Up to 2x collagen	scarce
Water	60-80%	60-80%
Organisation	More random	Organized
Orientation	Weaving pattern	Long axis orientation

Vascular Supply

There are two types of tendons: (1) tendons covered with paratenon, and (2) sheathed tendons. They mainly differ in vascular supply. In sheathed tendons a mesotenon (vincula) carries a vessel that supplies only one part of the tendon. Therefore, parts of the tendon are relatively avascular and their nutrition depends on diffusion. On the other hand, paratenon-covered tendons receive their blood supply from vessels entering the tendon surface and forming a rich capillary system. Because of the difference in the vasculature, paratenon-covered tendons heal better. As stated above, ligaments receive their blood supply from insertion sites.

There is still an ongoing debate about the efficiency of the blood supply to tendons during exercise. Experiments showed that although the increase in tendon blood flow is somehow restricted during exercise, there is no indication of any major ischemia in the tendon region. The question remains how blood flow to the tendon region is regulated. Several candidates as regulators of blood flow in skeletal muscle have been proposed, and it is possible that similar substances and metabolites are vasoactive also in the tendon region suca as bradykinin.

Insertion Sites

As tendons attach skeletal muscles to bony structures, two types of tendinous junction are to be distinguished – osteotendinous where tendon attaches to the bone and musculotendinous where it attaches to the muscle. Four distinct zones have been observed at the osteotendinous junction, with a gradual change between them. (1) The first zone is structurally similar to the tendon propter, but with smaller amounts of PG decorin. This zone is followed by (2) fibrocartilage, where mostly collagen type II and III are found, but also small amounts of types I, IX and X. Furthermore, there is less PGs aggrecan and decorin. In the third zone, (3) mineralized fibrocartilage is made up of mainly collagen type II, but large quantities of collagen X and aggrecan are also present. The fourth zone is (4) bone, build up mainly of collagen type I and minerals.

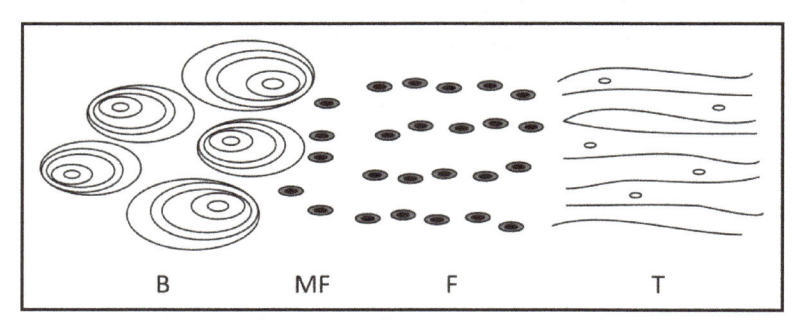

Diagram of a osteotendinous junction: B – bone;
MF – minarelized fibrocartilage; F – fibrocartilage; T – tendon.

At musculotendinous junction, muscle cells are involuted and folded to provide maximal surface for attachment where fibrils attach. Sarcomeres of the fast contracting muscles are shortened at the junction, which may reduce the force intensity within the junction.

Ligaments insert into bone in two ways: through indirect or direct insertions. In indirect insertions the superficial layer is continued at with the periosteum and the deeper layer anchores to bone via Sharpey's fibers. In direct insertions, fibers attach to bone at 90° angle. Four distinct zones have been observed, with a gradual change between ligament midsubstance, fibrocartilage, mineralized fibrocartilage, and bone.

Biomechanics of Tendons and Ligaments

Typical parameters describing the tendon/ligament mechanical properties are *strain*, which describes the elongation/deformation of the tendon (ΔL) relative to the normal length (L0); *stress*, the tendon force (Ft) relative to the tendon cross-sectional area (CSA), *stiffness*, the change in tendon length (ΔL) in relation to the force applied (ΔFt) and *modulus*, which describes the relation between tendon stress and tendon strain and represents the properties independently of the CSA. High modulus indicates stiffer tissue.

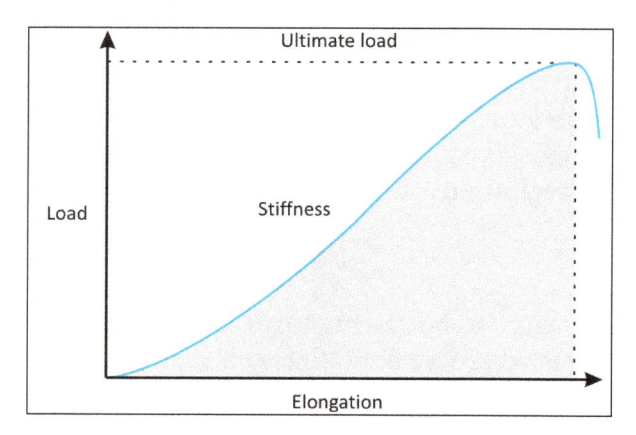

Structural properties of the bone-ligament-bone complex - A load/elongation curve; stiffness is represented by the slope of the curve; ultimate load is the highest load applied to the bone-ligament-bone complex before failure; the dashed area under the curve is the maximum energy stored by the complex.

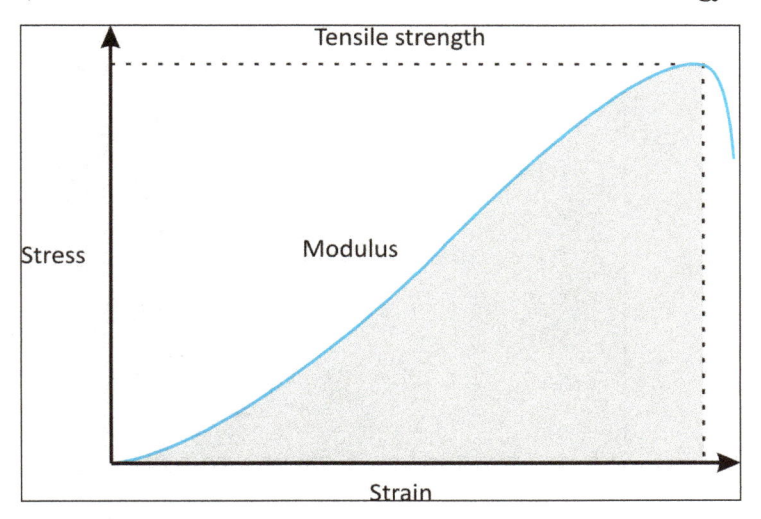

Mechanical properties of the bone-ligament-bone complex – A stress/strain curve; modulus is represented by the slope of the curve; tensile strength is the maximum stress of the bone-ligament-bone complex before failure; the dashed area under the curve represents the strain energy density.

The biomechanics of ligaments is similar to tendon biomechanics. The biomechanical properties of ligaments are described as either structural properties of the bone-ligament–bone complex or the material properties of the ligament midsubstance itself. Structural properties of the bone-ligament-bone complex depend on the size and shape of the ligament, therefore they are extrinsic measures. They are obtained by loading a ligament to failure and therefore represented as a load-elongation curve between two defined limits of elongation. Mechanical properties are intrinsic measures of the quality of the tissue substance and are represented by a stress-strain curve.

A tendon is the strongest component in the muscle-tendon-bone unit. It is estimated that tensile strength is about one-half of stainless steel (e.g. 1 cm^2 cross-section of a tendon can bear weight of 500-1000 kg).

Non-linear Elasticity and Viscoelasticity

There are three distinct regions of the stress/strain curve: (1) the toe region, (2) the linear region, and (3) the yield and failure region. In normal activity, most ligaments and tendons exist in the toe and somewhat in the linear region. This region is responsible for nonlinear stress/strain curve, because the slope of the toe region is not linear. The toe region represents "uncrimping" of the collagen fibrils. Since it is easier to stretch out the crimp of the collagen fibrils, this part of the stress strain curve shows a relatively low stiffness compared to linear portion. The toe region ends at about 2% strain when all crimpled fibers straighten. When all collagen fibrils become uncrimped, the collagen fibers stretch. The tendon deforms in a linear fashion due to the inter-molecular sliding of collagen triple helices. If strain is less than 4%, the tendon will return to its original length when unloaded, therefore this portion is elastic and reversible and the slope of the curve represents an elastic modulus. When a tendon/ligament is stretched beyond physiological limits, some fibrils begin to fail. Micro failure accumulates, stiffness is reduced and the ligament/tendon begins to fail. This occurs when intramolecular cross-links between collagen fibers fail. The tendon therefore undergoes irreversible plastic deformation. When the tendon/ligament is stretched to more than 8-10% of its original length, macroscopic failure.

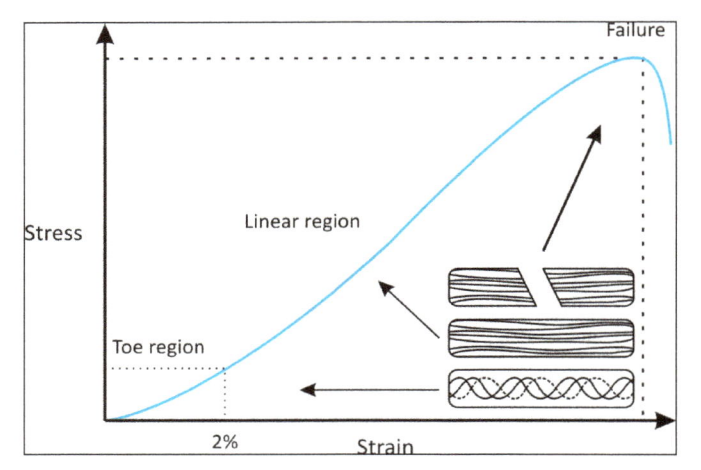

Viscoelasticity refers to time dependent mechanical behavior. In other words, the relationship between stress and strain is not constant but depends on the time of displacement or load. There are three major characteristics of a viscoelastic material of ligaments and tendons: creep, stress relaxation, and hysteresis or energy dissipation. *Creep* indicates increasing deformation under constant load. This is in contrast with the usual elastic material, which does not elongate, no matter how long the load is applied. *Stress relaxation* is a feature of a ligament or tendon meaning that stress acting upon them will be eventually reduced under a constant deformation. When a viscoelastic material is loaded and unloaded, the unloading curve is different from the loading curve. This is called *hysteresis*. The difference between the two curves represents the amount of energy that is dissipated or lost during loading. If loading and unloading are repeated several times, different curves are obtained. However, after about 10 cycles, the loading and unloading curves do not change anymore, but they are still different. In other words, the amount of hysteresis under cyclic loading is reduced and the stress-strain curve becomes reproducible. This behavior is called *pseudo-elasticity* to represent the nonlinearity of ligament/tendon stress strain behavior.

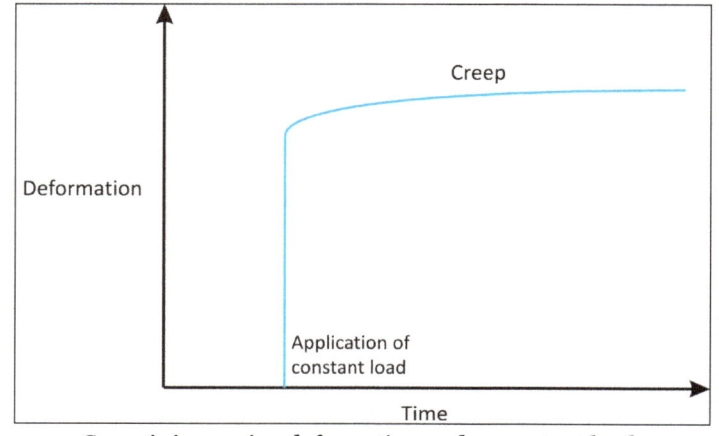

Creep is increasing deformation under constant load.

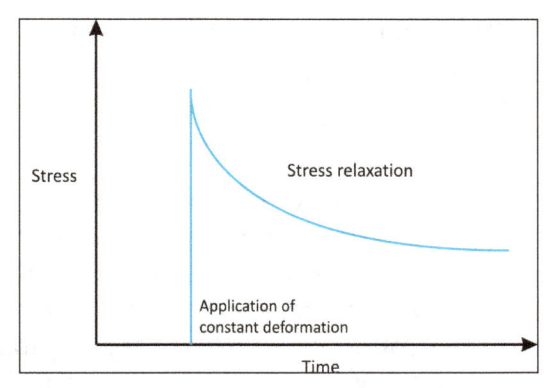

Stress relaxation - the stress will be reduced under a constant deformation.

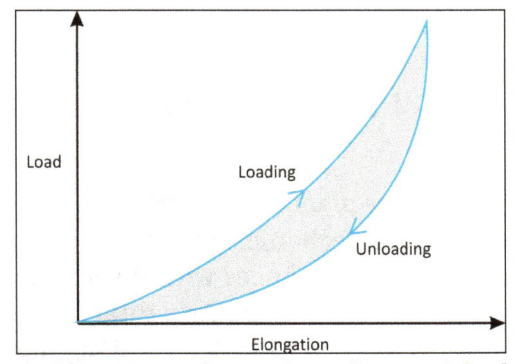

Hysteresis or energy dissipation – when tendon or ligament is loaded and unloaded, the unloading curve will not follow the loading curve. The energy is lost as heat (dashed area).

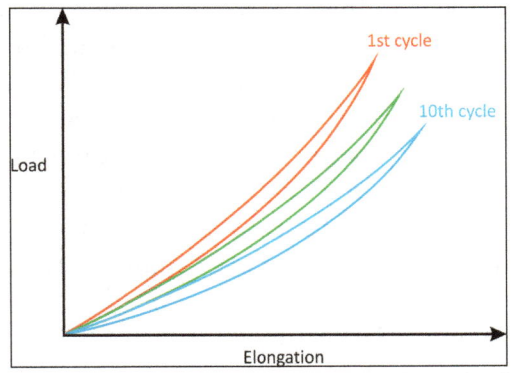

During cyclic loading and unloading, the stress/strain curve shifts to the right. After 10 repetitions, the curve becomes reproducible. The amount of hysteresis under cyclic loading is reduced.

The Influence of Loading and Gender on Tendon and Ligament Size

Ligaments and tendons are adapted according to changes in mechanical stiffness. However, changes occur slowly, partly due to the fact that tendons and ligaments are relatively avascular tissues. There is strong evidence that tendons undergo hypertrophy, at least after long-term mechanical loading.

Male runners were found to have about larger Achilles tendon cross-sectional areas than non-runners. Furthermore, greater cross-sectional area (CSA) of patella tendons in the leading leg of male athletes competing for at least 5 years in sports with a side-to-side difference was demonstrated; an almost 30% difference in the cross-sectional area of the proximal part of the tendon between the leading and non-leading leg was observed. When subjected to short-term loading, only certain parts of tendons hypertrophied. It appears that tendons undergo hypertrophy in response to both long- and short-term loading, but that short-term changes in CSA are relatively small and seemingly occur only in specific regions of the tendon.

Interestingly, findings described above seem to be gender specific since marked differences in tendon CSA were not consistently found between female athletes and sedentary controls. Some other studies do in fact indicate that the exercise related adaptation of the tendon tissue is lower when levels of estrogen are high but the mechanism of this is not clear. Similary, premenopausal women were found to have lower risk for developing lower leg tendinopathies than men. The risk for developing lower leg tendinopathy in women increases in the post-menopausal period and is probably influenced by hormone-replacement therapy and activity levels. The mechanism behind these observations is not clear.

The Effect of Aging and Immobilization Ligament and Tendon Structure and Function

With age there is an increase in the mechanical properties of ligaments and tendons up to the young adulthood when a decrease in the mechanical properties follows. Woo and colleagues tested femur-acl-tibia complex from young cadaver knees with the average age of 35 and older cadaver knees with the age of 76. They found that the linear structural stiffness of the ACL decreased both when tested at 30 degrees of knee flexion and when tested along the axis of the ligament complex.

Immobilization has a negative impact on tendons and ligaments. Corresponding to the reduction in mechanical properties, there is a reduction in the ligament structure. Immobilization has a more rapid effect on mechanical properties than increased load from exercise. It was established that during immobilization, the cross sectional area of the ACL is reduced, which is believed to be a consequence of a loss in collagen fibrils as well as glycosaminoglycan that form the ground substance of the ligament. In addition, there might be alterations in collagen fibril orientation reducing the ligament properties. Upon remobilization, it appeared that the mechanical properties normalized first, followed by the structural properties. It is also believed that structural loss at the ligament insertion site may take longer to be removed than changes in ligament substance.

Tendon and Ligament Injury Mechanisms

Tendon injury occurs because of direct trauma (i.e. penetrating, blunt, etc.) or indirect tensile overload. Acute tensile failure occurs if strain is more than 10%. However, lesser strain can cause tendon failure due to pre-existing chronic repeated insult and degeneration. Musculotendinous junction is the weakest link, especially during eccentric contractions. Maximum tension is created in forceful contractions. Furthermore, greater speed of eccentric contraction will increase the force developed. If the loading rate is slow, avulsion fracture is likely to occur. If loading is fast, tendon failure is more likely, especially if degenerated.

Tendon overuse injuries are a source of major concern in competitive and recreational athletes. It is estimated that 30% to 50% of all sport injuries are due to overuse. Studies from primary care show that 16% of general population suffers from shoulder pain, which rises to 21% in the elderly. The prevalence of Achilles tendinopathy in runners has been estimated at 11%. Tendinopathy of the forearm extensor tendons affects 1-2% of the population, most commonly occurring in the fourth and fifth decade of life. The overall prevalence of patellar tendinopathy among elite and non-elite athletes is high and varies between 3% and 45%. Quadriceps tendon and tibialis posterior tendon are also often affected. In the great majority of patients with spontaneous tendon rupture, the ruptured tendon shows degenerative lesions present before the rupture.

The term "tendinitis" has been widely used to describe a combination of tendon pain, swelling, and impaired performance. It is believed to be an inflammatory condition, although histopathological studies show degeneration rather than inflammation and therefore the term "tendinopathy" has been suggested as a more appropriate term. The term tendinopathy encompasses a spectrum of disorders, including lesions of the tenosynovium, the paratenon, the entesis, or tendon proper. Lesions can coexist and the tendon can tear partially or completely. Tendinopathies can be divided according to the duration of symptoms into acute (up to 2 weeks in duration), subacute (2-4 weeks), and chronic (over 6 weeks).

There are multiple theories for the mechanism of tendon degeneration: (1) mechanical, (2) vascular, (3) neural, and (4) alternative theory.

In the mechanical theory of tendon injury, the overload of the tendon tissue is blamed for the pathologic process. Towards the higher end of the physiologic range, a microscopic failure may occur within a tendon and repetitive microtrauma can lead to matrix and cell changes, altered mechanical properties of the tendon, and symptoms development. Non-uniform stress within a tendon may produce localized fiber degeneration and damage without a history of a specific injury. Studies have shown that cyclic mechanical stretching of cells can cause changes in cell morphology and alteration of both DNA and protein syntheses. In situ cell nucleus deformation does occur during tensile loading of tendons which may play a significant role in the mechanical signal transduction pathway in the affected tendon. The production of prostaglandin E2 (PGE2) in tendon fibroblasts increases in a stretching magnitude-dependent manner for which cyclooxygenase (COX) is responsible. Studies also showed that asymptomatic pathologic changes were common in the Achilles and patellar tendons in elite soccer players and that a greater number of hours per week resulted in a higher prevalence of patellar tendinopathy. However, "underuse" may also be the cause of tendon degeneration because the etiopathogenic stimulus for the degenerative cascade is the catabolic response of tendon cells to mechanobiological understimulation.

The vascular theory of tendinopathy suggests that tendons generally have poor blood supply, especially the Achilles tendon and those of tibialis posterior and supraspinatus muscle. The Achilles tendon should have a hypovascular region 2-6 cm proximal to its calcaneal insertion. In such tendons overuse may lead to injury.

However, studies on the Achilles blood flow show that blood supply along the whole tendon is in fact evenly distributed throughout the tendon, but is significantly lower at the distal insertion. Blood flow in the symptomatic tendons was significantly elevated as compared with the controls, demonstrated a similar vascular response to physical loading with a progressive decline in blood flow with increasing tension. Male gender, advancing age, and mechanical loading of the tendon are associated with diminished tendon blood flow. Therefore, vascular theory may be more important in the lesions of fibrocartilagenous entheses that are relatively avascular, and this may contribute to a poor healing response. Angiogenesis is mediated by angiogenic factors such as vascular endothelial growth factor (VEGF). VEGF is highly expressed in degenerative Achilles tendons, whereas its expression is nearly completely downregulated in healthy tendons. Several factors are able to upregulate VEGF expression in tenocytes: hypoxia, inflammatory cytokines, and mechanical load. Since VEGF has the potential to stimulate the expression of matrix metalloproteinases and inhibit the expression of tissue inhibitors of matrix metalloproteinases (TIMP), this cytokine might play a significant role in the pathogenetic processes during degenerative tendon disease.

The neural theory suggests that neurally mediated mast cell degranulation could release mediators such as substance P, which is contained in primary afferent nerves. Its quantity could be related to chronic pain. The increased amount of substance P in the subacromial bursa and nerve fibers immunoreactive to substance P were localized around the vessels of rotator cuff, especially in patients with the non-perforated rotator cuff injury. Inflammatory cytokines, proteinases, and cyclooxygenase enzymes, have been shown to be present in the subacromial bursa of patients with rotator cuff tear. However, neural theory does not explain why morphologically pathologic tendons are not always painful.

The alternative theory suggests that exercise induced localized hyperthermia may be detrimental to tendon cell survival. Tendons that store energy during locomotion, such as the equine superficial flexor digitorum tendon and the human Achilles tendon, suffer a high incidence of central core degeneration which is thought to precede tendon rupture. Studies have shown that the central core of equine tendon reaches temperatures as high as 45°C during high-speed locomotion, but temperatures above 42.5 °C are known to result in fibroblast death *In vitro*. Temperatures experienced in the central core of the tendon *In vivo* are unlikely to result in tendon cell death, but repeated hyperthermic insults may compromise cell metabolism of matrix components, resulting in tendon central core degeneration.

Although exact mechanism or their combination has not been determined yet, some factors influencing the development of tendinopathy have been. There is some evidence for genetic correlation, especially with target genes close to ABO gene on chromosome 9 like COL5A1 and TNC gene. Women seem to have less tendinopathy than men, especially prior to menopause. Although tendons do not degenerate with age as such, a reduction in proteoglycans and an increase in cross-links with increasing age make tendon stiffer and less capable in tolerating load. Decreased flexibility, training on harder surface, and even drugs such as corticosteroids and quinolone antibiotics have been reported to be associated with the development of tendinopathy.

Ligament injuries are classified into three grades. (1) Grade I injury – mild sprain. Clinically, there is minimal pain present over the injured ligament and no joint instability can be detected by clinical examination despite the microfailure of collagen fibers. (2) Grade II injury – moderate sprain or partial tear of the ligament. There is severe pain present and minimal instability detected by clinical testing. Ligament strength and stiffness decrease by 50%. (3) Grade III injury – a complete ligament tear. Most collagen fibers have ruptured and the joint is completely unstable. Another type of injury is ligament avulsion from its bony insertion. Midsubstance ruptures are more common in45 adults; avulsion injuries are more common in children. Avulsion occurs between unmineralized and mineralized fibrocartilage layers.

Pathophysiology of Tendon and Ligament Repair

The process of tendon healing follows a pattern similar to that of other healing tissues. There are three phases of healing: (1) hemostasis/inflammation, (2) reparative phase, and (3) remodeling and maturation phase. Ligament healing goes through the same stages as tendon healing. However, there are differences among different ligaments. A classic model for ligament healing is the rupture of medial collateral ligament of the knee (MCL). MCL has a good tendency to heal spontanelously. In contrast, the anterior cruciate ligament of the knee (ACL) does not show any tendency to heal spontaneously, which is believed to be the consequence of synovial fluid interrupting the healing process between the ruptured ends of the ligament. Therefore, an ACL reconstruction is a treatment of choice.

After the injury, the wound site is infiltrated by inflammatory cells. Platelets aggregate at the wound and create a fibrin clot to stabilize the torn tendon edges. The clot contains cells and platelets that immediately begin to release a variety of molecules, most notably growth factors (such as platelet-derived growth factor, transforming growth factor β, and insulin-like growth factor -I and –II) causing acute local inflammation. During this inflammatory phase that usually lasts three to five days, there is an invasion of extrinsic cells such as neutrophils and macrophages which clean up necrotic debris by phagocytosis and together with intrinsic cells (such as endotenon and epitenon cells) produce a second pool of cytokines to initiate the reparative phase.

In reparative phase (three to six weeks) large amounts of disorganized collagen are deposited at the repair site with granulation tissue formation, together with neovascularization, extrinsic fibroblast migration, and intrinsic fibroblast proliferation. After four days fibroblasts infiltrate the wound site and proliferate. They produce extracellular matrix, including large amounts of collagen III and glycosaminoglycan.

In the remodeling phase, there is a decrease in the cellular and vascular content of the repairing tissue, and an increase in collagen type I content and density. Eventually, the collagen becomes more organized, properly orientated, and cross-linking with the healthy matrix outside the injury takes place. Matrix metalloproteinase degrade the collagen matrix, replacing type II collagen with type I collagen. The remodeling stage can be divided into a consolidation and maturation phase. At the end of the consolidation phase, at about 10–12 weeks, and with the beginning of the maturation phase, the fibrous tissue is converted to a stronger scar tissue. Around the fourth week collagen fibers are being longitudinally reorganized so that they are aligned in the direction of muscle loading. During the next three months the individual collagen fibers form bundles identical to the original ones. After the healing process is complete, cellularity, vascularity, and collagen makeup will return to something approximating that of the normal tendon, but the diameters and cross-linking of the collagen will often remain inferior after healing. This phase lasts for months or years, usually between 6 weeks and 9 months or more. However, the tissue continues to remodel for up to 1 year. The structural properties of the repaired tendon typically reach only two thirds of normal, even years after injury.

There are slight differences in the way different tendons heal. Extrasynovial tendons can be easily influenced by growth factors and cytokines produced by extrinsic cells (e.g. paratenon), but intrasynovial tendons are more reliant on intrinsic cells (e.g. epitenon and endotenon).

Treatment of Tendon and Ligament Injuries

According to stages of healing response, a proper rehabilitation program time frame can be introduced. During the inflammatory phase of 3-5 days rehabilitation program should avoid excess motion because it can disrupt the healing process. During the repair phase a gradual introduction of motion can be introduced to prevent excessive muscle atrophy and prevent the diminishing of range of motion (ROM). Later progressive stress can be applied, however, tendons can require up to one year to get close to normal strength levels.

Proper postsurgical rehabilitation strategies are being debated. Rehabilitation protocols differ due to anatomical site, because different tendons have different healing characteristics. There is even a difference in the rehabilitation protocol between sheathed tendons and tendons that are not enclosed in sheaths. In sheathed tendons, early mobilization is crucial to prevent scar formation between tendon sheaths, therefore diminishing ROM. The response of healing tendons to mechanical load varies depending on anatomical location. Flexor tendons require motion to prevent adhesion formation, yet excessive force results in gap formation and subsequent weakening of the repair.

Immobilization and Early Remobilization

Ruptured and immobilized ligaments heal with a fibrous gap between the ruptured ends, whereas sutured ligaments heal without fibrous gap. The mechanical properties of scars are inferior to normal ligaments, which may lead to joint dysfunction by abnormalities in joint kinematics. In spite of this, many ligaments are not repaired routinely.

Protective immobilization may enhance tendon-to-bone healing compared with other post repair loading regimens like exercise or complete tendon unloading. In the repaired rotator cuff, immobilization has shown to be beneficial in tendon-to-bone healing. A complete removal of loading is detrimental to rotator cuff healing. However, immobilization is not a proper treatment for all repaired tendons; some require early passive motion.

Tendons requiring long excursions for function (e.g. the flexor tendons) are typically encased in synovial sheaths. To maintain gliding after injury, adhesions between the tendon surface and its sheath must be prevented. Passive mechanical rehabilitation methods have shown to be beneficial to prevent fibrotic adhesions.

The optimal time for the initiation of such treatment is about 5 days after tendon repair. Controlled loading can enhance healing in most cases, but a fine balance must be reached between loads that are too low (leading to a catabolic state) or too high (leading to micro damage).

Surgical Reconstruction

There is still a debate when ligament or tendon injuries should be treated conservatively and when surgical repair is indicated. In practice the "50% rule" is commonly used. The "50% rule" suggests that tendon/ligament injuries with structural involvement of less than 50% should be treated conservatively, but damage greater than 50% should be treated by surgical repair or reconstruction. This rule applies to a variety of orthopedic conditions, like partial fractural involvement of less than 50%, anterior cruciate ligament, partial-thickness injuries of the rotator cuff, and partial tears of the long head of the biceps tendon. However, there is very little evidence for accuracy, reproducibility, or predictive power and this rule has to be used with caution. It is maybe better to individualize the treatment according to a patient's clinical and physical status, expectations, and demands after the treatment.

The Role of Corticosteroid Injection Therapy

At the cellular level, anti-inflammatory and immunosuppressive actions of corticosteroids are the consequence of inhibition of cytokine-genes and pro-inflammatory mediators' synthesis, such as nitric oxide and prostaglandins. The immunosuppressive and anti-inflammatory actions of corticosteroids are mediated through the interference of two transcription factors: activating protein-1 (AP-1) and nuclear factor-κB (NF-κB). The exact mechanism by which corticosteroids inhibit the transcriptional activity of AP-1 is not fully understood. However, the activation of the cell by immune signals leads to degradation of IκB inhibitory protein from NF-κB, allowing nuclear translocation of NF-κB and consequently the transcription of multiple target genes. Corticosteroids induce the production of IκB and therefore provide efficient inactivation of NF-κB.

Besides the anti-inflammatory action, corticosteroids decrease the production of collagen and extracellular matrix proteins by the fibroblasts and enhance bone resorption. Furthermore, the production of extracellular matrix degrading enzymes MMP-3 (stromelysin-1), MMP-13 (collagenase-3), and MMP-1 (collagensae-1) in ligaments and other tissues is also suppressed. Whether this is beneficial when treating chronic tendon lesions is unknown, but some reports indicate the overexpression of MMPs in the Achilles tendinopathy.

Corticosteroids alter mechanical properties of tendons. Incubation of tendon fibrils in corticosteroids resulted in a significant reduction in tensile strength after only 3 days. It is possible, that corticosteroid injection affect the component of the extracellular matrix in a way that influences tensile strength. They may reduce decorin gene expression and inhibit the proliferation and activity of tenocytes, which leads to suppression in collagen production. However, the magnitude of reduction in collagen type 1 and decorin gene expression appeared to be smaller when corticosteroid treatment was combined with mechanical strain.

Recommendations for the use of local corticosteroid injections are still not clear. Application should be peritendinous rather than intratendinous due to the demonstrated deleterious effect of corticosteroid on tendon tissue. Short or moderate acting, more soluble preparations are recommended because in theory they cause fewer side effects (hydrocortisone, methylprednisolone). Local anesthetics are usually mixed with the corticosteroid injection for wider dispersion and more comfortable procedure; but some manufacturers warn against mixing because of theoretical risk of precipitation. Corticosteroid injections in "high strain" tendons, especially the Achilles tendon or patellar tendon, are discouraged due to the possible and well documented risk of tendon rupture. This therapy should be reserved only for chronic tendon injuries after the intensive use of other approaches for at least 2 months; injections should be peritendinous only. One study showed an increased rupture risk only when corticosteroids were injected intratendionously, but not when injected in peritendinous tissue. A maximum of three injections at one site should be given with a minimum interval between injections of 6 weeks. If two injections do not provide at least 4 week's relief, they should be discontinued.

Future Therapies to Improve Tendon and Ligament Healing

Injection of growth factors, especially those derived from activated thrombocytes, and tissue-engineering strategies, such as (1) the development of scaffold microenvironment, (2) responding cells, and (3) signaling biofactors are generating potential areas for additional prospective investigation in tendon or ligament regeneration. Tissue engendering is a promising field to enhance tendon and ligament repair. Nevertheless, significant challenges remain to accomplish a complete and functional tendon or ligament repair that will lead to a clinically effective and commercially successful application.

Skeletal Muscle Damage and Repair

Musculoskeletal injuries resulting in the necrosis of muscle fibers are frequently encountered in clinical and sports medicine and are the most common cause of severe long-term pain and physical disability, affecting hundreds of millions of people around the world and accounting for the majority of all sport-related injuries.

The annual direct and indirect costs for musculoskeletal conditions in the United States were estimated at USD $849 billion or 8% of the gross domestic product. Similarly, a study published examining musculoskeletal disorders in 23 European countries, reported that >44 million members of the European Union workforce had a long-standing health problem or disability that affected their ability to work and that musculoskeletal disorders accounted for a higher proportion of sickness absence from work than any other health condition. In 2009, the total cost of musculoskeletal disorders in European workforce was estimated at 240 billion a year.

Injured skeletal muscle can undergo repair spontaneously via regeneration; however, this process often is incomplete because the overgrowth of extracellular matrix and the deposition of collagen lead to significant fibrous scarring.

Muscle injuries therefore frequently result in significant morbidity, including early functional and structural deficits, contraction injury, muscle atrophy, contracture, and pain.

By neutralizing pro-fibrotic processes in injured skeletal muscle, it is possible to prevent fibrosis and enhance muscle regeneration, thereby improving the functional recovery of the injured muscle.

Muscle Structure and Mechanism of Action

A number of non-contractile connective tissue elements are necessary for the organization of the contractile muscle fibers into effective mechanical stress. Thus the fibers are bound together into fascicles by the fibroelastic perimysium; the ends of the muscle are attached to the bones by tendons and aponeuroses, and the whole muscle is held in its proper place by the connective tissue sheets called fasciae.

The arrangement of muscle fascicles, and the manner in which they approach the tendons, has many variations. In some muscles, the fascicles are parallel with the longitudinal axis and terminate at either end in flat tendons. In case of the converging fascicles to one side of a tendon the muscle is called *penniform,* like the semimembranosus muscle. If muscles converge to both sides of a tendon, they are called *bipenniform,* or if they converge to several tendons, they are called *multipenniform,* as in case of deltoid muscle. The nomenclature of striated muscle is based on different parameters describing their properties.

Table: Muscle nomenclature according to different parameters.

Muscle, named by	Muscle
Location	• Brachialis • Supraspinatus
Direction	• Rectus abdominis • Obliquus abdominis
Action	• Flexor hallucis • Extensor digitorum
Shape	• Deltoideus • Trapezius
Attachment points	• Sternocleidomastoideus • Omohyoideus

The arrangement of fascicles and the power of muscles are positively correlated. Those with comparatively few fascicles, extending the length of the muscle, have a greater range of motion but not as much power. Penniform muscles, with a large number of fascicles distributed along their tendons, have a greater power but a smaller range of motion (ROM).

Molecular basis of muscle contraction is in the interaction between *actin* and *myosin*, fuelled by ATP and initiated by the increase in $[Ca^{2+}]_i$. Skeletal muscle possesses an array of transverse T-tubules extending into the cell from the plasma membrane, through which the action potential is spread into the inner portion of the muscle fiber, followed by releasing a short puff of Ca^{2+} from the sarcoplasmic reticulum (SR) into the sarcoplasm. Ca^{2+} binds to troponin, a protein that normally blocks the interaction between actin and myosin. When Ca^{2+} binds, troponin moves out of the way and allows the contractile machinery to operate.

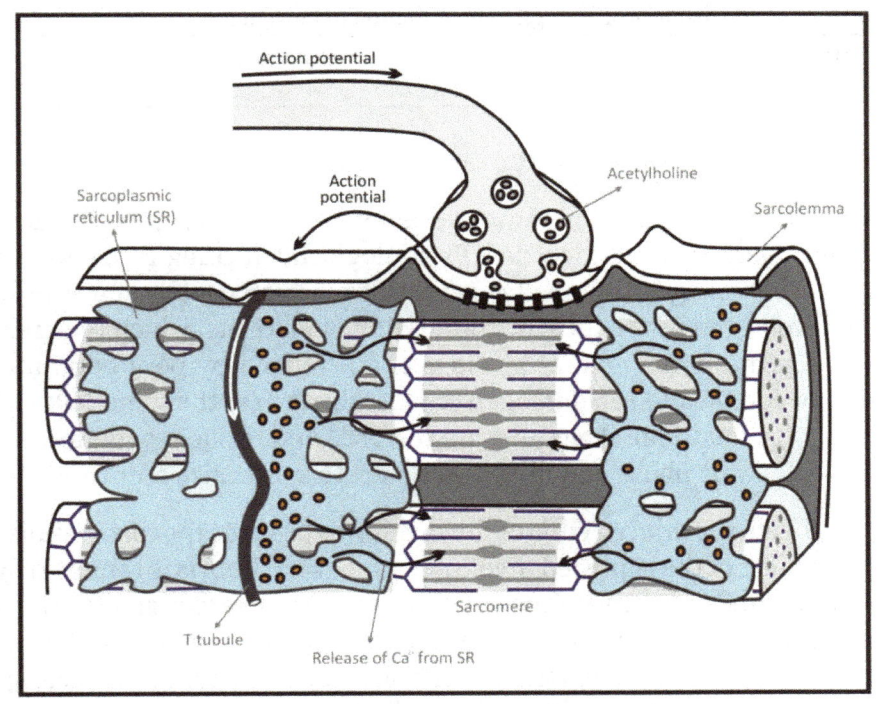

Molecular basis of muscle contraction.

Muscular Injury Mechanisms

Muscle injuries can be a consequence of a variety of causes: during the exercise, on the sports field, in the workplace, during surgical procedures, or in any kind of accidents. Regarding the mechanism, they are classified as direct and indirect. Direct injuries include lacerations and contusions, whereas the indirect class involves complete or incomplete muscle strain.

The current classification of muscle injuries distinguishes mild injuries from moderate and severe, based on the clinical symptoms. In a mild muscle injury, a strain or contusion is characterized by a tear of only a few muscle fibers with minor swelling and discomfort accompanied with no or only minimal loss of strength and restriction of movement. Moderate injury is represented by greater muscle damage with a clear loss of function, whereas a tear across the entire cross-section of the muscle resulting in a virtually complete loss of muscle function, is termed a severe injury.

Muscle strain injuries after eccentric contractions are the most common type of muscle injury in athletes and are especially common in sports that require sprinting or jumping. Submaximal lengthening contractions are used in everyday life, but it is well known that high-force lengthening contractions are associated with muscle damage and pain. Muscle strains are divided into three grades according to severity.

Table: Classification of muscle strains according to clinical manifestation.

Muscle strains classification according to clinical severity	
Grade	Clinical Manifestation
I	Tear of new muscle fibers with minimal swelling and discomfort Minimal loss of strength with almost no limitation of movements.
II	A greater damage of muscle Partial loss of strength and limitation of movements.
III	A severe tear across the whole section of the muscle Total loss of the muscle function.

Pathophysiology of Muscle Damage and Repair

The cellular and molecular mechanisms of muscle regeneration after injury and degeneration have been described extensively in recent decades. Physiologically, healing progresses over a series of overlapping phases. These stages include: (a) hemostasis, which usually starts with the formation of a blood clot and is followed by the local degranulation of platelets, which release several granule constituents; (b) the acute inflammatory phase is characterized by peripheral muscle fiber contraction, formation of edema and cell damagen and death; and (c) the remodeling phase that lasts from 48 hrs up to 6 wks; anatomic structures are restored and tissue regeneration occurs. Several cell types are involved in this phase and fibroblasts start to synthesize scar tissue.

Only local necrosis affects the injured ends of the myofibres because the torn sarcolemma is rapidly resealed, allowing the rest of the ruptured myofibres to survive. Debris is removed by macrophages that secrete growth factors and activate the satellite cells. These are regenerative mononucleated stem cells of muscle tissue that normally lie between the basal lamina and plasma membrane of the muscle fiber. First, they form myoblasts which then begin to produce muscle specific proteins and finally mature into muscle fibers with peripherally located nuclei.

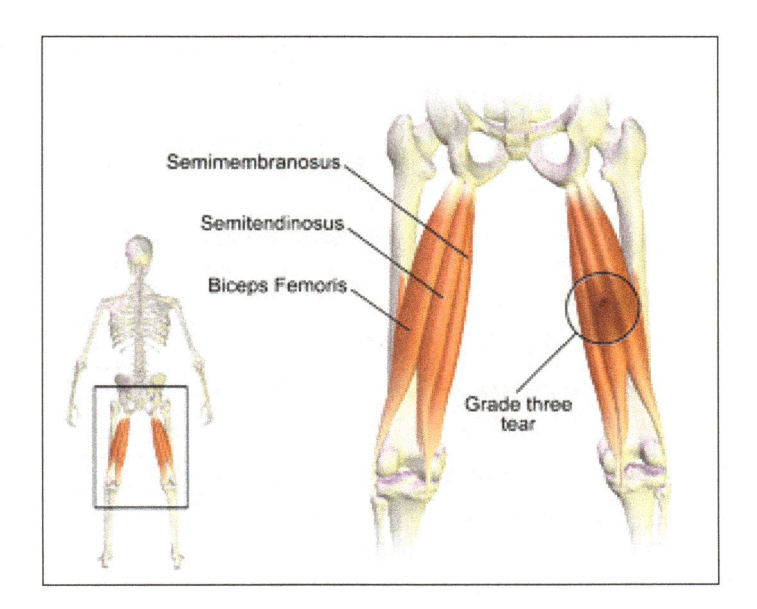

Semimembranosus
Semitendinosus
Biceps Femoris
Grade three tear

Role of satellite cells in muscle regeneration after acute injury. (a) quiescent satellite cells in a normal muscle just above sarcolemma; (b) mechanical stress and growth factors released from macrophages activate satellite cells that begin to express myogenic proteins which further stimulate proliferation; (c) in early differentiation phase, myoblasts express myogenin and MRF4, factors that promote further differentiation and the fusion of mononucleated cells; (d) in the late differentiation phase polynucleated myotubes begin to express factors that promote the final fusion and definite differentiation of myotubes into mature myofibres; (e) although muscle tissue is capable of self-regeneration, partial fibrosis contributes to function loss.

A typical feature during muscle differentiation is the variation in expression of various genes along with myogenic factors. Sequence-specific myogenic regulatory factors (MRFs) are expressed exclusively in skeletal muscle and regulate the process of muscle development. It is their role to govern the expression of multiple genes in myogenesis, from the engagement of mesodermal cells in the muscle lineage, to the differentiation of somatic cells and the terminal differentiation of myocytes into myofibres.

The MRFs consist of a group of transcription factors. They have been divided into two functional groups: The primary MRFs, MyoD, and Myf-5 required for the determination of skeletal myoblasts; and the secondary MRFs, myogenin and MRF4 that act later in the program, most likely as differentiation factors. Activated satellite cells first express either Myf-5 or MyoD followed soon by co-expression of Myf-5 and MyoD. After the proliferation, myogenin and MRF4 are expressed in cells and begin their differentiation program.

The cellular process required for degeneration and regeneration may be affected by alterations in the inflammatory response. Although strained skeletal muscle is capable of self-regeneration, the healing process is slow and often incomplete, resulting in strength loss and a high rate of reinjury at the site of the initial injury. Unfortunately, the muscle repair process involves a complex balance between muscle fiber regeneration and scar-tissue formation.

TGF-β and Myostatin – A Key Factors In Muscular Scarring

TGF-β is a cytokine with numerous biologic activities related to wound-healing, including fibroblast and macrophage recruitment, stimulation of collagen production, downregulation of proteinase activity, and increases in metalloproteinase inhibitor activity. There are three mammalian isoforms of TGF-β: TGF-β1, TGF-β2, and TGF-β3. All three isoforms are potentially produced by most cells active in wound-healing, with platelets being a major contributor. The major functions of TGF-β are listed in table:

Activity of TGF-β
Stimulation of mesenchymal cell proliferation.
Regulation of endothelial cells and fibroblasts.
Promotion of extracellular matrix production.
Stimulation of endothelial chemotaxis and angiogenesis.
Inhibition of macrophage and lymphocyte proliferation.
Inhibition of satellite cell differentiation.

TGF-β is a potent stimulator of fibrosis in the kidneys, liver, heart, and lungs and is closely associated with skeletal muscle fibrosis as well where it plays a significant role in both the initiation of fibrosis and the induction of myofibroblastic differentiation of myogenic cells in injured skeletal muscle. Many reports indicate that the overproduction of transforming growth factor TGF-β1 in response to injury and disease is a major cause of tissue fibrosis both in animals and humans.

Muscle-derived stem cells (MDSDs) are populations of stem cells that appear to be distinct from satellite cells and can differentiate into myofibroblasts after muscle injury. But myoblasts can also differentiate into fibrotic cells where TGF-β is a key factor that stimulates fibrotic differentiation.

Inhibition of TGF-β has been shown to decrease collagen deposition and scarring. For example, the application of neutralizing antibodies to TGF-β in rat incisional wounds successfully reduced cutaneous scarring.

However, it is not yet clear whether TGF-β acts alone or requires an interaction with other molecules during the development of muscle fibrosis. Recent studies have shown that myostatin may also be involved in fibrosis formation within skeletal muscle.

Over the last years, the TGF-β member myostatin (MSTN) has gained particular relevance because of its ability to exert a profound effect on muscle metabolism, by regulating the myofibre size in response to physiological or pathological conditions. Myostatin or GDF8 (Growth differentiation factor 8) is a TGF-β protein family member that inhibits muscle differentiation and growth and is expressed specifically in developing and adult skeletal muscle. It inhibits the activity of satellite cells during muscle regeneration due to its control of the movement of macrophages, and also inhibits the multiplication of myoblasts and their differentiation. In myogenic cells, myostatin induces down-regulation of Myo-D, an early marker of muscle differentiation, and decreases the expression of Pax-3 and Myf-5, which encode transcriptional regulators of myogenic cell proliferation. Its expression is restricted initially to the myotome compartment of developing somites and continues to be limited to the myogenic lineage at later stages of the development and in adult animals.

Table: Activity of myostatin.

Activity of myostatin.
Inhibition of satellite cell activity.
Control of macrophage movement.
Down-regulation of MyoD.
Inhibition of transcriptional regulators of proliferation.
Inhibition of myoblast multiplication in differentiation.
Regulation of myofibre size.

Myostatin loss-of-function due to naturally occurring mutations into its gene triggers muscle mass increase in cattle dogs, and humans as well. Jarvnien reported that the injection of a neutralizing monoclonal antibody to myostatin led to increased skeletal muscle mass in mice without side effects. This method was found to be safe in a subsequent clinical trial, although dose escalation was limited by cutaneous hypersensitivity restricting potential efficacy. Blocking of the MSTN signaling transduction pathway by specific inhibitors and genetic manipulations has been shown to result in a dramatic increase of skeletal muscle mass. In principle, blocking of MSTN signaling can be achieved by three different pharmacological strategies: blocking MSTN gene expression (knocking out, inactivating the MSTN gene by viral-based gene overexpression, and antisense technologies); blocking the synthesis of the MSTN protein; and blocking of the MSTN receptor (small molecules, specific blocking antibodies).

Therapeutic Standards and Controversies in Treatment of Muscle Injuries

Despite the clinical significance of muscle injuries, the current treatment principles for injured skeletal muscle lack a firm scientific basis and are based on performing RICE (Rest, Ice, Compression, and Elevation). These four methods are supposed to limit the hematoma formation, though there are no randomized studies confirming their true value in the management of soft tissue injuries.

The most convincing is the effect of "rest" on muscle regeneration. Limb immobilization prevents further retraction of the injured muscle and thereby greater discontinuity of the tissue, enlargement of hematoma, and the consequential scar tissue formation. Putting ice also limits the formation of the hematoma, additionally impairs inflammation, and accelerates early tissue regeneration. Concerns about the limited perfusion in the damaged muscle because of the limb compression are putting it under question while its elevation above the level of the heart follows the basic physiological principles as the hydrostatic pressure in the elevated tissue falls, followed by lesser interstitial fluid accumulation and the formation of edema. In this phase it is recommended to maintain the cardiovascular fitness without the risk for reinjury like cycling or swimming.

Although lacking scientific background, therapeutic ultrasound is a widely accepted adjuvant method for treating muscle injuries. Micro massage with high-frequency waves has a pain relieving effect and it is supposed to act proregeneratory, especially in the early phase after an injury. Despite promoting proliferation, therapeutic ultrasound does not seem to have a positive effect on the final outcome of muscle healing.

Another adjuvant therapeutic option for improving muscle repair is hyperbaric oxygen therapy (HBO), which has shown to have positive effects during the early phase of repair by accelerating the recovery of the injured muscle. However, not a single randomized prospective study has been performed on the treatment of severe skeletal muscle injuries by HBO, which might increase the sensation of pain in less severe forms of injuries like delayed onset muscle soreness (DOMS). In case of both mild and severe muscle injuries there is a lack of clinical studies confirming the real place of this therapeutic option in athletes.

The use of non-steroidal anti-inflammatory drugs (NSAID's) in the treatment of muscle injuries is common, but controversial. The most commonly prescribed are COX-2 inhibitors administered either via intramuscular, oral or transdermal route. While the first studies reported on the positive effects of NSAID's on muscle regeneration without compromising muscle contractility or stem cell proliferation, the more recent showed the importance of the inflammatory process after injury and by inhibiting it the NSAID's promote scar tissue formation. Incomplete muscle fiber regeneration and fibrotic infiltration can lead to long-term functional deficits and physical incapacitation. The use of glucocorticoids in case of muscle injuries is even more questionable as the elimination of the hematoma and necrotic tissue seems to be slower and biomechanical strength of the injured muscle reduced.

The identification of MRFs allows researchers a new and more detailed insight into the processes of muscle regeneration which is crucial for developing novel therapeutic targets. In recent years many studies using antifibrotic agents have been performed in patients with different heart and kidney diseases or systemic sclerosis. *In vitro* and *In vivo* studies showed important antifibrotic effects of platelet-rich plasma derived growth factors, recombinant proteins such as decorin, follistatin, γ-interferon, suramin, relaxin, and other biologically active agents like mannose-6-phosphate, N-acetylcysteine, and angiotensin-receptor blockers. Although none of these has yet been tested on humans, their promising effects may significantly alter the therapeutic options of muscle injuries in the future.

Articular Cartilage Damage and Repair

Cartilage comprises of inherited limited healing potential and thus remains a challenging tissue to repair and reconstruct. Traumatic and degenerative cartilage defects occur frequently in the knee joint and represent difficult clinical dilemma. Articular cartilage has a limited capacity to self-repair principally due to its avascular nature and the limited ability of mature chondrocytes to produce a sufficient amount of extracellular matrix. Untreated cartilage injuries therefore lead to the development of arthritis. Current first line treatment options for smaller and mid-sized lesions in lower-demand patients are debridement or lavage and bone marrow-stimulating techniques (microfracture) which promote a fibrocartilage healing response. On the other hand, restorative treatment options such as osteochondral autologous graft transplantation (OATS) are limited by the amount of donor tissue availability and the size and depth of the defect. Regenerative treatment techniques such as autologous chondrocyte implantation (ACI) are promising treatment options for large full thickness articular cartilage defects where cells from healthy non-weight bearing areas are multiplied *In vitro* and implanted into such defects. Opposed to the traditional reparative procedures (e.g. bone marrow stimulation – microfracture), which promote a fibrocartilage formation with lower tissue biomechanical properties and poorer clinical results, ACI is capable to restore hyaline-like cartilage tissue in damaged articular surfaces. This technique has undergone several advances and is constantly improving. Indeed, there are numerous studies exploring new biomaterials; applications of various growth factors; the synergistic effects of mechanical stimulation in terms of tissue engineering *In vitro*, *In vivo*, and in animal models in order to stimulate the formation of hyaline-like cartilage.

Cartilage Structure

Articular (hyaline) cartilage is a specific and well-characterized tissue with remarkable mechanical properties consisting of exclusively one cell type - chondrocytes which are embedded in the extracellular matrix (ECM). The principal function of articular cartilage is to withstand mechanical loads, facilitate smooth and perfect glide among articular surfaces, and enable painless and low friction movements of synovial joints. The articular cartilage is an aneural, avascular and alymphatic structure. The nutrition of chondrocytes occurs via diffusion between synovial fluid and cartilage matrix.

The only resident cells in articular cartilage (chondrocytes) contribute to only 1-5 % of tissue volume. The remaining 99 % represent the extracellular matrix (ECM) structural components that mainly consist of water, collagen, and proteoglycans (PGs). ECM works as a biphasic structure composed of a fluid phase (water and electrolytes) and solid phase consisting mainly of collagen and proteoglycans. The solid phase comprises of low permeability due to the high resistance of a fluid flow which causes a high rate of fluid pressurization and contributes to the load transmission of cartilage. Together, both solid and fluid phase establish the stiffness and viscoelastic properties of a cartilage.

Structural Layers

The structure of cartilage matrix varies with the depth; four different zones (superficial, transitional, radial, and calcified) are distinguished based upon the cell morphology, matrix composition, and collagen fibril orientation. Chondrocytes change their conformation from parallel to vertical in deep zones. Similarly, collagen fibers alignment becomes parallel in deeper zones of cartilage tissue. There is also an increase in the overall volume, water content, and overall biological activity in deeper zones.

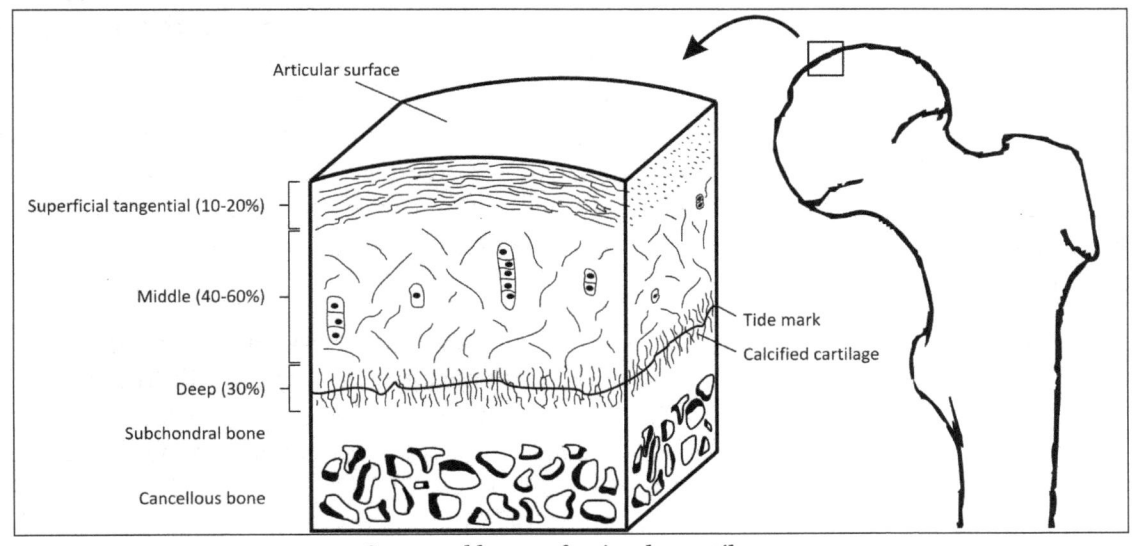

Structural layers of articuralar cartilage.

Chondrocytes are specialized cells and basic structural cells in the articular cartilage, which are sparsely spread within the matrix and altogether form only 1-5 % of cartilage volume. They are deprived of blood supply and obtain the nutrients by diffusion from synovial fluid.

The formation of cartilage tissue and maturation of chondrocytes follows a multi-step process called chondrogenesis. In general it comprises of mesenchymal stem cell proliferation and their differentiation into mature chondrocytes capable to synthesize structural components of ECM (type II collagen, PG and non-collagenous proteins) and to maintain its continuous formation and restoration.

Each step of chondrogenesis can be classified according to the expression of different sets of transcription factors, cell adhesion molecules and extracellular matrix components. Chondrocytes have no cell-to-cell contacts, are highly metabolically active (however, due to low overall cell volume the total activity appears low) and are exposed to low oxygen environment and anaerobic metabolism. Mature chondrocytes are in the continuous communication with ECM and hence respond to changes in ECM and regulate its metabolism.

Cartilage tissue is under constant impact of anabolic and catabolic cellular activity in response to extracellular environment and exposure to different cytokines and growth factors. Anabolic proteins such as tumor growth factor beta (TNF-beta), insulin growth factor (IGF-1), bone morphogenic protein (BMP), and fibroblast growth factor (FGF) stimulate matrix formation and promote the anabolic activity of chondrocytes. On the other hand, catabolic proteins such as tumor necrosis factor alpha (TNF-α) and interleukin 1 beta (IL-1β) inhibit protein synthesis and promote matrix degeneration. The constant equilibrium in the functioning of all signaling pathways is of crucial importance for the proper function and maintenance of cartilage tissue. The modern concept of cartilage tissue engineering is based on the imitation of the cartilage natural environment and the process of chondrogenesis to try to stimulate the formation of such a cartilage, which contains all the structural and biomechanical properties of native cartilage.

Extracellular matrix (ECM) is consists of water, collagen, and proteoglycans. All together water represents 60-85 % of the weight of the cartilage. The water content varies with the depth of the tissue; near the articular surface the water content is the highest and PG concentration is relatively low; vice versa is found in a deeper zone near subchondral bone, where the water content is the lowest but the PG concentration is the greatest. A high amount of water content in cartilage tissue is important for nutrition, lubrication, and for creating a low-friction gliding surface. In diseased cartilage such as osteoarthritis, the water content amounts to more than 90% as a result of matrix disruption and increased permeability. This leads to the decreased modulus of elasticity and reduction in load bearing capability.

Collagen is the main component of ECM. This fibrous protein represents 60 to 70% of the dry weight of the tissue. Type II collagen is the predominant collagen (90–95%) of ECM and provides a tensile strength to the articular cartilage. The high rate of cross-linkage between collagen molecules provides cartilages its resistance against traction forces. Other types of collagen molecules are also found in cartilage tissue in smaller amounts, these are types V, VI, IX, X and XI. Type IX and XI are most abundant in minor types collagen. Type XI participates in cross-linkage with type II collagen, integrins, and proteoglycans, whereas type XI is important in regulating the fibril diameter of type

II collagen. Collagen architecture varies through the depth of the tissue. On the sliding surface of entire cartilage (tangential zone) collagen fibers are oriented parallel to the cartilage surface.

Proteoglycans (PGs) are protein polysaccharides and form 10–20% dry weight of the articular cartilage. Their primary function is to provide compressive strength to cartilage tissue. In articular cartilage they can be classified in two major classes, large aggregating proteoglycan monomers (aggrecans) and small proteoglycan molecules (decorin, biglycan, and fibromodulin). PG are composed of glycosaminoglycans (GAG) subunits (chondroitin and keratin sulfate) which are bound to a central core protein via sugar bonds to form proteoglycan aggrecan, which is highly characteristic for hyaline cartilage. Aggrecan, 250 kDa protein represents more than 80 % of all PG molecules in cartilage tissue. It binds to hyaluronic acid to form high molecular weight aggregates with more than 3.5×10^6 kDa. In the cartilage tissue these aggregates are located within the collagen type II fibril network resulting in densely packed negative charge which interacts with water via hydrogen bond and causing electrostatic repulsion. This key feature enables cartilage tissue to resist deformation under compression and to withstand and redistribute mechanical.

Cartilage Lesions

Injuries to articular cartilage are observed with an increasing frequency in athletes. In particular participation in pivoting sports such as football, basketball, and soccer they are associated with a rising number of sport-related cartilage injuries. The exact incidence of the cartilage damage is not known since they mostly appear asymptomaticly. However, during a review of 25,124 and 31.516 knee arthroscopies the injury of articular cartilage was found in 60 - 63 %. The incidence of 5 – 11 % was reported for full-thickness cartilage lesions (ICRS grade III and IV). Additionally, cartilage injuries of the knee joint are often accompanied with other acute injures such as ligament and meniscal injuries, traumatic patellar dislocation, osteochondral injuries, etc.

The main symptom in patients with cartilage defects is the joint pain. Patients may also experience swelling and mechanical symptoms. Traumatic cartilage injury in the athletic population may progress to chronic pathological loading patterns such as joint instability and axis deviation. Although intact articular cartilage has the ability to adjust to the increasing weight bearing activity in athletes by increasing cartilage volume and thickness recent studies indicated that the degree of adaptation is limited. Any activity beyond a threshold value may therefore result in maladaptation and cartilage damage. It has been shown that high impact joint loading above the adaptation limit causes decreased PGs content and leads to increase of degradative enzymes release and chondrocytes apoptosis. Eventually, the integrity of functional weight bearing unit of cartilage is disrupted and leads to the loss of articular cartilage volume and stiffness, elevation of pressure and further articular cartilage damage in the long run.

Clinically, focal lesions are ranked according to the appearance of superficial zone of articular cartilage and are generally small (<1cm^2) and sub-chondral and therefore asymptomatic.

It is difficult to predict whether the chondral lesion will progress to the more extensive degradation. However, in animal studies it was observed that smaller defects have the potential of spontaneous healing while the inverse relationship to repair potential was revealed in larger defects. Once a patient becomes symptomatic due to cartilage damage, the lesion is likely to progress. A mechanical injury to articular cartilage can be acute, chronic, or acute and chronic. Cartilage loss often occurs after single or repeated impact loading due to trauma or misalignment. An increase in shear forces as a consequence of chronic abnormal loading of a joint surface results in irreversible changes in the biochemical composition of articular cartilage. Loading studies reported of significant swelling of articular cartilage (increased water content) and changes in the proteoglycans content only two weeks after abnormal loading.

Cartilage tissue has a limited intrinsic capacity of healing response after cartilage damage, thus cannot fully regenerate and often leads to secondary degenerative disease. Early recognized and treated cartilage lesions might therefore prevent the secondary damage and progression to the osteoarthritis. The main raisons for limited capacity to self-repair and regeneration seem to be the avascular nature of cartilage tissue and inability for clot formation, which is the basic step in the healing cascade. That is why progenitor cells in blood and bone marrow and resident chondrocytes are unable to migrate to sites of the cartilage lesion. Generally, intrinsic cartilage repair does not follow the main steps that usually occur after an injury in the other tissue: necrosis, inflammation, and repair or remodeling. Furthermore, mature chondrocytes own limited proliferative capacity and have the limited ability to produce a sufficient amount of extracellular matrix to cover the defect. However, several cells are mobilized to the cartilage surfaces after an injury and can produce the repair matrix, although this matrix is morphologically and mechanically inferior to the original native cartilage tissue. Such a spontaneous healing was observed in small sub-chondral defects of fetal lambs and partial healing was also detected in small (less than 3 mm diameter) full-thickness lesions in rabbits. However, larger cartilage defects of more than 6 mm rarely, if ever, show intrinsic healing potential but lead to progressive degenerative disease.

Partial and Full Thickness Defects

Cartilage lesions can be divided into partial thickness defects which do not penetrate the subchondral bone and do not repair spontaneously, and full thickness defects which do penetrate subchondral bone have a partial repair potential, depending on the size and locations of the defect. The nature of the partial thickness defects has been studied and it was observed that the cells adjacent to the wound margin undergo cell death. However, there is an increase in cell proliferation, chondrocyte cluster formation, and matrix synthesis, but this repair is short-lived and eventually fails to repair the defect. It was also documented that the cells from synovia can migrate to the lesion in the presence of growth factors and can fill the defect with repair tissue. Due to anti-adhesive properties of PG and the absence of fibrin matrix these cells usually fail to adhere to the surface of defect.

The potential of cartilage repair in full thickness lesions is due to breaching of subchondral bony plate which leads to local influx of blood and undifferentiated mesencyhmal cells and hematoma formation containing fibrin clot, platelet, red and white blood cells. The blood clot can only fill the smaller defects <2-3mm in diameter from the subchondral bone marrow. However, mobilized cells in the newly formatted blood clot are not capable to replace the defect with native hyaline cartilage, but produce fibrocartilage tissue, composed of higher collagen type I to collagen type II ratio and less proteoglycan, which has as mentioned already inferior properties compared to native hyaline cartilage. Several surgical techniques used the same attempt to treat full thickness defects such as micfrofracture which penetrate the subchondral bone in order to stimulate the clot formation and immobilize cells to the side of cartilage lesion.

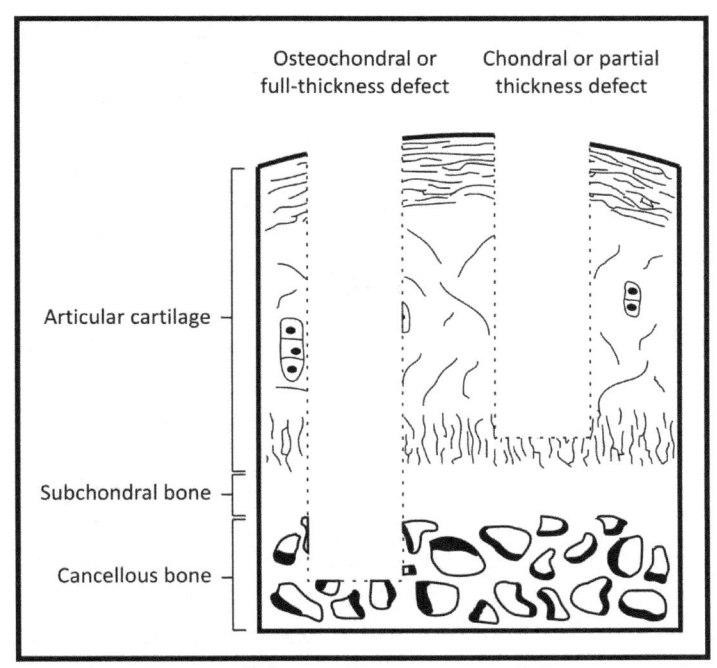

Partial and full thickness defects of articular cartilage.

Cartilage Lesion Classification

There are several classification systems to access cartilage lesion used in clinical practice. A number of elements are important in deciding what intervention might be the most helpful in trying to restore cartilage tissue such as: the size and area of cartilage damage, the depth of the damage, the degree of functional disability, patients' age, etc. However, not enough is known about a proper treatment of particular cartilage. Therefore, more objective data, methods and operative outcomes are required for good decision making regarding the treatment modalities since new procedures are rather expensive. Currently, the structural classifications such as Outerbridge and ICRS Classification are commonly used involving the examination of the extent and the depth of the cartilage lesion that helps surgeons to follow progression and improvement of the cartilage lesions.

Table: Classification of articular cartilage lesions - Outerbridge and ICRS classification.

	OUTERBRIDGE - description	ICRS - description
GRADE 0	Normal cartilage.	Normal cartilage.
GRADE 1	Cartilage with softening and swelling.	Nearly normal: soft indentation and superficial fissures and cracks.
GRADE 2	A partial-thickness defect (fibrillation or superficial fissures) less than 0.5-in diameter.	A partial-thickness defect: extending down to <50% of cartilage depth.
GRADE 3	Deep fissuring of the cartilage to the level of subhondral bone without bone exposed greater than 0.5-in diameter.	A partial-thickness defect: extending down to "/>50% of cartilage depth.
GRADE 4	Exposed subchondral bone.	Severely abnormal (through the subchondral bone).

The modified ICRS classification describes the defect macroscopically and correlates better with clinical outcome; grade 1 has good, grade 2-3 intermediate and grade 4 poor clinical results. However, along with the grade and depth, it is important to record the dimensions and position of the lesion (Modified ICRS Chondral Injury Classification System), to assess any bone loss or sclerotic change, the thickness of the surrounding cartilage and surrounding walls. Additionally, overall outcome depends also on patient's age, BMI index, the level of physical activity, etc.

Treatment of Articular Cartilage Lesions

The main goals of surgical management of cartilage defects are to reduce symptoms, restore cartilage congruence, prevent additional cartilage deterioration, and to maintain the function of the joint without the insertion of artificial implants. Surgical treatment options may be divided upon their expected outcome as palliative, reparative or restorative. Many procedures lead to the formation of fibro cartilaginous tissue with significantly inferior biochemical properties compared with those of hyaline cartilage. The newly formed scar tissue is unable to prevent a progression of a degenerative cartilage disease. The application of a specific surgical method is based on the patient's demand and the level of symptoms. For example, in lower demand patients with fewer symptoms the effective first-line treatments are palliative such as debridement and lavage. Similarly, reparative techniques are used in patients with moderate symptoms such as bone marrow stimulating procedures (drilling, abrasion arthroplasty, or microfracture) in effort to promote fibrocartilage formation. However, larger cartilage defects in higher demand patients (e.g. athletes with extreme weight bearing activity) with significant symptoms may not profit from standard treatment options, but should be advanced towards reparative treatment options such as autologous chondrocyte implantation (ACI) or osteochondral grafting.

Debridement and Lavage

The goals of palliative treatment options (debridement and lavage) are the reduction of the inflammatory response due to mechanical irritation, functional improvement, and pain relief. Debridement involves the smoothing of cartilage and meniscal surfaces, removing necrotic tissue, and refreshing edges of cartilage lesions. Likewise, the beneficial effect of lavage implies the reduction of inflammation; removal of free cartilage fragments due to an injury and potential calcium phosphate crystals. Although the effectiveness of such a method is short-termed since it does not apply the restoration of cartilage defects, it significantly reduces pain symptomatic and improves the functionality of the articular joint compared to the conservative therapy. It is primarily recommended for patients with lower daily physical load and specifically localized mechanical symptoms (e.g. meniscal tear). Rehabilitation time after surgery is short and allows immediate loading activities without restrictions.

Marrow Stimulating Techniques

Articular cartilage is deprived of its own blood supply; therefore traditional wound healing and clot formation is not possible. By opening up the subchondral bone plate, which separates the cartilage layer from the blood supply in bone marrow, hemorrhage can be induced to stimulate mesenchymal stem cells (MSCs), leukocytes, and growth on the side of the lesion as well as trigger remodeling and fibrocartilaginous cartilage repair. Bone marrow stimulating techniques are divided into drilling, microfracture, and abrasion, and are all based on the infiltration of blood products, fibrin clot formation, and fibrocartilage tissue repair.

Nowadays, microfracture is often used as a primary treatment option, and if not successful, more invasive cartilage repair methods are performed. The procedure is performed arthroscopically after a careful examination of articular cartilage surface and the quality of the cartilage. First, the focal chondral defects are debrided and the walls of the defect are smoothened. Any calcified cartilage is removed from the defect zone in order to prepare a better surface for the adherence of the clot and improved chondral nutrition through subchondral diffusion. Likewise, the walls of the lesion should be perpendicular to the defect to provide an area where the clot progenitor cell can form and adhere. After the initial preparation, the surgical awl is used to make multiple holes in the exposed subchondral bone. The holes should be placed 3-4mm from each other and should not connect. Subsequently, blood clot rich with bone marrow elements are formed which eventually undergoes the phase of remodeling and turns into fibrocartilage tissue. Such cartilage resembles the native cartilage, but it differs significantly in the structural, biochemical, and mechanical properties and mostly contains type I collagen, which is cartilage non-specific and results in poor mechanical properties and poorly integrates into the adjacent cartilage.

A major concern is therefore the longevity of a fibrocartilage to withstand the stress and mechanical load on an active knee joint. However, in follow-up studies 7-10 years after the surgery pain release and improved joint functionality was reported. Moreover, microfracturing seems to have similar clinical results as ACI. Another problem was recently reported with microfracture procedure whether it can decrease the success of further alternative procedures such as ACI. In the study patients allocated to bone stimulating technique showed similar results following ACI as those where only debridement alone was performed. Furthermore, in other study patients who previously underwent bone stimulating procedure showed a poorer outcome after ACI compared to those where only ACI alone had been performed.

Postoperative rehabilitation plays a key role in overall success of the treatment. Patients should undergo continuous passive motion physiotherapy for a period of 4 to 6 weeks and have the protected weight bearing. Following that period, patients are allowed an active range of motion exercises and progression to full weight bearing. However, no cutting, jumping or twisting sports are allowed until at least 4 – 6 months after surgery.

Osteochondral Autograft Transplantation (AOT)

Regeneration of damaged cartilage can be achieved with bone-cartilage transplants called osteochondral autograft transplantation (AOT). Nowadays, AOT is a well-established technique, but since the majority of the cartilage defects found in the knee joint are chondral rather than subchondral, there is a controversy regarding the overall usage of an osteochondral grafts and reaming in the healthy subchondral bone. The surgical procedure of AOT involves the removal of a full thickness hyaline cartilage attached to its underlying bone and the implantation of the osteochondral graft on the side of the lesion in a press-fit technique. Osteochondral autografts are usually harvested from non-weight bearing areas in order to avoid new damage or loss of function on the donor side. The site of the lesion should be prepared prior to implantation; any remaining cartilage is removed, the walls of the defect are made smooth and the tunnel of the same size as of the cartilage plug is drilled. However, the depth on the damage site should be 2 mm less than the plug size in order to achieve a favorable and stable position of the osteochondral graft and maintain an appropriate fit to the edges of the graft with surrounding intact cartilage. This helps to reduce shear stress on the border of the graft and ensures long-term success of the transplantation. Cartilage defects should not range more than 3cm2 due to a limited amount of donor tissue. For larger lesions several osteochondral plugs are used, therefore the procedure is called "mosaicoplasty".

The main advantage of osteohondral grafting is that it possesses the normal native hyaline cartilage and does not include fibrocartilage which develops in the microfrature technique. However, the disadvantages include donor side morbidity (pain and cartilage defect), technical difficulty to match the shape of the plug to the contour of the articular joint, residual gap between adjacent plugs, and the risk of osteochondral collapse. Postoperative rehabilitation contains the use of continuous passive motion machine and weight bearing restrictions for a period up to 6 weeks. Clinical results are satisfactory; they reported good to excellent results even 10 years after surgery in 79 - 92% patients. The effectiveness of the method depends on the site of injury and is the most successful in isolated injuries of the femur condyles.

Autologous Cartilage Implantation (ACI)

Autologous cartilage implantation represents a promising solution for the treatment of articular cartilage and enables permanent replacement of damaged cartilage tissue with its own native hyaline cartilage. The idea of an ACI is to harvest cartilage cells from the knee and grow them *In vitro* under specific laboratory conditions. Once millions of cells have been grown they are implanted into the area of cartilage defect. The procedure was first proposed by Brittberg in 1994 and has become more widespread so that it currently represents the most developed articular cartilage repair technique.

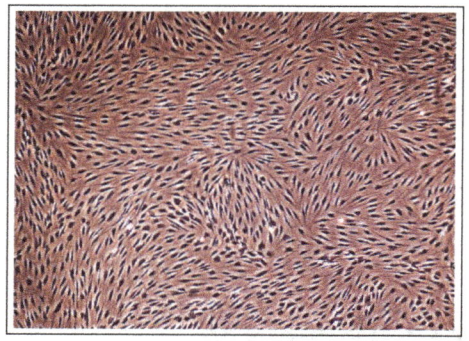

Proliferation of chondrocytes under monolayer culturing condition.

The original technique of ACI is a two-step procedure. The first step of ACI includes an arthroscopy to identify and access cartilage damage. Once the lesion is determined as suitable to perform the ACI procedure, the cartilage cells are harvested from the non-weight bearing zone in the knee. The chondrocytes are then isolated and grown in the tissue culture to allow them to multiply for several weeks. Once a sufficient number of cartilage cells has been obtained in the culture, the second surgery is scheduled. During the second surgery the cell suspension is re-injected into the cartilage defect underneath the periosteal patch. It is very important that the periosteal patch is carefully sutured in place and sealed with fibrin glue in order to prevent any leakage of newly implanted cell suspension. ACI is usually used in intermediate and high-demand patients who have failed arthroscopic debridement or microfracture. The technique can also be used for larger 2 – 10 cm^2 symptomatic lesions. Prior to the surgery, patients must understand and be well prepared to participate in intensive postoperative rehabilitation and should fit the following profile: (1) the cartilage damage is focal and not widespread arthritis, (2) presence of pain or swelling that limits everyday activities, (3) a stable knee with no associated ligament damage and (4) normal body mass index (BMI). The postoperative rehabilitation consists of non-weight bearing in addition to range of motion (ROM) exercises with the use of a CPM machine for 6 weeks. Due to two surgical procedures and larger open arthrotomy, pain relief and restoration of function may take as long as 12 to 18 months.

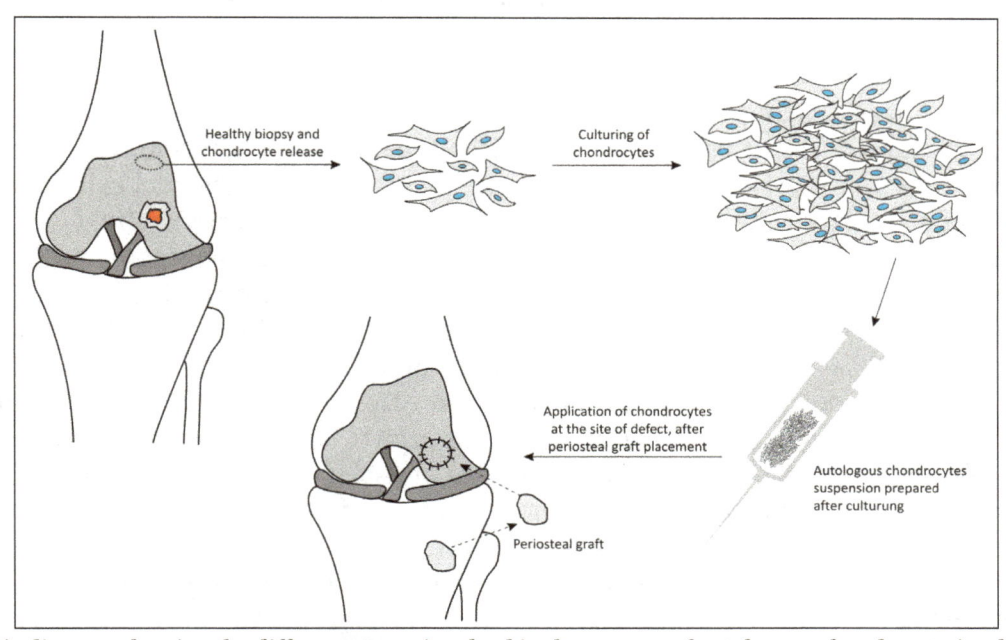

Schematic diagram showing the different stages involved in the process of autologous chondrocyte implantation.

The effectiveness of ACI varies and different levels of success were reported. Recently, ACI has been compared to microfracture technique. Both two and five years follow-up results, after patients were randomized for ACI or microfracture treatment of localized articular lesions of the knee joint, concluded that both methods had acceptable short-term results. There was no significant difference in macroscopic or histological results after two years. Similarly, after five years both methods provided satisfactory results in about 77 % of patients with no significant difference in clinical and radiographic results. Currently, it seems as ACI is as good or a slightly better technique compared to a less invasive, simpler, and cheaper surgical technique in short-term. On the other hand, the significant superiority of ACI over mosaicoplasty for the repair of articular defects in the knee was reported in prospective randomized controlled trails.

These results might not be surprising considering the traditional ACI (first generation ACI) encountered several problems. The most common complication with 10-25% incidence is periosteal hypertrophy due to scar tissue formation around the edge of the periosteal patch. In addition, the need of periosteum widens the donor site morbidity and extends the operation time. The periosteum has to be tightly and waterproof sutured to prevent the potential leakage of the cell suspension from the defect. Another frequent disorder is patch delamination due to incomplete bonding of the patch with surrounding tissue. There are several other disadvantages regarding this method: the growth of cartilage tissue is age-dependent (lower potential in the elderly), difficulty to harvest and isolate sufficient numbers of cells from a small amount of tissue removed, fast differentiation of chondrocytes during *In vitro* cultivation in monolayers (loss of phenotype, differentiation in fibroblast-like cells), etc. Reoperation rate as high as 42 % was reported by several authors.

Future Prospective for Cartilage Repair

Some of the problems have been avoided by using the collagen membrane instead of traditional periosteum patch. Anyway, the new technique (ACI-C) has still not solved the problem of watertight sutures and possible leakage. Nevertheless, in randomized control trial the comparison among the two procedures showed a lower re-operative rate in ACI-C, most probably due to the lesser extent of periosteum hypertrophy. The new concept of cartilage tissue preservation was developed using tissue engineering technologies, combining new biomaterials as a scaffold, and applying growth factors, stem cells, and mechanical stimulation. The recent development of so-called second regeneration ACI uses a cartilage-like tissue in a 3-dimensional culture system that is based on the use of biodegradable material which serves as a temporary scaffold for the *In vitro* growth and subsequent implantation into the cartilage defect. It has been shown *In vitro* that the application of 3-D environment promotes hyaline-like cartilage production and allows for mechanical stimulation. Several reports already described a superior role of the MACI (matrix/membrane autologous chondrocyte implantation) and CACI (collagen-covered autologous chondrocyte implantation) compared to the standard ACI procedure. Additionally, the modern concept of tissue engineering uses various types of growth factors which are the endogenous regulators of chondrogenesis and their logical choice of use and relative ease of application have been reported to promote cartilage development. Further studies are attempting to create the ideal scaffold and explore the synergistic effect of concomitant application of growth factors and mechanical loading. Finally, for clinical practice, single stage procedures appear attractive to reduce cost and patient morbidity.

Sprains and Strains of Sporting Injuries

Sprains and strains are some of the most common types of injuries in any sport. They involve the stretching or tearing of tissue. Sprains occur to ligaments (which connect bone to bone), while strains involve muscles or tendons (which connect muscle to bone).

How are Sprains and Strains Classified?

Sprains and strains are placed into three categories according to severity. They are classified as follows:

Grade I (Mild): Tissue is stretched.

- Slight swelling (hardly noticeable).
- Mild loss of range of motion (ability to move in various directions) and strength (0 – 25%).
- No decrease in stability.

Grade II (Moderate): Involves stretching and some tearing of tissue.

- Moderate swelling (may look "baseball" size).
- Usually includes some bruising.

- Moderate loss of range of motion and strength (25 – 75%).
- Some decrease in stability.

Grade III (Severe): Complete tearing of tissue.
- Significant swelling and bruising.
- Near complete loss of range of motion and strength (75 – 100%).
- Marked decrease in stability.

Range of motion and strength percentages are determined by comparing the injured body part to the uninjured side. Severity of injury is best determined by a physician or athletic trainer. Immediate first aid for all sprains and strains is Rest, Ice, Compression, and Elevation or R.I.C.E. After initial first aid is administered, prompt referral to an appropriate medical professional should be sought to ensure proper injury treatment.

Sprains and strains can be a big deal and lead to prolonged time away from sport, especially if not treated appropriately. Additionally, sprains and strains can mimic other more serious injuries. For example, young athletes are prone to growth plate injuries called Salter-Harris fractures.

"Growth plates are located near the ends of long, growing bones in children and gradually close as a child reaches skeletal maturity. "The growth plate in growing children is weaker than the nearby ligaments and tendons. Therefore, the growth plate will become injured under lower forces than those that would injure a tendon or ligament".

Young athletes with Salter-Harris fractures will be very tender over the growth plate. They may have bruising and are often reluctant to bear weight. A careful physical exam is the best way to confirm this diagnosis although x-rays are often helpful as well. Even if the initial x-rays are negative, repeat studies can sometimes reveal subtle fractures. There are complications of growth plate injuries that are undiagnosed, untreated, or treated incorrectly. This confirms the importance of seeking the advice of a qualified medical professional with experience in dealing with these injuries even when it looks like it is "just a sprain".

Initially, the inability to bear weight (about 4 steps) after the injury or tenderness over any bone should prompt an evaluation that includes x-rays.

"Within a few days, any continued significant pain, continued reluctance to bear weight, or significant swelling and bruising may warrant re-evaluation and possibly an x-ray. Any other unusual symptoms such as numbness, loss of pulses near the injured area, discoloration, out of proportion pain, or rashes would indicate the need for further evaluation".

Sport-related Concussion

A concussion is a type of traumatic brain injury. Concussion is caused by a strong impact to the head that leads to problems with thinking or other neurological symptoms. Concussions can occur in any sport when there is a blow to the head, neck, or body that sends a strong force to the head.

The symptoms of concussion include headache, cognitive problems such as mental fogginess or changes in memory, problems with balance and coordination, behavioral changes such as irritability, and slowed reaction time. Although most concussions are not associated with loss of consciousness, temporary loss of consciousness can occur.

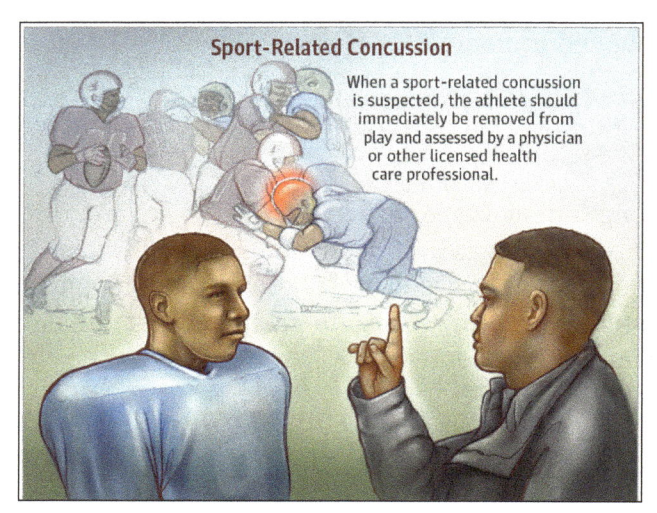

Sport-Related Concussion

When a sport-related concussion is suspected, the athlete should immediately be removed from play and assessed by a physician or other licensed health care professional.

Evaluation

In cases of suspected sport-related concussion, athletes should immediately be removed from play and assessed by a physician or other licensed health care professional. Assessment begins with evaluation for serious signs of injury such as severe headache, neck pain, double vision, weakness or tingling in the arms or legs, vomiting, seizure, or decreased level of consciousness. If any of these "red flags" are present, emergency transportation to a medical facility may be needed.

If no "red flags" are present, then a more detailed evaluation for concussion may be performed on the sidelines or in the locker room. There is no single test that can definitively diagnose concussion, and various tools are available to aid in diagnosis. One instrument that is commonly used by health care professionals is the Sport Concussion Assessment Tool—5th Edition (SCAT5). The SCAT5 involves questions about symptoms; brief testing of cognitive functions such as memory and concentration; and a screening neurological examination that includes evaluation of eye movements, balance, and coordination.

Head imaging is not needed to diagnose concussion but may be used to rule out other causes of brain injury. Neuropsychological testing may be conducted for more detailed assessment of mental processes such as memory, reaction time, and cognitive processing speed.

Management and Return to Play

New problems can arise during the first 24 to 48 hours after a concussion, so the athlete should not be left alone during this time and medical care should be urgently sought if symptoms worsen. Repeat concussions are most likely to occur in the first several days after a concussion and can cause serious injury, so athletes should not rush to return to play.

The general approach to recovery from concussion involves both physical and mental rest for the first few days after the injury, followed by gradual increases in activity over time (graduated return to activity). If concussion-related symptoms worsen at any point as activity level is being increased, then the athlete should return to the prior level of activity. Typically, after 24 to 48 hours of rest, daily activities should be slowly reintroduced for short periods (ie, 5-15 minutes) and then increased as long as concussion symptoms do not worsen. Mental activities and schoolwork should be gradually resumed as tolerated. Once the athlete is able to complete usual daily activities without concussion-related symptoms, light aerobic activity (such as brisk walking) can be resumed. If this is well tolerated, running or other noncontact training exercises can be added, followed later by light resistance exercises. The decision to ultimately return to play should be individualized, and athletes should be cleared by a health care professional before returning to full contact practice or regular play.

In most cases, concussion-related symptoms usually resolve by 10 to 14 days after the concussion. If symptoms persist for longer, additional evaluation and treatment may be needed. Treatment for prolonged symptoms may include symptom-limited aerobic exercise, physical therapy, balance training, and psychological interventions such as cognitive behavioral therapy.

Knee Injuries

Some of the most common knee injuries include fractures, dislocations, sprains, and ligament tears.

Many knee injuries can be successfully treated with simple measures, such as bracing and rehabilitation exercises. Other injuries may require surgery to correct.

Anatomy

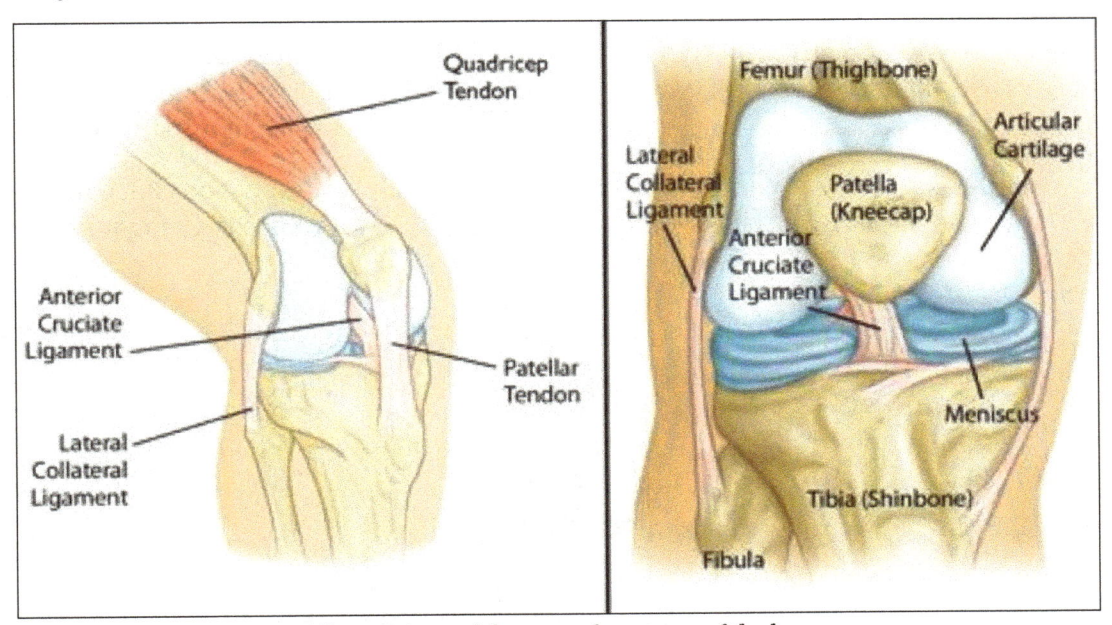

Different views of the normal anatomy of the knee.

The knee is the largest joint in the body, and one of the most easily injured. It is made up of four main things: Bones, cartilage, ligaments, and tendons.

- Bones: Three bones meet to form your knee joint: your thighbone (femur), shinbone (tibia), and kneecap (patella).

- Articular cartilage: The ends of the femur and tibia, and the back of the patella are covered with articular cartilage. This slippery substance helps your knee bones glide smoothly across each other as you bend or straighten your leg.

- Meniscus: Two wedge-shaped pieces of meniscal cartilage act as "shock absorbers" between your femur and tibia. Different from articular cartilage, the meniscus is tough and rubbery to help cushion and stabilize the joint. When people talk about torn cartilage in the knee, they are usually referring to torn meniscus.

- Ligaments: Bones are connected to other bones by ligaments. The four main ligaments in your knee act like strong ropes to hold the bones together and keep your knee stable.
    - Collateral ligaments: These are found on the sides of your knee. The medial collateral ligament is on the inside of your knee, and the lateral collateral ligament is on the outside. They control the sideways motion of your knee and brace it against unusual movement.
    - Cruciate ligaments: These are found inside your knee joint. They cross each other to form an "X" with the anterior cruciate ligament in front and the posterior cruciate ligament in back. The cruciate ligaments control the back and forth motion of your knee.

- Tendons: Muscles are connected to bones by tendons. The quadriceps tendon connects the muscles in the front of your thigh to your patella. Stretching from your patella to your shinbone is the patellar tendon.

Common Knee Injuries

Your knee is made up of many important structures, any of which can be injured. The most common knee injuries include fractures around the knee, dislocation, and sprains and tears of soft tissues, like ligaments. In many cases, injuries involve more than one structure in the knee.

Pain and swelling are the most common signs of knee injury. In addition, your knee may catch or lock up. Many knee injuries cause instability — the feeling that your knee is giving way.

Fractures

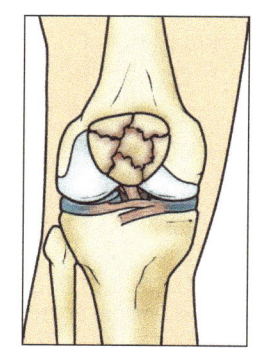

The most common bone broken around the knee is the patella. The ends of the femur and tibia where they meet to form the knee joint can also be fractured. Many fractures around the knee are caused by high energy trauma, such as falls from significant heights and motor vehicle collisions.

Dislocation

A dislocation occurs when the bones of the knee are out of place, either completely or partially. For example, the femur and tibia can be forced out of alignment, and the patella can also slip out of place. Dislocations can be caused by an abnormality in the structure of a person's knee. In people who have normal knee structure, dislocations are most often caused by high energy trauma, such as falls, motor vehicle crashes, and sports-related contact.

Anterior Cruciate Ligament (ACL) Injuries

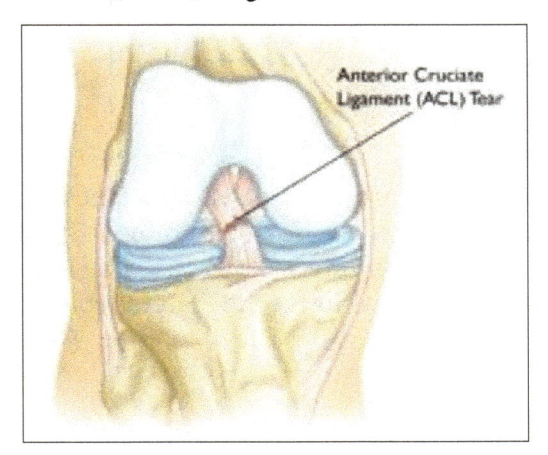

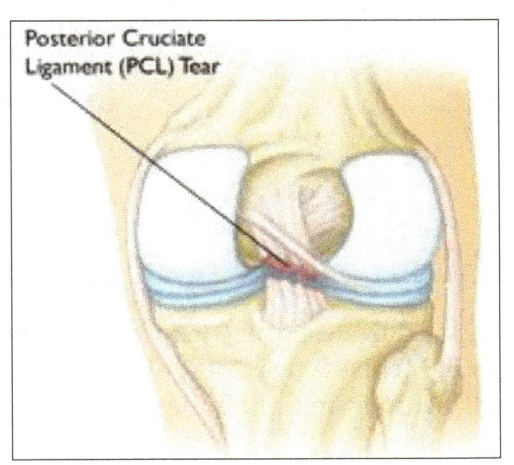

The anterior cruciate ligament is often injured during sports activities. Athletes who participate in high demand sports like soccer, football, and basketball are more likely to injure their anterior cruciate ligaments. Changing direction rapidly or landing from a jump incorrectly can tear the ACL. About half of all injuries to the anterior cruciate ligament occur along with damage to other structures in the knee, such as articular cartilage, meniscus, or other ligaments.

Posterior Cruciate Ligament (PCL) Injuries

The posterior cruciate ligament is often injured from a blow to the front of the knee while the knee is bent. This often occurs in motor vehicle crashes and sports-related contact. Posterior cruciate ligament tears tend to be partial tears with the potential to heal on their own.

Collateral Ligament Injuries

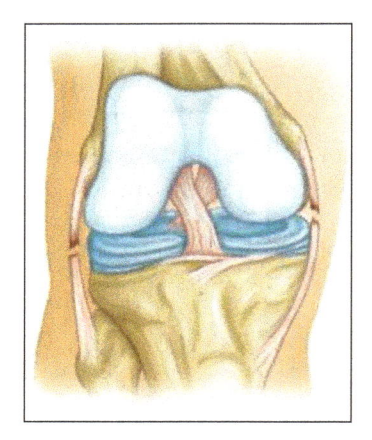

Injuries to the collateral ligaments are usually caused by a force that pushes the knee sideways. These are often contact injuries. Injuries to the MCL are usually caused by a direct blow to the outside of the knee, and are often sports-related. Blows to the inside of the knee that push the knee outwards may injure the lateral collateral ligament. Lateral collateral ligament tears occur less frequently than other knee injuries.

Meniscal Tears

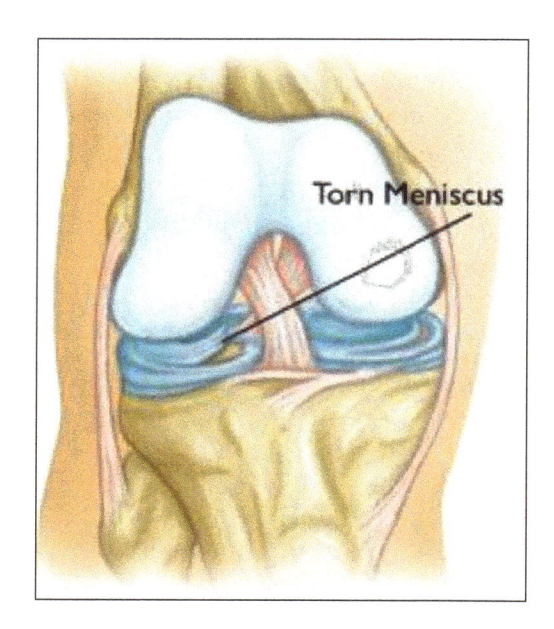

Sudden meniscal tears often happen during sports. Tears in the meniscus can occur when twisting, cutting, pivoting, or being tackled. Meniscal tears may also occur as a result of arthritis or aging. Just an awkward twist when getting up from a chair may be enough to cause a tear, if the menisci have weakened with age.

Tendon Tears

The quadriceps and patellar tendons can be stretched and torn. Although anyone can injure these tendons, tears are more common among middle-aged people who play running or jumping sports. Falls, direct force to the front of the knee, and landing awkwardly from a jump are common causes of knee tendon injuries.

Hip Tendonitis

Hip tendonitis is inflammation and degeneration in the tendons, the thick cords that attach muscle to the hip bone, typically due to overuse.

The iliac muscle starts in the hip bone, and the psoas muscle starts in the lower spine. These muscles come together in a tendon at the top of the femur, and this is where tendonitis in the hip occurs giving it the scientific name iliacus tendonitis or iliopsoas tendinitis.

Causes of Hip Tendonitis

Hip tendonitis typically occurs when the tendon is under abnormal stress from activity that you are not used to doing. Hip tendonitis is a degenerative injury that causes disorientation in the tendon fibers. Because blood supply in the tendons is poor, they are slow to heal.

Other causes of hip tendonitis include:

- Sudden progression of exercise without adequate training.
- Repetitive stress related to overuse.

Risk Factors for Hip Tendonitis

Risk factors for hip tendonitis include:

- Specific sports — People who participate in sports such as running, cycling or high kicking are at a higher risk for developing hip tendonitis. Also sports that require squatting or lifting weights put you at higher risk.
- Rapidly increasing training — People who rapidly increase intensity and duration of training are at a higher risk for developing hip tendonitis.

Symptoms of Hip Tendonitis

The most common symptom of hip tendonitis is pain that develops gradually over time.

Other symptoms of hip tendonitis include:

- Tenderness on the hip where the tendon starts.
- Hip stiffness in the morning or after long periods of rest.

- Pain that lessens as you warm up but intensifies later in the day.
- Discomfort when contracting the muscles in the hip.

Diagnosis of Hip Tendonitis

Your primary care, orthopedist or sports medicine doctor can diagnose hip tendonitis during a full physical examination. You will be assessed for range of motion, joint stability and flexibility. Your physician will also look for torn or ruptured tendons in the hip and discuss training that led to the injury.

In some cases, the physician will order an x-ray or MRI to determine if there is a severe tear or a hip fracture that is causing the pain.

Diagnosis of Tendon Injury

Many athletes with groin pain have tried prolonged rest and various treatment regimens and received differing opinions regarding the cause of their pain. The rehabilitation specialist is often given a nonspecific referral of "groin pain" or "anterior hip pain," the cause of which can be as simple as a tight iliopsoas (which may require stretching) or as complex as athletic pubalgia.

Athletic pubalgia is defined as an injury to the rectus abdominis insertion onto the pubic symphysis, often accompanied by injury to the conjoined tendon insertion and the adductor longus attachment to the pelvis. The distinctive feature of this disorder is subtle pelvic instability and accompanying compromise of the transversalis fascia, eventually leading to incompetency of the posterior inguinal wall. The exact structures involved are not always clear unless surgery is performed, and overlapping conditions may exist. A muscle imbalance between the adductor muscles and abdominal muscles may be the underlying cause of athletic pubalgia, but this has yet to be proven.

Adductor Muscle Strains

The adductors of the hip joint include 6 muscles: the adductor longus, magnus, and brevis and the gracilis, obturator externus, and pectineus. All these are innervated by the obturator nerve, with the exception of the pectineus, which receives innervation from the femoral nerve. The primary function of this muscle group is adduction of the thigh in open chain motions and stabilization of the lower extremity and pelvis in closed chain motion. The adductor longus is most commonly injured during sporting activity. Its lack of mechanical advantage may make it more susceptible to strain. An important anatomic consideration in groin pain is the local distribution of cutaneous nerves in the inguinal region. Akita examined the cutaneous branches of the inguinal region in 27 male adult cadavers. The ilioinguinal nerve and cutaneous branches were present in 49 of 54 half specimens, and genitofemoral cutaneous branches were present in 19 of 54. The cutaneous branches of the ilioinguinal nerve traverse around the spermatic cord and are distributed to the skin of the dorsal surface of the scrotum. The ilioinguinal nerve and the genital branch of the genitofemoral nerve are considered the most critical sensory nerves, and they likely play a key role in the chronic pain produced by groin injuries.

Adductor muscle strains can result in missed playing time for athletes in many sports. Adductor muscle strains are frequently encountered in ice hockey and soccer. These sports require a strong eccentric contraction of the adductor musculature during competition. Adductor muscle strength has recently been linked to the incidence of adductor muscle strains. Specifically, the strength ratio of the adduction:abduction muscle groups has been identified as a risk factor in professional ice hockey players. Intervention programs can lower the incidence of adductor muscle strains but not prevent them altogether. Proper injury treatment and rehabilitation should be implemented to limit the amount of missed playing time and avoid surgical intervention.

An adductor strain is defined as an injury to the muscle-tendon unit that produces pain on palpation of the adductor tendons or its insertion on the pubic bone with or without pain during resisted adduction. Adductor strains are graded as a first-degree strain if there is pain but minimal loss of strength and minimal restriction of motion. A second-degree strain is defined as tissue damage that compromises the strength of the muscle but does not include complete loss of strength and function. A third-degree strain denotes complete disruption of the muscle tendon unit and loss of muscle function. A thorough history, clinical examination, magnetic resonance imaging (MRI), bone scan, and radiograph can be useful in differentiating groin strains from athletic pubalgia, osteitis pubis, hernia, hip flexor strain, intra-articular hip abnormalities, rectal or testicular referred pain, piriformis syndrome, lumbar disc pathology, or a fracture of the pelvis or the lower extremities. More obscure etiologies may include genitourinary infections, avascular necrosis of the hip, or soft tissue tumors.

The exact incidence of adductor muscle strains in most sports is unknown because athletes often play through minor groin pain and the injury goes unreported. In addition, overlapping diagnoses can skew the incidence. Groin strains accounted for 10% of all injuries in elite ice hockey players. Molsa reported that groin strains accounted for 43% of all muscle strains in elite Finnish ice hockey players. The incidence of groin strains in a single National Hockey League (NHL) team was 3.2 strains per 1000 player-game exposures. In a larger study of 26 NHL teams, Emery reported that the incidence of adductor strains in the NHL increased from 2003 to 2009. The rate of injury was greatest during the preseason compared with regular and postseason play. Prospective soccer studies in Scandinavia showed a groin strain incidence rate of 10 to 18 injuries per 100 soccer players. Giza reported that 9.5% of all professional US male soccer players incurred a groin strain in the 2002 season. Ekstrand and Gillquist documented 32 groin strains in 180 male soccer players, representing 13% of all injuries over the course of 1 year. Despite their prevalence, adductor muscle strains are not isolated to these 2 sports.

Risk Factors

Previous studies have shown an association between strength or flexibility and musculoskeletal strains in various athletic populations. Ekstrand and Gillquist found decreased preseason hip abduction range of motion in soccer players who subsequently sustained groin strains, compared with uninjured players. This finding is in contrast to the data on professional ice hockey players that found no relationship between passive or active abduction range of motion (adductor flexibility) and adductor muscle strains. Adductor muscle strength has been associated with a subsequent muscle strain. Tyler found that preseason hip adduction strength was 18% lower in NHL players who subsequently sustained groin strains, compared with the uninjured players. The hip adduction:abduction strength ratio was also significantly different between the 2 groups. Injured players had less adduction strength. In the players who sustained a groin strain, preseason adduction: abduction strength ratio was lower on the side that subsequently sustained a groin strain (as compared with the uninjured side). Adduction strength was 86% of abduction strength on the uninjured side but only 70% of abduction strength on the injured side. Conversely, a study on adductor strains in ice hockey players found no relationship between peak isometric adductor torque and the incidence of adductor strains. Unlike the Tyler study, this study had multiple testers using a handheld dynamometer, which could increase the variability in strength testing and decrease the likelihood of finding strength differences.

Emery and colleagues' results demonstrated that players who practiced during the off-season were less likely to sustain a groin injury, as were rookies in the NHL. The final risk factor was the presence of a previous adductor strain. Tyler also linked pre-existing injury as a risk factor to recurrent injury for 4 of the 9 groin strains (44%). This is consistent with Seward, who reported a 32% recurrence rate for groin strains in Australian Rules football.

Arnason conducted a multivariate prospective analysis in 306 professional male soccer players in Iceland and determined that the predictor risk factors were previous groin strains (odds ratio = 7.3, $P = .001$) and decreased range of motion in hip abduction (odds ratio = 0.9 [1°], $P = .05$). It has become increasingly apparent that groin strains and athletic pubalgia have continued to rise in hockey, soccer, and American football.

Intervention

Tyler were able to demonstrate that strengthening the adductor muscle group could be an effective method for preventing adductor strains in professional ice hockey players. Before the 2000 and 2001 seasons, professional players were strength tested, and 33 of 58 players were classified as at risk—that is, abduction: abduction strength ratio of less than 80%. These players were placed on an intervention program consisting of strengthening and functional exercises aimed at increasing adductor strength. The injuries were tracked over the course of the 2 seasons: 3 adductor strains occurred in games. The incidence was 0.71 adductor strains per 1000 player-game exposures and accounted for approximately 2% of all injuries. In the previous 2 seasons before the intervention, there were 11 adductor strains (incidence of 3.2 per 1000 player-game exposures), accounting for approximately 8% of all injuries. This was significantly lower than the incidence reported by Lorentzon, who found adductor strains to account for 10% of all injuries in ice hockey players. Of the 3 players injured in the Tyler study, none had sustained a previous adductor strain on the same side. One player had bilateral adductor strains at different times during the first season. The Tyler study suggests that adductor strengthening can be an effective method for preventing adductor strains in professional ice hockey players.

Table: Adductor strain postinjury program.

Phase 1: Acute	First 48 hours after injury: RICE (rest, ice, compression, elevation).
	Nonsteroidal anti-inflammatory drugs.
	Massage.
	Transcutaneous electrical nerve stimulation.
	Ultrasound.
	Submaximal isometric adduction with knees bent → with knees straight progressing to maximal isometric adduction, pain free.
	Hip passive range of motion in pain-free range.

	Nonweightbearing hip progressive resistance exercises without weight in antigravity position (all except abduction): pain free, low load, high repetition.
	Upper body and trunk strengthening.
	Contralateral lower extremity strengthening.
	Flexibility program for noninvolved muscles.
	Bilateral balance board.
Clinical milestone	Concentric adduction against gravity without pain.
Phase 2: Subacute	Bicycling/swimming.
	Sumo squats.
	Single-limb stance.
	Concentric adduction with weight against gravity.
	Standing with involved foot on sliding board moving in frontal plane.
	Adduction in standing on cable column or resistance band.
	Seated adduction machine.
	Bilateral adduction on sliding board moving in frontal plane (ie, simultaneous bilateral adduction).
	Unilateral lunges (sagittal) with reciprocal arm movements.
	Multiplane trunk tilting.
	Balance board squats with throwbacks.
	General flexibility program.
Clinical milestone	Lower extremity passive range of motion equal to that of the uninvolved side and involved adductor strength at least 75% that of the ipsilateral abductors.
Phase 3: Sports- specific training	Phase II exercises with increase in load, intensity, speed and volume.
	Standing resisted stride lengths on cable column to simulate skating.
	Slide board.
	On ice kneeling adductor pull together.
	Lunges (in all planes).
	Correct or modify ice skating technique.
Clinical milestone	Adduction strength at least 90-100% of the abduction strength and involved muscle strength equal to that of the contralateral side.

Table: Adductor strain injury prevention program.

Warm-up	Bike.
	Adductor stretching.
	Sumo squats.
	Side lunges.
	Kneeling pelvic tilts.
Strengthening program	Ball squeezes (legs bent to legs straight).
	Different ball sizes.
	Concentric adduction with weight against gravity.
	Adduction in standing on cable column or elastic resistance.

	Seated adduction machine.
	Standing with involved foot on sliding board moving in sagittal plane.
	Bilateral adduction on sliding board moving in frontal plane (ie, simultaneous bilateral adduction).
	Unilateral lunges with reciprocal arm movements.
Sports-specific training	On ice kneeling adductor pull together.
	Standing resisted stride lengths on cable column to simulate skating.
	Slide skating.
	Cable column crossover pulls.
Clinical goal	Adduction strength at least 80% of the abduction strength.

Despite the identification of risk factors and strengthening intervention for ice hockey players, adductor strains continue to occur in most sports. The high incidence of recurrent strains could be due to incomplete rehabilitation or inadequate time for complete tissue repair. Hagglund studied 12 elite male soccer teams to determine if prior injury served as a risk factor for a recurrence in a subsequent consecutive season. They determined that those players who sustained a previous hamstring, groin, or knee injury were 2 to 3 times more likely to incur a recurrence in the following season. Interestingly, no such relationship was found with ankle sprains. Homlich found that an 8- to 12-week active strengthening program consisting of progressive resistive adduction and abduction exercises, balance training, abdominal strengthening, and skating movements on a slide board proved more effective in treating chronic groin strains, whereas a passive physical therapy program of massage, stretching, and modalities was ineffective in treating chronic groin strains.

An increased emphasis on strengthening exercises may reduce the recurrence rate of groin strain. Tyler developed an adductor muscle strain injury program progressing the athlete through the phases of healing, which, anecdotally, seems to be effective. This type of treatment regime combines modalities: passive treatment immediately followed by an active training program emphasizing eccentric resistive exercise. This method of rehabilitation has been supported.

A comprehensive 20-minute alternative warm-up program was recently developed to address the rise in groin-related injuries in adult male professional soccer players in US Major League Soccer. This 20-minute program was used 2 to 3 times per week during the 2004 season. Active players (N, 315) were prospectively and randomly enrolled into 1 of 2 groups: Group 1 participants (n, 106) served as the groin injury prevention group; Group 2 participants (n, 209) served as the matched control group (age, sex, skill) and continued with their usual preseason and warm-up training. The groin injury prevention program was a combination of dynamic stretching, core strengthening, and pelvic proprioceptive exercises to encourage a neutral pelvis during dynamic activities using the lumbar paraspinals, multifidus, rectus abdominus, transversus, internal and external obliques, abductors, adductors, and hip external and internal rotators. During the season, certified athletic trainers recorded all groin injuries into a central database. The overall incidence of groin injuries occurring in the 2004 season was 10.9%; in Group 1 (intervention), 0.44 injuries per 1000 hours; and in Group 2 (control), 0.61 injuries per 1000 hours. The incidence of athletes requiring groin surgery in the intervention group was 0.13 per 1000 hours, compared with the control group incidence of 0.18 per 1000 hours ($P>.05$). The groin injury prevention program was successful in reducing injury by 28%, when compared with the control group ($P<.05$).

Athletic Pubalgia

Athletic pubalgia occurs with weakening of the rectus abdominis, pyramidalis, internal and external obliques, transversus abdominis muscles, and the tendons. This is where inguinal hernias occur: the inguinal canal. When an inguinal hernia occurs because of weakening of the abdominal wall, a hernia may be felt. In the case of an athletic pubalgia, there is weakening or tears in the abdominal wall muscles but no palpable hernia. Fon described athletic pubalgia as an incipient hernia, based on the findings of a posterior bulge found in 80% to 85% of surgeries. This is analogous to a classic inguinal hernia where the absence of striated muscle at the posterior inguinal wall and the passage of the spermatic cord predispose the abdominal wall to weakness. In athletic pubalgia, the anatomically thin transversalis fascia that forms part of the posterior wall is injured. Joesting defines the athletic pubalgia as an actual tear in the transversalis fascia in the posterior inguinal wall between the internal inguinal ring and the pubic tubercle, typically 3 to 5 cm long. Lynch and Renstrom also localized the pathology to the posterior inguinal wall.

Athletic pubalgia is a common cause of chronic groin pain in athletes. Most often seen in soccer and ice hockey players, athletic pubalgia can be encountered in a variety of sports and in a variety of age groups. Despite several reports of athletic pubalgia in women, it is almost exclusively found in men. It is largely a clinical diagnosis of exclusion, with a history of chronic groin pain that is nonresponsive to treatment. Physical examination findings are subtle, and most tests do not definitively confirm the diagnosis. Nonoperative treatment of athletic pubalgia does not often result in resolution of symptoms. Surgical intervention results in a pain-free return of full activities in a majority of cases.

The symptoms of athletic pubalgia are characterized by pain during sports movements—particularly, twisting and turning during single-limb stance. This pain usually radiates to the adductor muscle region and origin and to the testicles, often difficult for the patient to pinpoint. There may be excessive anterior pelvic tilting and an internal rotation of the ilium on the symptomatic side concomitant with the adductor pathology. Following sports activity, the athlete may be stiff and sore, and after competition, mobility and practice can be difficult. Physical exertion that increases intra-abdominal pressure, such as coughing or sneezing, can cause pain. Pain resolution after a sports herniorrhaphy may be due to the nerve decompression during the surgical procedure itself.

Imaging

Groin pain has been investigated through plain radiograph, dynamic ultrasound, bone scan, computed tomography scanning, and MRI. Although MRI findings such as bone marrow edema, adductor muscle strain, and hernias have been described in athletes with chronic groin pain, there has been a paucity of attention to a direct association between clinical findings and the on-field functional performance. Slavotinek published a report analyzing the association of preseason clinical findings and functional outcomes throughout the season with 52 Australian football players: Preseason MRI showed pubic bone marrow edema in 19 (37%) and linear parasymphysial T2 hyperintensity in 16 (31%). Groin pain restricted training during the season in 22 (42%), and 9 (17%) missed at least 1 game. Preseason pain ($P =.0004$), pubic bone tenderness ($P =.02$), and linear parasymphysial T2 hyperintensity ($P =.01$) were directly associated with restricted training capacity during the subsequent season. Of 39 athletes with groin tenderness, 16 (41%) had linear parasymphyseal T2 hyperintensity on MRI (largely paracortical in location), of whom 11 (69%)

experienced training restriction. The 16 athletes with groin tenderness and a T2 hyperintense line were more likely to experience training restriction ($P = .01$) than were other athletes in the study. Continued advancement in imaging techniques may allow the clinician to identify high-risk individuals and institute preventative intervention before the development of symptoms.

Sports Hernia

A sports hernia is a painful, soft tissue injury that occurs in the groin area. It most often occurs during sports that require sudden changes of direction or intense twisting movements.

Although a sports hernia may lead to a traditional, abdominal hernia, it is a different injury. A sports hernia is a strain or tears of any soft tissue (muscle, tendon, and ligament) in the lower abdomen or groin area.

Because different tissues may be affected and a traditional hernia may not exist, the medical community prefers the term "athletic pubalgia" to refer to this type of injury. The general public and media are more familiar with "sports hernia".

Anatomy

The soft tissues most frequently affected by sports hernia are the oblique muscles in the lower abdomen. Especially vulnerable are the tendons that attach the oblique muscles to the pubic bone. In many cases of sports hernia, the tendons that attach the thigh muscles to the pubic bone (adductors) are also stretched or torn.

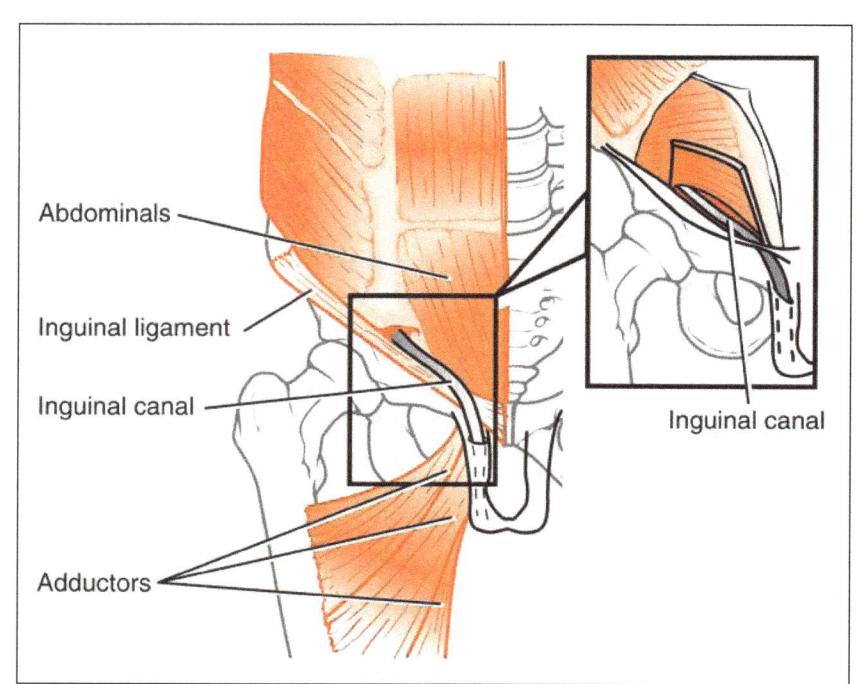

Sports hernias often occur where the abdominals and adductors attach at the pubic bone.
Traditional hernias occur in the inguinal canal.

Cause

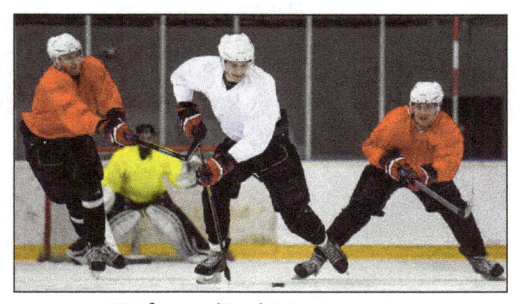

Technotr/E+/Getty Images.

Sports activities that involve planting the feet and twisting with maximum exertion can cause a tear in the soft tissue of the lower abdomen or groin.

Sports hernias occur mainly in vigorous sports such as ice hockey, soccer, wrestling, and football.

Symptoms

A sports hernia will usually cause severe pain in the groin area at the time of the injury. The pain typically gets better with rest, but comes back when you return to sports activity, especially with twisting movements.

A sports hernia does not cause a visible bulge in the groin, like the more common, inguinal hernia does. Over time, a sports hernia may lead to an inguinal hernia, and abdominal organs may press against the weakened soft tissues to form a visible bulge.

Without treatment, this injury can result in chronic, disabling pain that prevents you from resuming sports activities.

During your first appointment, your doctor will talk to you about your symptoms and how the injury occurred. If you have a sports hernia, when your doctor does a physical examination, he or she will likely find tenderness in the groin or above the pubis. Although a sports hernia may be associated with a traditional, inguinal hernia, in most cases, no hernia can be found by the doctor during a physical examination.

Physical Tests

To help determine whether you have a sports hernia, your doctor will likely ask you to do a sit-up or flex your trunk against resistance. If you have a sports hernia, these tests will be painful.

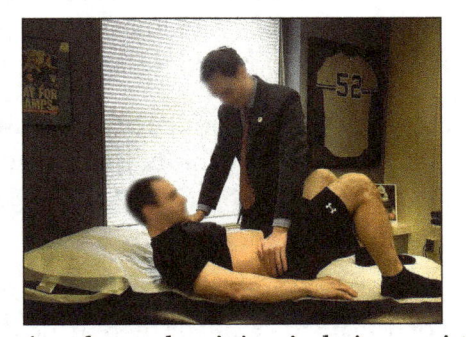

A common sign of sports hernia is pain during a resisted sit-up.

Imaging Tests

After your doctor completes a thorough exam, he or she may order x-rays or magnetic resonance imaging (MRI) scans to help determine whether you have a sports hernia. Occasionally, bone scans or other tests are recommended to rule out other possible causes of the pain.

Shin Splints

Shin splints is a common complaint, especially among participants of running sports. The term 'shin splints' is colloquially used to describe shin pain along the inside or front edges of the shin. Shin splints are the most common cause of painful shins.

There are two regions where you can suffer shin splints:

- Anterior Shin Splints,
- Posterior Shin Splints.

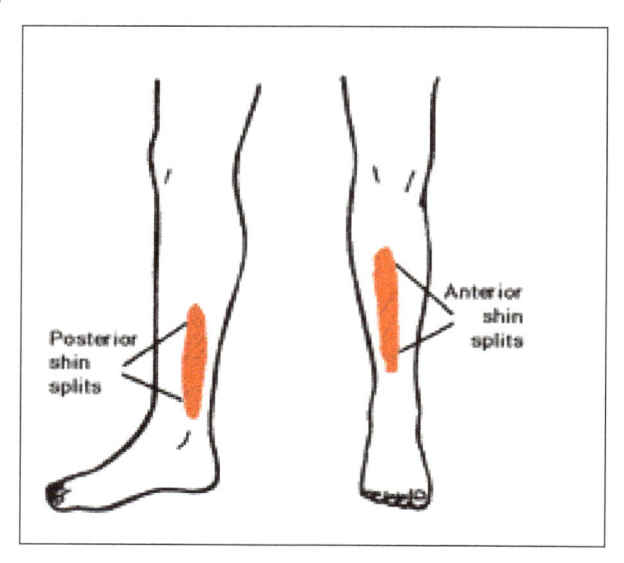

Anterior Shin Splints

Anterior shin splints are located on the front (or anterior) part of the shin bone and involve the tibialis anterior muscle. The tibialis anterior lifts and lowers your foot. It lifts your foot during the swing phase of a stride. Then, it slowly lowers your foot to prepare your foot for the support phase.

If your anterior shin pain increases when lifting your toes up while keeping heels on the ground – you are likely to suffer from anterior shin splints. Medically anterior shin splints can also be referred to as anterior tibial stress syndrome (ATSS).

Posterior Shin Splints

Posterior shin splints are located on the inside rear (or medial/posterior) part of the shin bone and involve the tibialis posterior muscle. The tibialis posterior lifts and controls the medial aspect of your foot arch during the weight bearing support phase. When your tibialis posterior is weak or lacks endurance your arch collapses (overpronation), which creates torsional shin bone stresses.

If you feel pain along the inside rear of your shin bone – you are likely to suffer from either posterior shin splints or tibia stress fractures. Medically, posterior shin splints and tibial stress fractures can also be referred to as medial tibial stress syndrome (MTSS).

Causes of Shin Splints

Shin splints are caused by overstraining of your muscles where they attach to your shin.

The most common cause is overuse or overtraining associated with poor foot and leg biomechanics. Shin splints can be caused by a number of factors which are mainly biomechanical (abnormal movement patterns) and errors in training.

Overtraining/Overloading

- Increasing your training too quickly.
- Running on hard or angled surfaces.
- Insufficient rest between loads.

Biomechanical

- Overpronation of your feet.
- Oversupination of your feet.
- Decreased flexibility at your ankle joint.
- Poor hip-knee-leg muscle control (dynamic alignment).
- Poor buttock control at in the stance phase.
- Poor core stability.
- Tight calf muscles, hamstrings.
- Weak quadriceps, foot arch muscles.

Equipment

- Inappropriate footwear.

What Structures are Injured?

Generally shin pain arises from a combination of three structures:

- Muscles.
- Tenoperiosteum.
- Shin bone (tibia).

Muscle

As a result of repeated overuse, one or more of your muscles in the lower leg may become injured through excessive loading stress. This can result in muscle tenderness, inflammation or knots.

The most common muscles that cause shin splints are tibialis anterior (anterior shin splints) and tibialis posterior (posterior shin splints).

Tenoperiosteum

All bones are covered in a 'shell', called periosteum. The tendons, which connect the muscle to the bone, attach on to this periosteum. This zone at which the tendon meets the bone is known as tenoperiosteum.

Almost all cases of 'shin splints' have some element of inflammation of the tenoperiosteum. Inflammation of different tendons leads to pain in different areas of the shin.

Bone

Damage to the shin bone usually concentrates in the lower one-third of the shin bone (tibia). The bone damage may be mild, such as a simple stress reaction, or may be a severe stress fracture. Except in the worst cases, bone damage is not visible on normal x-rays. A bone scan or MRI may be recommended if your physiotherapist or doctor need to exclude or confirm a bone injury.

Symptoms of Shin Splints

- Shin splints cause dull, aching pain in the front of the lower leg.
- Depending on the exact cause, the pain may be located along either side of the shinbone or in the muscles.
- The area may be painful to the touch.

The Four Stages of an Overuse Injury

Your physiotherapist will guide you with respect to how much exercise you can do. Here are some basic guidelines until you seek your physiotherapist's opinion:

Stage 1: Discomfort that disappears during warm-up

Injury identification and treatment in stage one allows continuing activity as long as the injury does not worsen. Professional guidance is recommended to confirm your diagnosis and to implement treatment strategies to ensure that your condition does not deteriorate.

Stage 2: Discomfort that may disappear during warm-up but reappears at the end of activity

At stage two, the activity may continue at a modified pain-free level while being treated. Professional assessment and treatment is highly recommended and must continue until you have completely resumed normal activity and training levels.

Stage 3: Discomfort that gets worse during the activity

If the injury progresses to stage three, the activity must immediately cease. Professional guidance is very highly recommended to confirm diagnosis and ensure that the condition has not progressed into bone stress fractures. A thorough rehabilitation program is recommended to gradually return to your desired activity and exercise levels.

Stage 4: Pain or discomfort all the time

All activity must immediately cease. Professional guidance is essential to exclude stress fractures or more significant tibia fractures. Potentially, you may need to be non-weight bear on crutches or in an air cast. Please book an appointment with your healthcare professional who has a special interest in shin pain to fully investigate and rehabilitate you based on their assessment.

How is Shin Splints Diagnosed?

Shin splints are usually diagnosed based on your medical history and a physical examination by your physiotherapist. In some cases, an X-ray or other imaging studies such as bone scans or MRI can help identify other possible causes for your pain, such as a stress fracture.

Shoulder Injuries

Shoulder injuries are frequently caused by athletic activities that involve excessive, repetitive, overhead motion, such as swimming, tennis, pitching, and weightlifting. Injuries can also occur during everyday activities such washing walls, hanging curtains, and gardening.

Warning Signs of a Shoulder Injury

If you are experiencing pain in your shoulder, ask yourself these questions:

- Is your shoulder stiff? Can you rotate your arm in all the normal positions?
- Does it feel like your shoulder could pop out or slide out of the socket?
- Do you lack the strength in your shoulder to carry out your daily activities?

If you answered "yes" to any one of these questions, you should consult an orthopaedic surgeon for help in determining the severity of the problem.

Common Shoulder Injuries

Most problems in the shoulder involve the muscles, ligaments, and tendons, rather than the bones. Athletes are especially susceptible to shoulder problems. In athletes, shoulder problems can develop slowly through repetitive, intensive training routines.

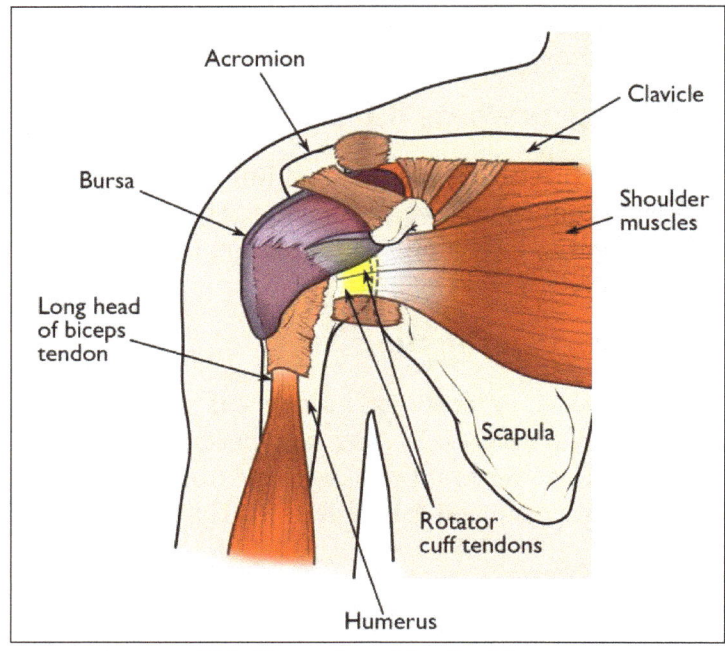

This illustration of the shoulder highlights the major components of the joint.

Some people will have a tendency to ignore the pain and "play through" a shoulder injury, which only aggravates the condition, and may possibly cause more problems. People also may underestimate the extent of their injury because steady pain, weakness in the arm, or limitation of joint motion will become almost second nature to them.

Orthopaedic surgeons group shoulder problems into the following categories:

Instability

Sometimes, one of the shoulder joints moves or is forced out of its normal position. This condition is called instability, and can result in a dislocation of one of the joints in the shoulder. Individuals suffering from an instability problem will experience pain when raising their arm. They also may feel as if their shoulder is slipping out of place.

Impingement

Impingement is caused by excessive rubbing of the shoulder muscles against the top part of the shoulder blade, called the acromion.

Impingement problems can occur during activities that require excessive overhead arm motion. Medical care should be sought immediately for inflammation in the shoulder because it could eventually lead to a more serious injury.

Rotator Cuff Injuries

The rotator cuff is one of the most important components of the shoulder. It is comprised of a group of muscles and tendons that hold the bones of the shoulder joint together. The rotator cuff muscles provide individuals with the ability to lift their arm and reach overhead. When the rotator cuff is injured, people sometimes do not recover the full shoulder function needed to properly participate in an athletic activity.

Shoulder Injuries in the Throwing Athlete

Overhand throwing places extremely high stresses on the shoulder, specifically to the anatomy that keeps the shoulder stable. In throwing athletes, these high stresses are repeated many times and can lead to a wide range of overuse injuries.

Although throwing injuries in the shoulder most commonly occur in baseball pitchers, they can be seen in any athlete who participates in sports that require repetitive overhand motions, such as volleyball, tennis, and some track and field events.

Anatomy

Your shoulder is a ball-and-socket joint made up of three bones: your upper arm bone (humerus), your shoulder blade (scapula), and your collarbone (clavicle).

The head of your upper arm bone fits into a rounded socket in your shoulder blade. This socket is called the glenoid. Surrounding the outside edge of the glenoid is a rim of strong, fibrous tissue called the labrum. The labrum helps to deepen the socket and stabilize the shoulder joint. It also serves as an attachment point for many of the ligaments of the shoulder, as well as one of the tendons from the biceps muscle in the arm.

Strong connective tissue, called the shoulder capsule, is the ligament system of the shoulder and keeps the head of the upper arm bone centered in the glenoid socket. This tissue covers the shoulder joint and attaches the upper end of the arm bone to the shoulder blade.

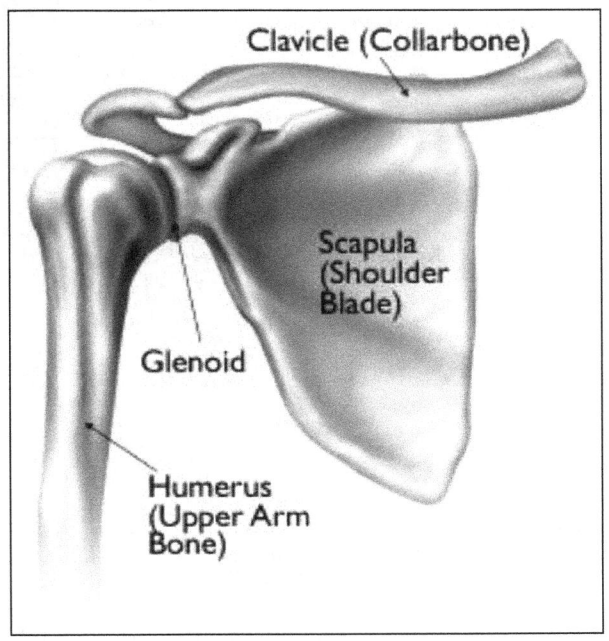

The bones of the shoulder.

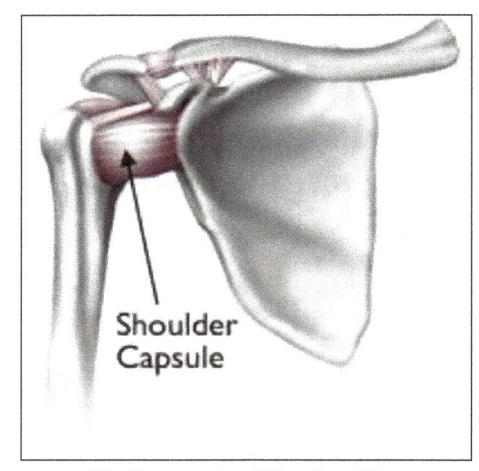

The ligaments of the shoulder.

Your shoulder also relies on strong tendons and muscles to keep your shoulder stable. Some of these muscles are called the rotator cuff. The rotator cuff is made up of four muscles that come together as tendons to form a covering or cuff of tissue around the head of the humerus.

The biceps muscle in the upper arm has two tendons that attach it to the shoulder blade. The long head attaches to the top of the shoulder socket (glenoid). The short head attaches to a bump on the shoulder blade called the coracoid process. These attachments help to center the humeral head in the glenoid socket.

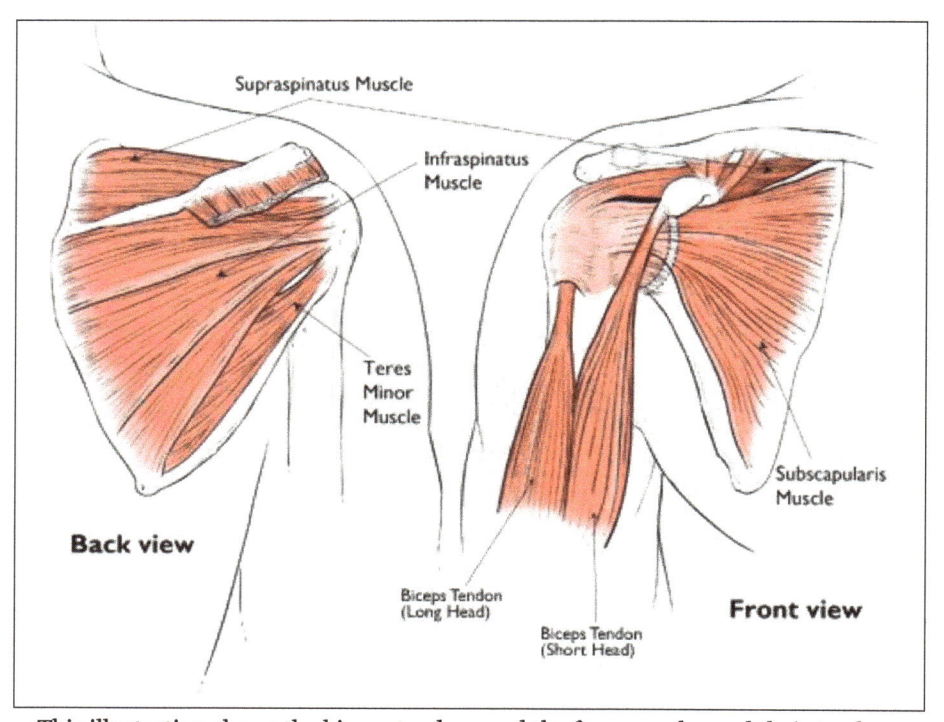

This illustration shows the biceps tendons and the four muscles and their tendons that form the rotator cuff and stabilize the shoulder joint.

In addition to the ligaments and rotator cuff, muscles in the upper back play an important role in keeping the shoulder stable. These muscles include the trapezius, levator scapulae, rhomboids, and serratus anterior, and they are referred to as the scapular stabilizers. They control the scapula and clavicle bones — called the shoulder girdle — which functions as the foundation for the shoulder joint.

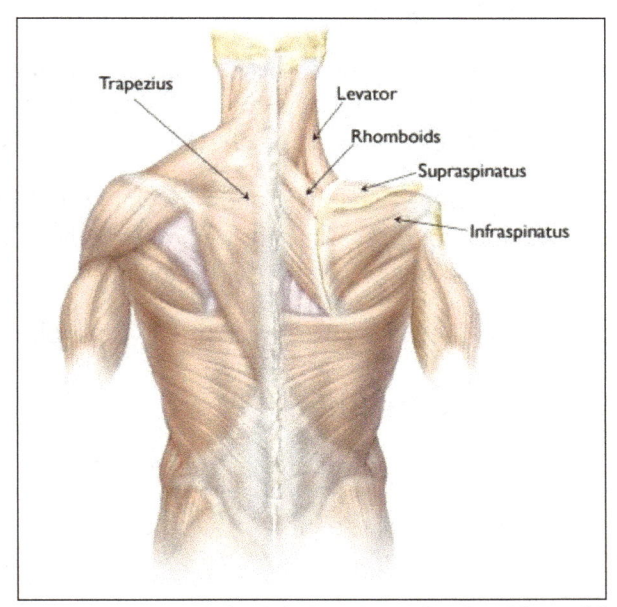

Muscles in the upper back help to keep the shoulder stable, particularly during overhead motions, like throwing.

Cause

When athletes throw repeatedly at high speed, significant stresses are placed on the anatomical structures that keep the humeral head centered in the glenoid socket.

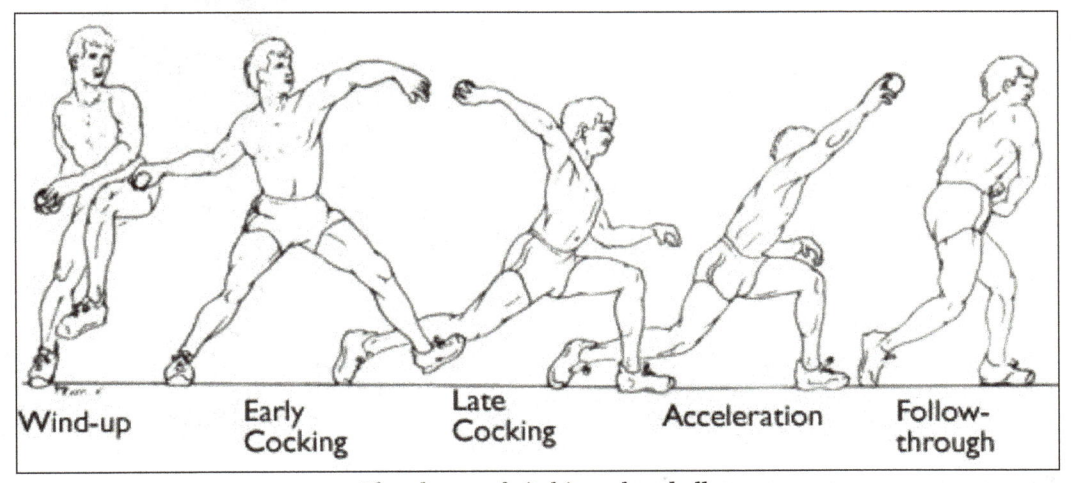

The phases of pitching a baseball.

Of the five phases that make up the pitching motion, the late cocking and follow-through phases place the greatest forces on the shoulder.

- Late-cocking phase: In order to generate maximum pitch speed, the thrower must bring the arm and hand up and behind the body during the late cocking phase. This arm position of extreme external rotation helps the thrower put speed on the ball, however, it also forces the head of the humerus forward which places significant stress on the ligaments in the front of the shoulder. Over time, the ligaments loosen, resulting in greater external rotation and greater pitching speed, but less shoulder stability.

- Follow-through phase: During acceleration, the arm rapidly rotates internally. Once the ball is released, follow-through begins and the ligaments and rotator cuff tendons at the back of the shoulder must handle significant stresses to decelerate the arm and control the humeral head.

When one structure such as the ligament system becomes weakened due to repetitive stresses, other structures must handle the overload. As a result, a wide range of shoulder injuries can occur in the throwing athlete.

The rotator cuff and labrum are the shoulder structures most vulnerable to throwing injuries.

Common Throwing Injuries in the Shoulder

SLAP Tears (Superior Labrum Anterior to Posterior)

In a SLAP injury, the top (superior) part of the labrum is injured. This top area is also where the long head of the biceps tendon attaches to the labrum. A SLAP tear occurs both in front (anterior) and in back (posterior) of this attachment point.

Typical symptoms are a catching or locking sensation, and pain with certain shoulder movements. Pain deep within the shoulder or with certain arm positions is also common.

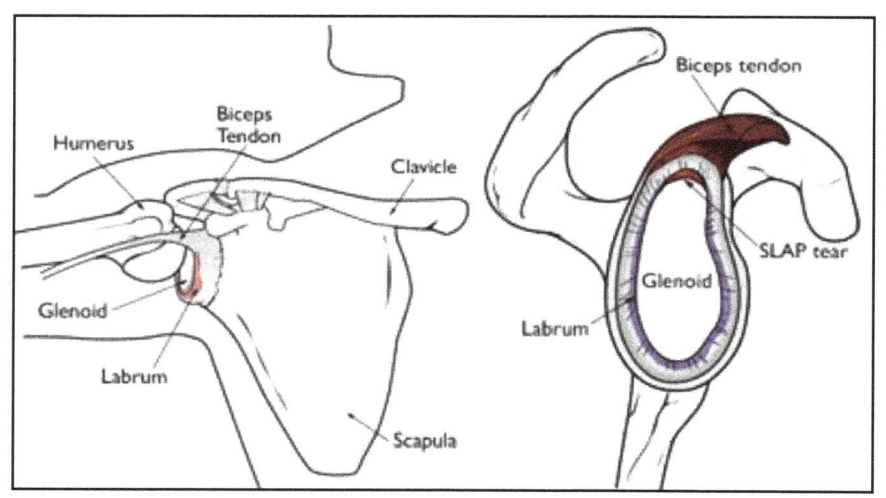

(Left) The labrum helps to deepen the shoulder socket.
(Right) This cross-section view of the shoulder socket shows a typical SLAP tear.

Bicep Tendinitis and Tendon Tears

Repetitive throwing can inflame and irritate the upper biceps tendon. This is called biceps tendinitis. Pain in the front of the shoulder and weakness are common symptoms of biceps tendinitis.

Occasionally, the damage to the tendon caused by tendinitis can result in a tear. A torn biceps tendon may cause a sudden, sharp pain in the upper arm. Some people will hear a popping or snapping noise when the tendon tears.

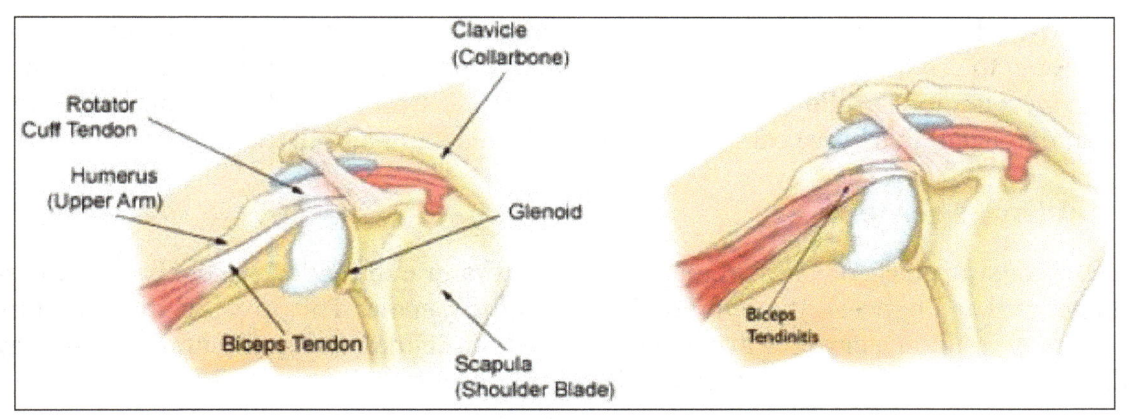

(Left) The biceps tendon helps to keep the head of the humerus centered in the glenoid socket.
(Right) Tendinitis causes the tendon to become red and swollen.

Rotator Cuff Tendinitis and Tears

When a muscle or tendon is overworked, it can become inflamed. The rotator cuff is frequently irritated in throwers, resulting in tendinitis.

Early symptoms include pain that radiates from the front of the shoulder to the side of the arm. Pain may be present during throwing, other activities, and at rest. As the problem progresses, pain may occur at night and the athlete may experience a loss of strength and motion.

Rotator cuff tears often begin by fraying. As the damage worsens, the tendon can tear. When one or more of the rotator cuff tendons is torn, the tendon no longer fully attaches to the head of the humerus. Most tears in throwing athletes occur in the supraspinatus tendon.

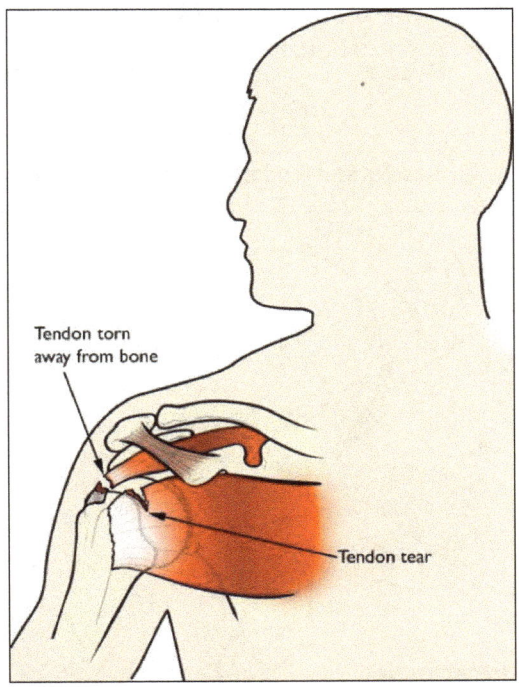

Rotator cuff tendon tears in throwers most often occur within the tendon.
In some cases, the tendon can tear away from where it attaches to the humerus.

Problems with the rotator cuff often lead to shoulder bursitis. There is a lubricating sac called a bursa between the rotator cuff and the bone on top of your shoulder (acromion). The bursa allows the rotator cuff tendons to glide freely when you move your arm. When the rotator cuff tendons are injured or damaged, this bursa can also become inflamed and painful.

Internal Impingement

During the cocking phase of an overhand throw, the rotator cuff tendons at the back of the shoulder can get pinched between the humeral head and the glenoid. This is called internal impingement and may result in a partial tearing of the rotator cuff tendon. Internal impingement may also damage the labrum, causing part of it to peel off from the glenoid.

Internal impingement may be due to some looseness in the structures at the front of the joint, as well as tightness in the back of the shoulder.

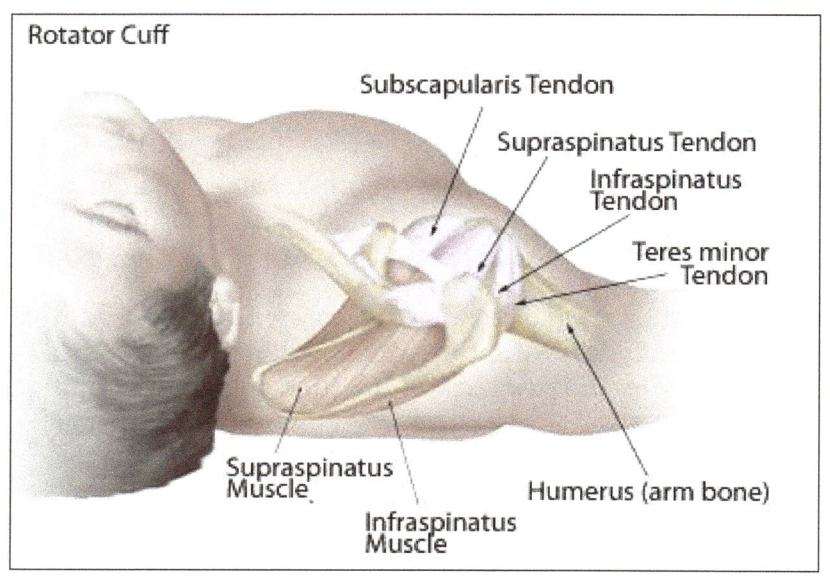

The muscles and tendons of the rotator cuff.

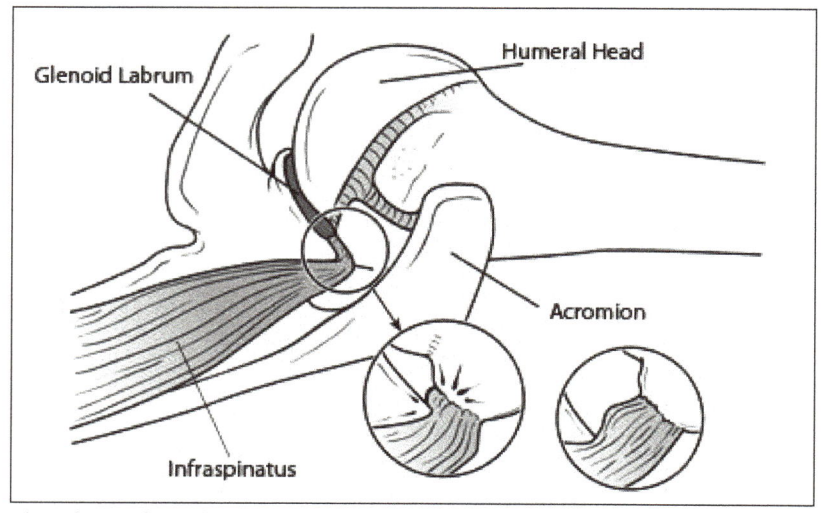

This illustration shows the infraspinatus tendon caught between the humeral head and the glenoid.

Instability

Shoulder instability occurs when the head of the humerus slips out of the shoulder socket (dislocation). When the shoulder is loose and moves out of place repeatedly, it is called chronic shoulder instability.

In throwers, instability develops gradually over years from repetitive throwing that stretches the ligaments and creates increased laxity (looseness). If the rotator cuff structures are not able to control the laxity, then the shoulder will slip slightly off-center (subluxation) during the throwing motion.

Pain and loss of throwing velocity will be the initial symptoms, rather than a sensation of the shoulder "slipping out of place". Occasionally, the thrower may feel the arm "go dead". A common term for instability many years ago was "dead arm syndrome".

Glenohumeral Internal Rotation Deficit (GIRD)

As mentioned above, the extreme external rotation required to throw at high speeds typically causes the ligaments at the front of the shoulder to stretch and loosen. A natural and common result is that the soft tissues in the back of the shoulder tighten, leading to loss of internal rotation.

This loss of internal rotation puts throwers at greater risk for labral and rotator cuff tears.

Scapular Rotation Dysfunction (SICK Scapula)

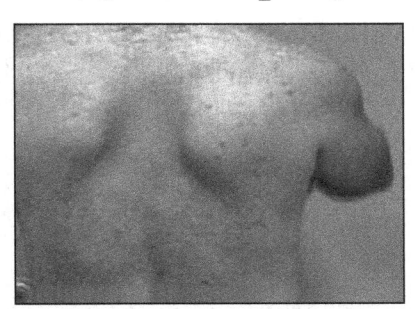

Abnormal positioning of the scapula on the right side.

Proper movement and rotation of the scapula over the chest wall is important during the throwing motion. The scapula (shoulder blade) connects to only one other bone: the clavicle. As a result, the scapula relies on several muscles in the upper back to keep it in position to support healthy shoulder movement.

During throwing, repetitive use of scapular muscles creates changes in the muscles that affect the position of the scapula and increase the risk of shoulder injury.

Scapular rotation dysfunction is characterized by drooping of the affected shoulder. The most common symptom is pain at the front of the shoulder, near the collarbone.

In many throwing athletes with SICK scapula, the chest muscles tighten in response to changes in the upper back muscles. Lifting weights and chest strengthening exercises can aggravate this condition.

Medical History and Physical Examination

The medical history portion of the initial doctor visit includes discussion about your general medical health, symptoms and when they first began, and the nature and frequency of athletic participation

During the physicial examination, your doctor will check the range of motion, strength, and stability of your shoulder. He or she may perform specific tests by placing your arm in different positions to reproduce your symptoms.

The results of these tests help the doctor decide if additional testing or imaging of the shoulder is necessary.

Imaging Tests

Your doctor may order tests to confirm your diagnosis and identify any associated problems.

- X-rays: This imaging test creates clear pictures of dense structures, like bone. X-rays will show any problems within the bones of your shoulder, such as arthritis or fractures.

- Magnetic resonance imaging (MRI): This imaging study shows better images of soft tissues. It may help your doctor identify injuries to the labrum, ligaments, and tendons surrounding your shoulder joint.

- Computed tomography (CT) scan: This test combines x-rays with computer technology to produce a very detailed view of the bones in the shoulder area.

- Ultrasound: Real time images of muscles, tendons, ligaments, joints, and soft tissues can be produced using ultrasound. This test is typically used to diagnose rotator cuff tears in individuals who are not able to have MRI scans.

Muscle Injuries

Muscle lesions are the most common category of injuries in athletes and comprise approximately 10% to 55% of all injuries. The majority of muscle injuries (>90%) are contusions or strains, while lacerations are much less common. The most severe types can produce chronic pain, dysfunction, recurrence, and even compartment syndrome. A thorough understanding of these types of injuries is needed, since appropriate injury management may determine the difference between an early return to sport and a delayed return.

Basic Anatomy and Physiology of Skeletal Muscle

Skeletal muscle is a composite of multiple muscle fibers (myofibers) arranged in bundles within a connective tissue network. At the basic level, each myofiber contains a contractile element called the myofibril. Actin and myosin protein filaments are arranged in repeating units within the myofibril to form the sarcomere, which extends from Z-line to Z-line within the myofibril. The sarcomere is the basic unit of the myofibril and gives skeletal muscle its distinctive striated appearance.

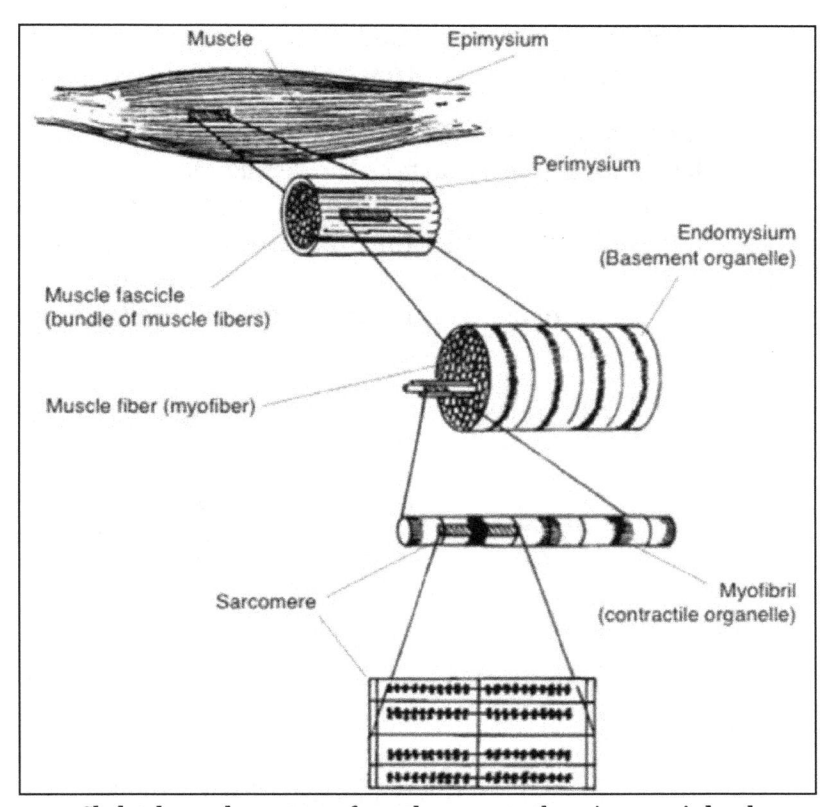

Skeletal muscle anatomy from the gross to the microscopic level.

Each myofiber is surrounded by a sarcolemma (plasma membrane) and is further enclosed by a basement membrane that forms the endomysium. The endomysium is contiguous with the perimysium, which surrounds the muscle bundles. Ensheathing the muscle in its entirety is the tough epimysium, which is made up of multiple fascicles.

Myofibers are attached at both ends of the muscle to tendons and tendon-like fascia, forming what are known as myotendinous junctions (MTJs). These MTJs are necessarily durable, with the ability to resist forces of up to 1000 kg, which can be experienced during activity and locomotion.

Muscle Fiber Type

Skeletal muscle is often characterized as either fast-twitch (type II) or slow-twitch (type I). This distinction is a function of the length of time for the motor unit to reach peak tension and has important clinical significance. Type I fibers rely predominantly on aerobic metabolism (long-distance running), whereas type II fibers are dependent on anaerobic metabolism (sprinting). Type II muscle fibers can generate greater muscular contraction but fatigue more rapidly than type I fibers. Type II muscle fibers are also more prone to injury, since they play a larger role during high-speed and power activities, such as sprinting, football, basketball, soccer, and weight lifting.

Pathophysiology of Muscle Injury

Muscle injury tends to occur through 2 main mechanisms: (1) the muscle is subjected to a sudden large direct, compressive force, resulting in a contusion or (2) the muscle is subjected to an excessive tensile force, resulting in injury to the myofibers and possible rupture, commonly near the MTJ. For a strain injury to occur, the muscle must be stretched beyond its resting length.

Muscle contusions can occur in any muscle group subjected to a direct blow. Strains, however, tend to occur in muscles that cross 2 joints, such as the rectus femoris, the hamstrings, and the gastrocnemius muscles. Muscles that cross 2 joints can generate higher levels of tension by passive joint positioning, as compared with muscles that only cross a single joint. Once muscle injury has occurred, healing progresses through 3 distinct phases, regardless of the etiology (contusion, strain, or laceration). These phases are: (1) destruction, (2) repair, and (3) remodeling.

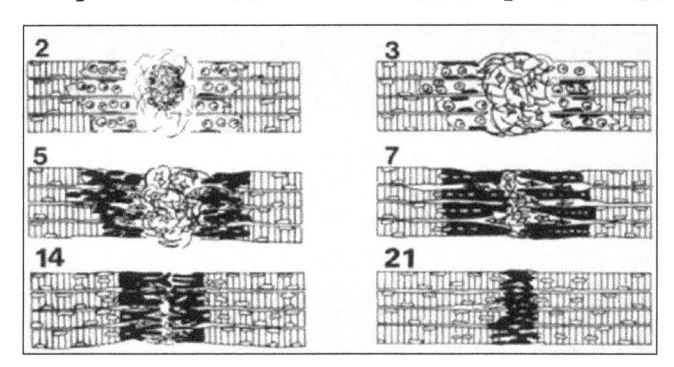

Schematic of skeletal muscle healing. Day 2: Necrotic muscle tissue is removed by macrophages while fibroblasts form scar tissue in the central zone (CZ). Day 3: Satellite cells are activated within the basal lamina cylinders in the regeneration zone (RZ). Day 5: Myoblasts fuse into myotubes in the RZ and scar tissue in the CZ is now denser. Day 7: Regenerating muscle cells migrate into the CZ and begin to pierce through the scar. Day 14: The scar of the CZ is reduced in size, and the regenerating myofibers close the CZ gap. Day 21: The interlacing myofibers are virtually fused with little intervening connective tissue (scar) in between.

Destruction (Inflammatory) Phase (First Week after Injury)

This is characterized by rupture of the myofibers, hematoma formation, and inflammation. During muscle injury, the sarcoplasm is disrupted, leading to local necrosis; this process is limited from spreading along the length of the myofiber by the contraction band. This band restricts access to the plasma membrane defect, which, in conjunction with lysosomal vesicles, allows for plasma membrane repair (ie, resealing of the sarcolemma). Muscle injury also results in local blood vessel injury and subsequent hematoma formation between the myofiber stumps. This sequence initiates an inflammatory cascade in which macrophages play an early, primary role.

Repair (Weeks 2-6 After Injury) and Remodeling Phase (Week 7-Several Months After Injury)

These stages aid in myofiber regeneration as well as connective tissue scar formation. The degree of motor recovery will be determined by the balance struck between muscle healing and fibrosis.

Muscle Regeneration

Satellite cells are undifferentiated cells located between the sarcolemma and the basal lamina of each myofiber that play an integral role in the regeneration of muscle. During the adult stages of development, these cells lay quiescent until the time of injury when they re-enter the cell cycle. Satellite cells can proliferate and mature into myoblasts, which can form multinucleated myotubes and ultimately myofibers. The ends of the ruptured myofibers are typically prevented from reuniting completely by the scar tissue that forms during healing. In this scenario, the ends of the repaired fibers attach to the extracellular matrix of the scar by adhesion molecules at the MTJs.

Scar Formation

The process of scar formation begins almost immediately following injury. Inflammatory cells degrade the blood clot while fibrin/fibronectin cross-links form an initial extracellular matrix (ECM) that functions as an initial scaffold to support a reparative response. Immature scar tissue is predominantly composed of type III collagen, which is susceptible to reinjury. With time, the addition of type I collagen significantly increases the tensile strength of the connective tissue scar. Neoangiogenesis and regeneration of intramuscular neural units are also critical steps that occur during the repair phase. In cases of excessive fibroblast proliferation, exuberant scar tissue can form; this may be seen in rerupture or major trauma.

Classification of Muscle Injuries

A consensus classification system for muscle injury currently does not exist. A simple system classifies muscle injuries (strains or contusions) as mild, moderate, or severe based on clinical criteria. Mild muscle injuries (first degree/grade I) present with minor swelling and discomfort with little or no loss of strength or range of motion, which represents minimal tearing of muscle fibers. Moderate muscle injuries (second degree/grade II) are associated with loss of motor function (ie, inability to fully contract the muscle group and limited range of motion). Severe (third degree/grade III) muscle injuries have complete loss of motor function, indicating complete rupture of the muscle.

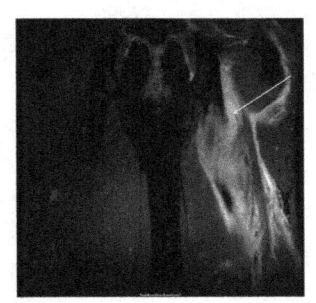

Coronal MRI T2 fat-suppressed image demonstrating high-grade acute muscle strain of the left proximal hamstring.

Coronal MRI T2 fat-suppressed image demonstrating low-grade muscle strain of the left biceps femoris.

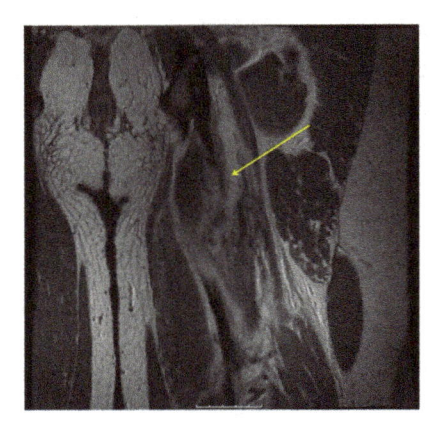

Coronal MRI T1-weighted image of the same injury.

Complications of Muscle Injuries

Myositis Ossificans (Posttraumatic Calcific Metaplasia)

Myositis ossificans can occur in any muscle group but is most common in the quadriceps and the brachialis. The incidence is highest in contact sports where protection is limited. Individuals with bleeding disorders may also be at increased risk. The cause of myositis ossificans is not known; myoblasts may be the cause response to bone morphogenetic protein (BMP) signaling. Additionally, endothelial precursor cells contribute to all stages of heterotopic ossification in animals. Clinical factors including early vigorous massage and excessive mobilization may also contribute. However, full motion and return to normal activity may occur despite heterotic bone exostosis.

Optimal treatment and prevention are unknown. No data exist to support indomethacin for myositis ossificans prevention. Surgical excision may be necessary for symptomatic myositis ossificans. Surgical timing is critical—a year-long wait from the time of injury may be necessary to ensure full maturation of the lesion and thereby minimize recurrence.

Tennis Elbow

Lateral epicondylitis, also known as "Tennis Elbow", is the most common overuse syndrome in the elbow. It is a tendinopathy injury involving the extensor muscles of the forearm. These muscles originate on the lateral epicondylar region of the distal humerus. In a lot of cases, the insertion of the extensor carpi radialis brevis is involved.

It should be remembered that only 5% of people suffering from tennis elbow relate the injury to tennis. Contractile overloads that chronically stress the tendon near the attachment on the humerus are the primary cause of epicondylitis. It occurs often in repetitive upper extremity activities such as computer use, heavy lifting, forceful forearm pronation and supination, and repetitive vibration. Despite the name you will also commonly see this chronic condition in other sports such as squash, badminton, baseball, swimming and field throwing events. People with repetitive one-sides movements in their jobs such as electricians, carpenters, gardeners also commonly present with this condition.

Clinically Relevant Anatomy

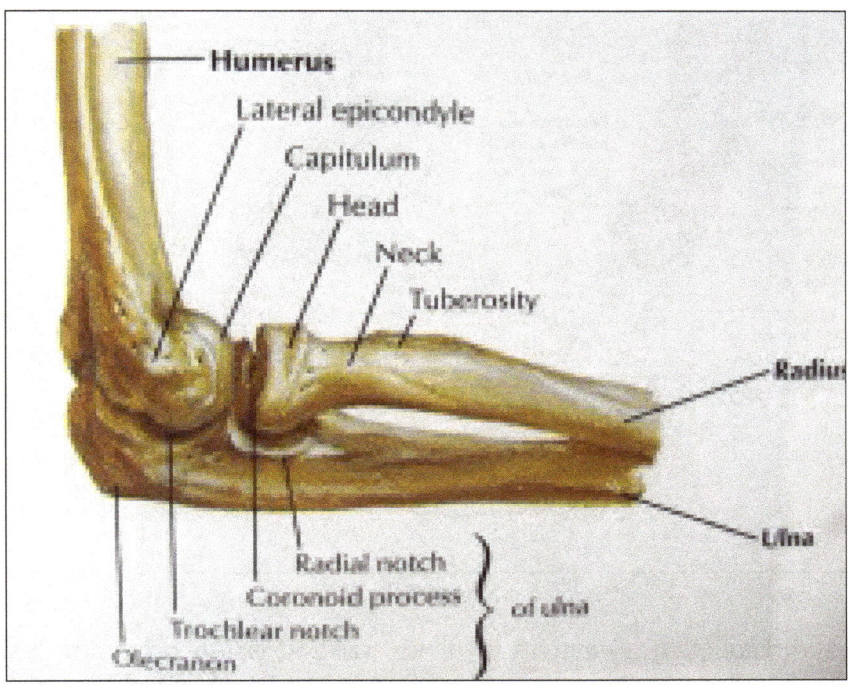

Bony Anatomy of the elbow.

The elbow joint is made up of three bones: The humerus (upper arm bone), the radius and ulna (two bones in the forearm). At the distal end of the humerus there are two epicondyles, one lateral (on the outside) and one medial (on the inside).

The area of maximal tenderness is usually an area just distal to the origin of the extensor muscles of the forearm at the lateral epicondyle. Most commonly, the extensor carpi radialis brevis (ECRB) is involved, but others may include the extensor digitorum, extensor carpi radialis longus (ECRL), and extensor carpi ulnaris.

The radial nerve is also in close proximity to this region, and divides into the superficial radial nerve and the posterior interosseous nerve.

Lateral epicondylitis is classified as an overuse injury that may result in hyaline degeneration of the origin of the extensor tendon. Overuse of the muscles and tendons of the forearm and elbow together with repetitive contractions or manual tasks can put too much strain on the elbow tendons. These contractions or manual tasks require manipulation of the hand that causes maladaptions in tendon structure that lead to pain over the lateral epicondyle. Mostly, the pain is located anterior and distal from the lateral epicondyle.

Epicondylitis occurs at least five times more often and predominantly occurs on the lateral rather than on the medial aspect of the joint, with a 4:1 to 7:1 ratio. It affects 1-3% of the population, with those 35-50 years old most commonly being affected. If a patient is <35, it is important to consider differential diagnosis (growth plate disorder, referral from the cervical spine. If a patient is >50, consider OA, referred cervical spine pain. In a study, of 200 tennis players aged >30, 50% had symptoms of tennis elbow at some stage.

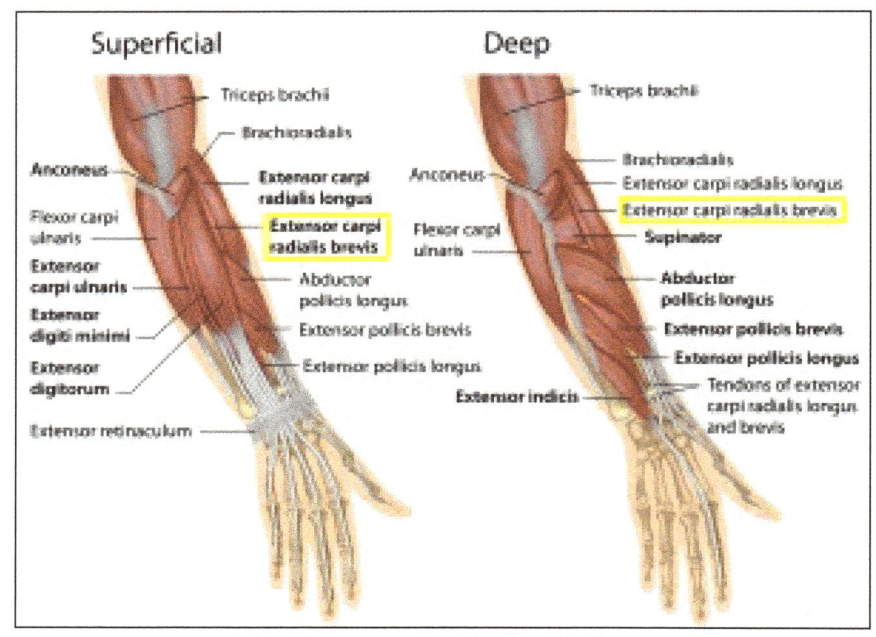

Muscular anatomy of the lateral elbow.

This injury is often work-related, any activity involving wrist extension, pronation or supination during manual labour, housework and hobbies are considered as important causal factors. Lateral epicondylitis is equally common in both sexes. Between the ages of 30-50 years the disease is most prevalent. Obtaining of the condition at the both lateral epicondyle is rare, the dominant arm has the greatest chance of the occurrence of lateral epicondylitis. Twenty percent of cases persist for more than a year.

A systematic review identified 3 risk factors: handling tools heavier than 1 kg, handling loads heavier than 20 kg at least 10 times per day, and repetitive movements for more than 2 hours per day. Other risk factors are overuse, repetitive movements, training errors, misalignments, flexibility problems, ageing, poor circulation, strength deficits or muscle imbalance and psychological factors.

There are several opinions concerning the cause of lateral epicondylitis:

Inflammation

Although the term epicondylitis implies the presence of an inflammatory condition, inflammation is present only in the earliest stages of the disease process.

Microscopic Tearing

- Nirschl and Pettrone attributed the cause to microscopic tearing with formation of reparative tissue (angiofibroblastic hyperplasia) in the origin of the extensor carpi radialis brevis (ECRB) muscle. This micro-tearing and repair response can lead to macroscopic tearing and structural failure of the origin of the ECRB muscle.

- That microscopic or macroscopic tears of the common extensor origin were involved in the disease process, was postulated by Cyriax in 1936.

- The first to describe macroscopic tearing in association with the histological findings were Coonrad and Hooper.

- Histology of tissue samples shows "collagen disorientation, disorganisation, and fibre separation by increased proteoglycan content, increased cellularity, neovascularisation, with local necrosis". Nirschl termed these histological findings bangiofibroblastic hyperplasia. The term has since been modified to bangiofibroblastic tendinosis. He noted that the tissue was characterised by disorganized, immature collagen formation with immature fibroblastic and vascular elements. This grey, friable tissue is found in association with varying degrees of tearing involving the extensor carpi radialis brevis.

Degenerative Process

The histopathological features of 11 patients who had lateral epicondylitis were examined by Regan. They determined that the cause of lateral epicondylitis was more indicative of a degenerative process than an inflammatory process. The condition is degenerative with increased fibroblasts, vascular hyperplasia, proteoglycans and glycosaminoglycans, and disorganized and immature collagen. Repetitive eccentric or concentric overloading of the extensor muscle mass is thought to be the cause of this angiofibroblastic tendinosis of the ECRB. Epicondylitis is a degenerative condition in which increased fibrolastic activity and granulation tissue formation occur within the tendon.

Hypovascularity

Because this tendinous region contains areas that are relatively hypovascular, the tendinous unit is unable to respond adequately to repetitive forces transmitted through the muscle, resulting in declining functional tolerance.

Clinical Presentation

The most prominent symptom of epicondylitis lateralis is pain, this pain can be produced by palpation on the extensor muscles origin on the lateral epicondyle. The pain can radiate upwards along the upper arm and downwards along the outside of the forearm and in rare cases even to the third and fourth fingers. Furthermore it is also often seen that the flexibility and strength in the wrist extensor and posterior shoulder muscles are deficient.

According to Warren, there are four stages on the development of this injury with regard to the intensity of the symptoms:

- Faint pain a couple of hours after the provoking activity.
- Pain at the end of or immediately after the provoking activity.
- Pain during the provoking activity, which intensifies after ceasing that activity.
- Constant pain, which prohibits any activity.

Furthermore it is also often seen that the flexibility and strength in the wrist extensor and posterior shoulder muscles are deficient. At least patients report weakness in their grip strength or difficulty carrying objects in their hand, especially with the elbow extended. This weakness is due to finger extensor and supinator weakness. Some people have a sense of paralysis but this is rare.

Symptoms last, on average, from 2 weeks to 2 years. 89% of the patients recover within 1 year without any treatment except perhaps avoidance of the painful movements.

Assessment

A thorough assessment and examination are key elements in ensuring that the correct treatment plan is implemented, enhancing the recovery process. The assessment should also include elements to exclude a differential diagnosis.

Subjective Assessment

- Onset of pain 24-72hours after provocative activity involving wrist extension.
- Pain may radiate down forearm as far as the wrist and hand.
- Difficulty with lift and grip (Pain+/- weakness).
- Changes in biomechanical factors- new tennis racquet, wet ball, overtraining, poor technique, shoulder injury.

Objective Assessment

- Pain and point tenderness over lateral epicondyle and 1-2cm distal to epicondyle.
- Pain and weakness on resisted wrist extension.
- Weakness on grip strength testing (Dynamometer).
- Pain and decreased movement on passive elbow extension, wrist flexion and ulnar deviation and pronation.
- Weak elbow extensors and flexors.

Differential Diagnosis

- Radial Tunnel Syndrome.
    - Pain in the posterolateral area of the forearm.
    - Pain sometimes spreads to the dorsal side of the wrist.
    - Parasthesia.
    - Weakness (overuse injuries of the musculoskeletal system).
- Posterior Interosseus Syndrome.
    - Pain.
    - Weakness involving wrist extension and finger extension.
    - Motor deficits.
- Elbow osteoarthritis.
    - Pain.
    - Loss of range of motion.

- Fractures.
    - Distal Radial Fractures.
    - Radial Head Fracture.
    - Olecranon Fracture.
- Cervical Radiculopathy.
    - Radiating arm pain corresponding to the dermatomes.
    - Neck pain.
    - Parasthesia.
    - Muscle weakness in myotome.
    - Reflex impairment/loss.
    - Headaches.
    - Scapular pain.
    - Sensory and motor dysfunction in upper extremities and neck.
- Cervical Disc Disease.
- Cervical Myofascial Pain.
- Cervical Spondylosis.
- Fibromyalgia.
- Medial Epicondylitis.

Diagnostic Procedures

The diagnose starts with asking about the activity level, occupation risk factors, recreational sports participation, medication and other medical problems. During the physical exam, the medicine will feel the structure of the elbow and other joints. Also the nerves, muscles, bones and skin are examined. It's important to know which activities cause symptoms and where on your arm the symptoms occur.

Investigations

Investigations are usually not performed in the straightforward case of lateral elbow pain. However, in longstanding cases, plain X-ray (AP and lateral views) of the elbow may show osteochondritis dissecans, degenerative joint changes or evidence of heterotopic calcification.

Ultrasound examination may prove to be a useful diagnostic tool in the investigation of patients with lateral elbow pain. Ultrasound may demonstrate the degree of tendon damage as well as the presence of a bursa.

- X-rays: These may be taken to rule out arthritis of the elbow. 16% calcification along lateral epicondyle.

- Magnetic Resonance Imaging (MRI): If the symptoms are related to a neck problem, an MRI scan may be ordered. This will show if there is a possible herniated disk or arthritis in your neck. Both of these conditions often produce arm pain. MRI- 100% thickening.

- Electromyography (EMG): An EMG is used to rule out nerve compression. Many nerves travel around the elbow, and the symptoms of nerve compression are similar to those of tennis elbow.

Outcome Measures

- Pain reported outcome measures.
  - Numeric Pain Rating Scale (NPRS).
  - Visual Analogue Scale (VAS).
- Self-reported Questionnaires.
- The Upper Limb Functional Index (ULFI).
- Patient Rated Tennis Elbow Evaluation (PRTEE).
- QuickDASH (Disabilities of the Arm Shoulder and Hand).
- Patient Specific Functional Scale (PSFS): Although the PSFS has not yet been validated for lateral epicondylalgia, it has been shown to be valid, reliable and responsive to change in other conditions such as knee dysfunction, cervical radiculopathy, acute low back pain, mechanical low back pain, and neck dysfunction (Pain ICC = 0.89-0.99, Function ICC = 0.83-0.99, Total ICC = 0.89-0.99).

Examination

The diagnosis of lateral epicondylitis is substantiated by tenderness over the ECRB or common extensor origin. By the following methods, the therapist or physiotherapist should be able to reproduce the typical pain:

- To examine the severity of the tennis elbow, there is a dynamometer and a Patient-rated Tennis Elbow Evaluation Questionnaire (PrTEEQ). The dynamometer measures grip strength. The PrTEEQ is a 15-item questionnaire, it's designed to measure forearm pain and disability in patients with lateral epicondylitis. The patients have to rate their levels of tennis elbow pain and disability from 0 to 10, and consists of 2 subscales. There is the pain subscale (0 = no pain, 10 = worst imaginable) en the function subscale (0 = no difficulty, 10 = unable to do).

- Cozen's test: Cozen's test is also known as the resisted wrist extension test. The elbow is stabilized in 90° flexion. The therapist palpates the lateral epicondyle and the other hand positions the patient's hand into radial deviation and forarm pronation. Then the patient is asked to resist wrist extension. The test is positive if the patient experiences a sharp, sudden, severe pain over the lateral epicondyle.

- Chair test: The patient grasps the back of the chair while standing behind it and attempts to lift the chair by using a three finger pinch (thumb, index long fingers) and the elbow fully extended. The test is positive when pain occurs at the lateral epicondyle.

- Mills test: The patient is seated with the upper extremity relaxed at side and the elbow extended. The examiner passively stretches the wrist in flexion and pronation. Pain at the lateral epicondyle or proximal musculotendinous junction of wrist extensors is positive for lateral epicondylitis.

- Maudsley's test: The examiner resist extension of the third digit of the hand, while palpating the lateral epicondyle. A positive test is indicated by pain over the lateral epicondyle.

- The coffee cup test (by Coonrad and Hooper): While doing a specific activity such as picking up a full cup of coffee or a milk bottle. The patient is asked to rate their pain on a scale of zero to ten.

Sports Specific Injuries

Overuse and strain injuries are most common. An overuse injury results from excessive wear and tear on the body, especially in areas subject to repeated activity. Ankle, knee, shoulder and elbow joints are most prone to overuse injuries. A strain injury is where fibers in a muscle or tendon tear as a result of over-stretching.

Many sports injuries can be avoided by suitable conditioning and sufficient warm-up and cool-down before and after.

Athletics Injuries

Avid athletic professionals as well as amateurs may encounter debilitating pain and injuries from over-training, rough competition or plain accidental damages. Athletic injury is common to all athletes and can happen at any time without warning. Athletics injuries can even occur without notice, even up to few days later and may affect your performance until you have fully recovered. With physiotherapy treatment you can resume training and get back in the game quicker. The benefits of rehabilitation and recuperation through physiotherapy are well worth looking into.

Athletics Injuries and Treatment Options

Sports and other athletic injuries usually occur when athletes are not careful during their sport of choice. In the event of an athletics injury, first aid may only be the first step in recovery. Causes of and symptoms such as sprains, muscle aches, overworked tendons or ligaments and other muscular damage can be treated efficiently with physiotherapy. Physiotherapy sessions will focus on special exercise and manual therapy treatments as well as recovery plans and workout schedules to provide relief from pains. Whether you are a professional or an amateur athlete, we can plan and provide proper care you need to get out and do what you love doing.

Avoiding Stress and Injury

Athletics injury occurs when carelessness and other factors come in to play with their sport. Wearing proper sports attire and wearing it correctly can help to prevent such injuries. Excessive amounts of stress can hold you back from your full potential. This extra stress can cause aches, pains, discomfort and even the inability to think while exercising. This is when an athlete is in greatest danger of hurting themselves and others by accidental causes. In the event that you are harmed or feel pain after sporting activities, you should visit us for evaluation and to discuss how we can serve you to solve your problems and get you on the right track to recovery.

Cricket Injuries

It is common for injuries to occur in the game of cricket. As a cricket player, avoiding injuries is something every player would like to possibly do. Here are the most common injuries sustained by these players, along with the symptoms and physiotherapy treatments for each injury.

Knee Injuries

The player most prone to knee injuries is a bowler. In a single cricket season, as many as 60% of the bowlers will suffer a knee injury. One common injury that happens to bowler is a torn meniscus, ACL or Collateral Ligaments. The symptoms are pain, swelling, stiffness and weakness. Players need physiotherapy treatment and a mix of ice packs, knee brace or action knee strap.

Shoulder Injuries

Batters and bowlers are prone to shoulder injuries, which include dislocated shoulder, frozen shoulder and a shoulder separation. The symptoms of such injuries include pain, swelling, stiffness and weakness. To work through these symptoms, players will need physiotherapy treatment and hot/cold therapy packs.

Lower Back Injuries

The most common player to receive lower back pain is a bowler. The back pain occurs mainly in younger, faster bowlers as they have more mobility than their older counterparts. Back injuries could be anything from a herniated disc, back strain or spondylolysis. The symptoms of such injuries include pain, stiffness and weakness. Treatment involves a strengthening and stabilizing exercise program with manual therapy.

Every part of the body in fact is prone to injury for cricket players. The best way to avoid an injury through is by warming up properly before any game. Today's Cricketers are actually becoming more fit and able to stave unwanted injuries which keep them out of a game. A typical warm up should increase blood flow and oxygen to muscles and range of motion of joints reducing the risk of tearing the muscles. Once off the field, keep your muscles warm by putting on a warm up outfit too.

To avoid any injury on the field, make sure you wear the proper gear, such as a mouth guard, proper headgear, shoes and protective pads. Keeping the field free from stones or water is important.

Cycling Injuries

The joy of cycling comes from a love of fresh air, good exercise and enjoyment of the sights along the road. Unfortunately, after a cycling injury the pleasure of getting on a bike and enjoying the freedom of the ride is overtaken by pain and discomfort. The good news is that latest sports injury healing techniques are designed to quickly identify the type of injury and apply the appropriate treatment.

Leg Cramps

Many cyclists experience leg cramps after spending long hours on a bicycle. The muscles repeatedly pump and contract, causing stiffness and an aching feeling. If the condition is chronic and hinders the ability to enjoy a ride, physiotherapy can bring relief and help avoid reoccurance.

Knee Pain

Some cycling injuries occur as the result of climbing steep elevations. In some cases this can be prevented by ensuring that appropriate gears are selected and that the bike is suited for elevated terrain. You should check the seat height and handlebar levels are suitable. But even with the proper equipment, warm up and stretching routines, injuries may still occur. The knee area receives stress from weight bearing pressure and could sustain significant injury.

Back Injuries

Some of the most serious cycling injuries involve trauma to the back and spinal cord. Particularly on a long ride, a cyclist may be hunched over the handlebars for long periods of time. Add this to a sudden bump in the road and the entire back region experiences a jolt. Good posture may help prevent some of the strain but physiotherapy is the best cure for back injuries. In many cycling injuries, back and spinal cord problems are some of the most painful and chronic conditions.

Warming up before a ride and taking precautions to not over-stress the body are important practices to prevent injuries.

Endurance Sports Injuries

Athletes who participate in endurance sports are subject to injuries different from those suffered by other athletes. Most of these endurance sports injuries are the direct result of pushing the body to its limits over a long period of time. For example, shin splints and various forms of tendonitis are common among long-distance runners and triathletes, while rotator cuff injuries are common with rowers.

When an athlete participates in an endurance sport, the continual, intense strain on the body almost inevitably leads to injury. To reduce such injuries, endurance athletes should undergo extensive training to ensure they're using their bodies correctly and to build the necessary strength and endurance to stand up to the intensity of long-term physical exertion. Warming up is important to prepare the body by loosening tight muscles and lowering the risk of strain and tearing.

In general, the best way to treat endurance injuries is prevention. Injuries of this kind are most often caused when the athlete pushes himself too far or too hard after insufficient training or warm-up. Even when pushing endurance to its limits with this kind of extreme sport, it's important to treat the body properly.

When endurance injuries do occur, correct treatment is also vital to ensure proper healing of the injured muscles, tendons or ligaments. Physiotherapy is an important element of recovery. A skilled physiotherapist can help restore an injured athlete to full performance levels.

Physiotherapy for endurance sports injuries can take a variety of approaches, including stretching regimens, weightlifting, application of heat and cold, manual therapy and other techniques to help rebuild and strengthen injured muscles.

Field Hockey Injuries

Field hockey is a tough sport requiring skill, fitness and the ability to make quick changes in direction. As a result, field hockey has a high percentage of impact injuries. Some common field hockey injuries are:

ACL (Anterior Cruciate Ligament) Rupture

The ACL is an important ligament as it helps to stabilise the knee. ACL ruptures are common field hockey injuries, especially in women and can occur when the knee is twisted during a change in direction. This type of injury causes knee pain, swelling, instability and difficulty walking. A loud pop may be heard at the time of injury. If this happens you should stop play immediately, apply the RICE formula (Rest, Ice, Compression and Elevation) and seek medical attention as soon as possible. Rehabilitation with physiotherapy is always needed to help return to the hockey field.

Meniscus Tears

The menisci are made up of two rings of cartilage – the medial meniscus and the lateral meniscus. Their function is to absorb shock in the knee. Constant twisting of the knee can cause pain, swelling, difficulty bearing weight and inability to bend the knee. When this happens you should stop play and apply the RICE formula as above. Physiotherapy will be needed to help you return to future games, but in severe cases surgery may be necessary, followed by rehabilitation.

Ankle Sprain

This is a very common field hockey injury which occurs when the ankle turns over causing the sole of the foot to turn inward. Damage is usually to the ligaments on the outside of the ankle. Symptoms are ankle pain, swelling, stiffness, bruising and an inability to bear weight. Using the RICE formula followed by physiotherapy, is the best form of treatment.

Hamstring Strain

Sudden, sharp pain at the back of the leg while sprinting or quickly changing direction can signal a hamstring strain. Other symptoms are pain while stretching the muscle, swelling and bruising. There are different grades of hamstring strains, with symptoms ranging from mild to severe. In severe cases, walking is greatly limited and crutches may be needed. Treatment consists of the RICE formula followed by physiotherapy.

Groin Strain

A tear or rupture to any of the muscles on the inner side of the thigh constitutes a groin strain. This type of field hockey injury results in groin pain, ranging from mild to severe, grade 1 being mild, 2 moderate and 3 severe. Tightness may be felt in the groin area as well as pain when squeezing the legs together. In a grade 3 strain, a lump or a gap in the muscle may be felt. Rest and ice along with physiotherapy are needed to help you return to the field.

These are just some of the ways that players can be injured while playing field hockey. In many cases, injury can be prevented by warming up properly before play and cooling down afterward. Also, wearing protective gear will go a long way in avoiding some of the contusions and fractures that occur during this sport.

Football Injuries

Football injuries cover a wide array of complaints and involve every part of the body. From concussions (head trauma) to plantar fasciitis (foot pain at the bottom of the heel), football players are prone to them all. Some of the most common football injuries are:

ACL (Anterior Cruciate Ligament) Tears

Knee pain, swelling and tenderness on the inner side of the knee are the usual symptoms of this common soccer injury. There may also be difficulty walking or straightening the knee. The athlete needs to stop all activity when this happens and apply ice to the knee. Taping and elevating will help to reduce swelling. ACL tears always require surgery and physiotherapy to restore function, range of motion and strength. The athlete may have to wear a brace to stabilise the knee following surgery.

Concussions

This can occur from a sudden blow to the head during a fall or during play. Concussions may be mild or severe and symptoms may range from confusion to loss of consciousness. In every instance, medical attention should be sought as even mild concussions can have serious consequences later on.

Hamstring Pull or Tear

This is a common football injury and can range from minor strains to serious rupture of the hamstring muscle. It is characterised by sudden, sharp pain at the back of the thigh that may disrupt your movement. Straightening the leg all the way will also be difficult. This type of football injury can be avoided by warming up properly before play and by keeping the leg muscles strong and flexible. If you do suffer a hamstring injury, you need to rest the leg and apply ice until the swelling subsides. A physiotherapist can help you stretch and strengthen your muscles to decrease recovery time, improve performance and prevent injury.

Patellofemoral Pain Syndrome

This term refers to pain under and around the kneecap and is also called Runner's knee. Because the patella can move in different directions, inadequate muscle strength, overuse or improper balance can affect the patella and cause knee pain. A player suffering from this type of pain needs to rest from soccer and do some type of low-impact sport such as swimming. A proper rehabilitation program is necessary to stretch and strengthen the muscles surrounding the knee and help prevent re-injury.

Shin Splints

This is a type of football injury that manifests itself in generalised pain along the inside of the shin bone. Shin pain can be caused by trauma, repeated stress on the leg as a result of over-training or excessive running on hard surfaces. Beginners are prone to this type of football injury as their muscles, bones and joints are used to the effects of high-impact sports. Proper warm-up and cool down are important to preventing this type of injury, as well as stretching and strengthening of the calf muscles. Also, if you over-pronate in your feet, you may be advised by your physiotherapist to wear orthotic lifts in your shoes. Resting from football and getting yourself under the care of a capable physiotherapist are the best steps you can take to correct this problem.

Golf Injuries

Repetitive injuries are quite common in golf and usually occur in the soft tissues (muscles, ligaments and tendons) of the lower back, shoulders and wrists. Many injuries can be avoided with proper conditioning and by improving your swing mechanics. Some of the major golf injuries are:

Low Back Strains

These may result from a sudden force applied to the ligaments of the lower back due to poor swing mechanics. Poor conditioning of the body, lack of flexibility and repetitive strain can lead to injury and low back pain. An injury of this type can be treated with restricted and light activity including stretching and strengthening exercises. Your physiotherapist can perform a proper assessment, then set up an individual program designed especially for you to help you return to golf. Not only will your body be less likely to break down, but will also have increased efficiency improving your game.

Torn Rotator Cuff

The rotator cuff consists of a group of muscles and their tendons that help to stabilise the shoulder and allow arm movements. A torn rotator cuff is a severe golf injury and can seriously limit shoulder movement and strength. Other symptoms are shoulder pain, which is worse at night, and weakness in the shoulder. Raising the arm overhead becomes difficult. A torn rotator cuff potentially requires surgery, followed by rehabilitation.

Shoulder Tendonitis, Bursitis and Impingement Syndrome

These are golf injuries that may result from overuse. Tendonitis is inflammation of a tendon; bursitis is inflammation of the bursa – the fluid-filled sacs between the tendon and skin or tendon and bone. Tendonitis can lead to impingement syndrome as the muscles and tendons become inflamed and swollen. Repetitive overhead arm motions may irritate the muscles, tendons and tissues over time leading to inflammation and impingement.

Symptoms of this condition are slow onset of pain, and shoulder or upper arm pain at night when lying on the affected side. Pain may also be felt with abduction of the arm (moving the arm out to the side) or raising the arm overhead. Shoulder pain at the front or the side is also common and may radiate down to the elbow and forearm. Treatment involves rest, icing and the use of anti-inflammatory medications. Physiotherapy is needed to help return to golf.

Golfer's Elbow (Medial Epicondylitis)

This is an overuse injury often experienced by golfers as a result of small tears occurring in the tendons of the forearm. Elbow pain occurs on the inside of the elbow as opposed to tennis elbow where pain occurs on the outside. Pain increases when flexing the wrist and when grasping objects. Treatment should begin with the RICE method to decrease pain, swelling and inflammation. Your physiotherapist will prescribe exercises to stretch and strengthen the flexor muscles, manual therapy will also be used to break down any scar tissue. A wrist splint may also prove helpful. Recurrence of this injury is quite common, therefore you may be advised not to return to golf too quickly.

Many golf injuries can be avoided with proper conditioning, warm-up and cool down before and after the game.

Martial Arts Injuries

Martial arts in its different forms carry with it the risk of injury, ranging from mild to severe. Seasoned martial arts performers stand a higher chance of sustaining a catastrophic injury due to the competitive nature of the sport. Amateurs are more likely to suffer contusions, sprains and strains. Before beginning martial arts or any type of sport it is wise to consult with your physician to see if you can withstand rigorous training. Some major martial arts injuries are:

Contusions and Lacerations

Inherent close contact puts these among the most common martial arts injuries. First aid treatment consists of ice and bandaging depending on the nature of the bruise or cut.

Sprains and Strains

Injury to ligaments and muscles can occur from over-stretching of the ligaments or tears to the muscle and tendons. Legs and the cervical spine are most affected, with men having a higher incidence than women. Rest, ice, compression and elevation (RICE) are helpful in relieving these conditions, followed by physiotherapy.

Knee Injuries

Knee injuries can result from forceful kicking and sudden changes in direction with the knee bent. Karate, judo and Thai kick boxers are all prone to this type of injury. ACL (anterior cruciate ligament) injuries are quite common for the reasons mentioned. An ACL injury causes sharp knee pain, swelling and difficulty bearing weight. RICE can be used to decrease pain and swelling, but you should get to your physiotherapist quickly as possible for an assessment. Surgery may be required in some cases.

Dislocations and Fractures

These are quite common in most martial arts, especially where grappling or throwing is involved. Fractures to the fingers and toes as well as the long bones of the forearm and legs are common. Dislocations to the shoulders, fingers and toes may also be sustained. RICE, medical attention and physiotherapy are vital to enable you to return to martial arts.

Back Injuries

These occur in martial arts where lifting and twisting, and falling is involved (e.g. throwing in judo). Back pain, decreased movement and stiffness are some of the symptoms. Rest and ice are helpful, but it is important to see your physiotherapist in order to rule out any other form of injury. Physiotherapy is needed for pain management and to improve flexibility and strength.

Severe Injuries

These are life-threatening and encompass a wide array of injuries such as thoracic trauma, stomach trauma involving internal organs, spinal cord injury, cervical neck injury (whiplash), testicular injury, head injuries resulting in neurological damage, and many more. These all require immediate medical attention, and in some instances the player may not be able to return to martial arts.

Participating in Martial arts is a great way to keep fit, improve concentration and discipline while at the same time learning how to defend oneself and others. However, it can be dangerous and demanding. In order to stave off the risk of injury, it is wise to constantly improve flexibility, strength and endurance. Physiotherapy can help you do this,

Rugby Injuries

Rugby is a tough, fast-moving sport that incurs a number of injuries from tackling and scrummaging. Many rugby injuries can be avoided with the use of protective gear but others may be unavoidable. Some of the more common rugby injuries are:

Contusions and Lacerations

These represent a high percentage of rugby injuries and can be easily treated with ice and bandaging.

Muscle Strains

These can result from sudden force applied to the ligaments during tackle. Poor conditioning, lack of flexibility and overuse can lead to muscle pain. An injury of this type can be treated with rest and light activity including stretching and strengthening exercises. Your physiotherapist can perform a proper assessment, and then set up a program designed especially for you to help you return to rugby.

Fractures

Fractures, usually of the clavicle (collar bone), are quite common among rugby players. Falling onto an outstretched arm or coming into contact with another player can lead to this type of fracture. There is extreme pain in the clavicle, swelling and a bony deformity. This injury calls for immediate medical attention. The bone may have to be immobilised in a sling or bandage. In some cases surgery may be needed. Physiotherapy is needed once the bone has healed.

Meniscal Injuries

The menisci are bands of cartilage that act as shock absorbers to the knee and help distribute weight evenly between the tibia (shinbone) and the femur (thighbone). During tackles the medial meniscus is more likely to be injured as forces are impacted from the outside of the knee. Twisting of the knee may also lead to a meniscal tear. Symptoms are knee pain on the inner surface of the joint. Swelling usually occurs within a day or two of the injury and it may be difficult to bend the knee fully or bear weight. The athlete should stop play and use the RICE formula (Rest, Ice, Compression, Elevation). Consulting with a physiotherapist is necessary to set up a rehabilitation program to help you return to rugby.

ACL (Anterior Cruciate Ligament) Injuries

This type of knee injury occurs through a twisting force when the foot is firmly planted on the ground, or it can occur as a result of direct trauma during rugby tackle. There may be an audible pop at the time of the injury, followed by knee pain, swelling and tenderness on the inner side of the knee. It may be difficult to walk or straighten the knee. With this type of knee injury, the athlete should stop the activity immediately and apply the RICE protocol. Surgery is almost always needed. Physiotherapy may be started beforehand in order to strengthen the knee and reduce swelling.

Ankle Sprains

Sprained ankles are another common rugby injury and are caused by the stretching and tearing of ligaments. This is a painful condition requiring rest from play. Other symptoms are swelling, inflammation, difficulty walking and decrease in the elasticity of the ligament. A serious ankle sprain can be more painful and take a longer time to heal than a broken bone. The RICE formula is always helpful but once the pain and swelling subside the athlete should seek physiotherapy in order to promote flexibility and strength.

Running Injuries

Running injuries result from:
- Wearing improper footwear.
- Over-training.
- Under training.
- Not warming-up or cooling down properly.

To avoid running injuries, athletes should pay attention to the above factors as well as preparing their bodies to meet the physical challenges of running.

Some common injuries sustained while running are:

Metatarsalgia

Metatarsalgia manifests itself in pain and inflammation in the ball of the foot. Wearing shoes with soles that are too thin or inflexible can lead to this foot injury. Pain in the forefoot is most pronounced when the person tries to bear weight or push off. Rest and icing are helpful followed by physiotherapy for stretching and strengthening exercises.

Achilles Tendonitis

This is a common, painful condition experienced by runners. It is characterised by pain to the back of the heel which increases with exercise and decreases when the exercise stops. There is also difficulty walking or rising up on the toes.

The best treatment for Achilles tendonitis is to rest and ice the injured foot until the pain goes away. Rehabilitation is necessary to toughen the tendon and stretch and strengthen the calf muscles.

The Iliotibial Band Injury

This is the thick sheath of connective tissue that runs from the hip bone (femur) down the outside of the thigh and attaches to the outside of the shin bone (tibia). It acts to extend (straighten) the leg and abduct the hip (move it sideways). As this band passes over the bony part on the outside of the knee, it causes friction which leads to pain. Iliotibial band syndrome is sometimes referred to as runner's knee. Major symptoms are a burning sensation on the outside of the knee, or along the entire sheath and worsening pain when the foot strikes the ground.

The athlete can rest and apply cold therapy to the knee to reduce pain. A rehabilitation program will prevent the rolling action during the stance phase which is responsible for the friction injury. Minimising downhill running or eliminating it altogether can speed up recovery.

Shin Splints

This condition occurs at the front inside of the shin bone and results in pain at the start of exercise, fading away as the session progresses and returning when the activity ceases. Pain is usually felt when the toes or foot are bent downwards. There may also be lumps or bumps felt over the area. Treatment involves rest to allow the injury to heal. Icing and anti-inflammatory medications are also helpful.

A physiotherapist will perform a gait analysis to determine if you over-pronate (sole of the foot turns outward) or over-supinate (sole turns inward). Both of these conditions cause problems for runners as the foot does not absorb shock during running.

Faulty movement patterns or weaknesses at the hip and knee are frequently responsible for biomechanical problems at the foot/ankle.

Skiing Injuries

Skiing injuries are quite common, especially among occasional skiers. Most injuries occur as a result of falls; concussions, shoulder injuries and fractures being common as skiers lose control. Other common skiing injuries are ACL (anterior cruciate ligament) and thumb injuries. Many skiing injuries can be avoided by embarking on a conditioning program before you begin the season and by wearing protective gear.

Concussions

These may be mild or severe and may occur from a fall or direct blow to the head. A concussion occurs when the brain moves violently in the skull as a result of the trauma. Someone who sustains a mild concussion while skiing may appear disoriented, confused and may suffer memory loss. In severe cases there may be headaches, stiff neck, bleeding from the nose or ears, dizziness, blurred vision and even loss of consciousness. Any of these signs require immediate medical attention. Even mild cases should be reported as more severe effects could be felt later.

Skier's Thumb

Also known as gamekeepers' thumb, this is a common skiing injury that causes pain and a premature end to a skiing trip. This injury takes place at the MCP (metacarpophalangeal) joint at the base of the thumb and involves the UCL (ulnar collateral ligament). This type of skiing injury usually occurs when a skier's thumb is forced into abduction (movement away from the index finger) and hyperextension (moving backward) against the ski pole during a fall or other impact. For a simple strain or tear, icing and casting to immobilise the joint work best. However, if there is a complete tear, fracture or instability of the MCP joint, surgery may be necessary. Physiotherapy will follow to restore joint mobility, strength and stability. It is important to treat a thumb injury promptly; if neglected, it may become chronic and arthritis and instability will develop.

Knee Injuries

Medial collateral ligament (MCL) injuries occur most commonly among beginning and immediate skiers due to faulty biomechanics. Knee pain, swelling and tenderness are the usual symptoms. This type of skiing injury responds well to conservative treatments with RICE (Rest, Ice, Compression and Elevation) and physiotherapy. However, in some instances, your doctor may decide to perform surgery.

Most advanced skiers who become injured while skiing may suffer an anterior collateral injury (ACL) of the knee. This may occur in conjunction with a MCL injury and can be disabling. There may be an audible pop at the time of the injury, followed by knee pain, swelling and tenderness on the inner side of the knee. It may be difficult to walk or straighten the knee. With this type of knee injury, the athlete should stop the activity immediately and apply the RICE protocol. If you are not a high-powered athlete, your doctor may decide to operate and recommend physiotherapy before surgery to ensure the best results. A knee brace is often recommended for stability.

Squash Injuries

The game of squash is a high-impact, fast moving one that lends itself to a lot of injuries, some of which may be severe. Apart from the injuries that can occur from moving around the court, players also become injured from contact with the ball, their opponent's racquet and even the wall. Players need to be very fit in order to avoid being injured while playing squash. Some of the most common squash injuries are muscle, tendon and ligament sprains and eye injuries.

Achilles Tendonitis

This is one of the most common squash injuries that affect either the heel or the mid-point of the Achilles tendon just above the heel. It may be an acute injury or chronic and healing can be slow because of the poor blood supply to this portion of the leg. Symptoms are gradual onset of pain which starts with exercises and lessens as exercises progresses. Pain usually subsides with rest. Achilles tendonitis can become chronic if the athlete does not rest or seek help at first onset.

Achilles tendonitis is an overuse injury that can be caused by increase in activity, less recovery between activities and exercising in flat shoes which puts stress on the tendon. The condition can be prevented by warming up thoroughly before play and stretching properly afterward. Wearing shoes that provide adequate cushion is also helpful. Proper rehabilitation is necessary if you sustain this type of squash injury in order to prevent from becoming chronic. The athlete should apply the RICE (Rest, Ice, Compression, Elevation) formula at the first sign of injury.

Ankle Sprains

These are another common squash injury and are caused by the stretching and tearing of ligaments. This is a painful condition requiring rest and rehabilitation. Other symptoms are swelling, inflammation, difficulty walking, and decrease in the elasticity of the ligament. A serious ankle sprain can be more painful and take a longer time to heal than a broken bone. The RICE formula is always helpful but once the pain and swelling subside the athlete should seek physiotherapy in order to promote flexibility and strength.

Squash injuries occur more among older players than younger ones. Lack of conditioning, experience playing the game and reduced reaction times may all contribute to injuries. By taking certain common sense precautions these injuries can be avoided. Players should be careful of their surroundings, wear proper footwear and protective eyewear, warm up and cool down thoroughly and maintain strength and flexibility. Finally, if you do become injured while playing squash, stop playing immediately and seek assistance.

Swimming Injuries

On the surface it would appear that swimming injuries are rare compared to that of other sports. After all, swimming is touted to be one of the best and safest forms of exercise. The fact is that injuries do occur among novices as well as competitive swimmers. The main areas that are injured while swimming are the shoulder and the knee. These injuries are generally known as swimmers shoulder and breast-stroke knee respectively. However, muscle cramps also occur as well as injuries of the back and neck.

Swimmers perform a vast number of overhead arm movements during the course of their training. It follows therefore that the shoulders are subjected to tremendous stress and micro-traumas can result. These micro-traumas develop into a number of syndromes: rotator cuff tendonitis, biceps tendonitis and subacromial tendonitis. Overuse and instability are the main causes of swimmers shoulder followed by faulty mechanics, sudden increases in training load or intensity and the use of hand paddles.

Symptoms of swimmers shoulder are deep shoulder pain felt at night or it may only be felt in a painful arc between the shoulder and the waist. If there is an impingement, pain may increase over time, as opposed to sudden pain if there is a tear. At the first sign of swimmers shoulder, an evaluation should be done by a physiotherapist so that rehabilitation can begin before the condition worsens. Rest and ice in the beginning are helpful. Rehabilitation will initially focus on stretching exercises to improve joint mobility and isometric exercises (muscle contracts without movement) for strengthening. You should cease from overhead training and from using hand paddles.

Knee injuries involving increased stress on the medial collateral ligament (that stabilises the knee), may occur in young as well as more experienced swimmers. The capsule and the patella (kneecap) can also be injured while swimming. Weak vastus medialis (the inner thigh muscle which is part of the quadriceps), poor mechanics and decreased hamstring flexibility can contribute to these swimming injuries. Rest and icing to reduce pain and inflammation, followed by physiotherapy will help you return to swimming.

Muscle cramps while swimming can be fatal. They can be mild or painful and occur mostly in muscles that cross two joints, example the calf muscle. Cramps may occur as a result of poor conditioning, muscle fatigue, dehydration or performing a new activity. If a cramp occurs while swimming you should flip over on your back, raise the leg high and massage the location, while using one arm to paddle to the poolside/shore.

The back, neck and upper spine can also become injured while swimming as a result of being over stretched during the breast stroke and from repetitive motions during the frontward strokes. To avoid back pain while swimming, you should examine your technique. Sudden, jerky movements can put strain on your neck and upper spine. Wearing a life vest or other flotation device can help you maintain proper form while swimming. If back injury does occur, you should rest from the activity, apply ice and seek physiotherapy treatment. Specially designed exercises to stretch and strengthen the muscles may be what you need.

Tennis Injuries

The game of tennis is one that requires endurance, flexibility and overall fitness. Many people become injured while playing tennis either from a sudden impact or from overuse of muscles and joints. Beginners are very likely to suffer injury. Some common overuse injuries are:

Tennis Elbow (Lateral Epicondylitis)

This is a common repetitive injury that leads to elbow pain however it may also be caused by sudden impact. Symptoms are pain on the outside of the elbow which may radiate down the forearm. Lifting heavy objects may also cause elbow pain. The RICE (rest, ice, compression, elevation) method is helpful in relieving pain and inflammation. Physiotherapy is recommended for flexibility and strengthening so that you can return to playing tennis.

Rotator Cuff Tendonitis

This is a tennis injury that results from repeated overhead movements. This causes inflammation in the tendons of the rotator cuff muscles, leading to shoulder pain and weakness with overhead movements or pain at night, especially when lying on the affected shoulder. Rest and icing are the first forms of treatment followed by physiotherapy exercises for strengthening. In severe cases, surgery may be necessary.

Wrist Tendonitis

Inflammation of the tendons of the thumb may occur when someone starts playing tennis for the first time but it can also be an overuse injury. Injury to the arm, poor technique or improper equipment may also lead to this type of tennis injury. Wrist pain is felt in the front of the wrist and if you make a fist with the thumb inside, there would most likely be pain. Rest and icing should be employed to allow the inflammation to heal. Stretching and strengthening exercises will be helpful to allow you to return to tennis.

Sprained Wrist

A sprained wrist may occur from a fall on an outstretched hand. This causes stretching or tears to the ligaments of the wrist. Pain, tenderness and swelling over the wrist will be seen. If you experience these symptoms you should rest from the activity and apply ice. Once the symptoms have subsided you should contact your physiotherapist for a rehabilitation program.

Ankle Sprains

During a game, a tennis player is required to stop, start or make sudden changes in direction. This can result in stretching or tearing of the ligaments of the ankle leading to ankle sprain. Sometimes a loud "snap" or "pop" may be heard at the time of injury, followed by pain, swelling and tenderness over the site. Applying the RICE treatment should be your first course of action. Rest is needed to take the strain off the ankle and ice helps to relieve pain and inflammation. Compression of the ankle with a bandage and elevation of the foot while sitting and lying helps to reduce oedema or swelling. Physiotherapy will help with rehabilitation and your return to tennis in a short time.

ACL (Anterior Cruciate Ligament) Injuries

ACL injuries are quite common among tennis players for the reasons mentioned above. The ACL is one of the two major ligaments that help to stabilise the knee. When this is injured, knee stability is compromised, and knee pain, swelling and difficulty walking result. The first thing to do is use the RICE method, then seek out physiotherapy.

Weight Training Injuries

Weight training is a demanding activity that calls for concentration, commitment and overall health and fitness. It is not a high-impact sport like rugby or football, yet injuries can occur if a person is not careful.

Some Common Weight Training Injuries

- Rotator cuff injuries: Inflammation of the four muscles and tendons that stabilise the shoulder and help to move the arm. Shoulder pain, weakness and numbness are common. Rest, ice and anti-inflammatory medications are the first line of treatment followed by physiotherapy.

- Tennis elbow: This may arise from triceps exercise. Symptoms are pain on the outside of the elbow, weakness when attempting to lift, elbow pain when gripping or using the wrist. Treatment calls for rest from lifting, then physiotherapy for stretching and strengthening injuries.

- Thoracic outlet syndrome (TOS): The thoracic outlet is the area between the rib cage and collar bone. Compression of the subclavian artery and brachial plexus as they pass through a narrow space between the armpit and the arms leads to this syndrome. Symptoms include neck and shoulder pain, feeling of cold, numbness and tingling of the fingers and a weak grasp. Rest and physiotherapy are indicated to strengthen the shoulder muscles, improve range-of-motion and posture. If this is not successful, you may need surgery.

- Low back pain: Causes are improper form during lifting, weakness of the surrounding muscles and using too much weight. Rest and physiotherapy are vital to help the person return to weight-training.

Weight training injuries occur for the following reasons:

- Improper stretching: Over-stretching of muscles, tendons and ligaments can lead to weight-training injuries. Proper stretching relaxes the muscles, increases flexibility and eliminates soreness.

- Inadequate warm up: Exercising on a cold, stiff muscle can lead to muscle strains and ligament sprains. To get the most out of your workout, warm-up with a few high-rep, low-intensity exercises first.

- Over-training: Sessions should be no more than an hour. Rest between sets and between workouts. Using weight that is too heavy adds up as over-training.

- Incorrect technique: This can tear or injure a muscle. Avoid twisting and turning while lifting and do not lock your joints.

- Cheating: Using momentum in order to handle heavy weight can cause you to drop the weight and injure yourself or someone else.

Injuries suffered during weight-training can be far-reaching and complex.

Yoga Injuries

Yoga has increased popularity over the years as a form of exercise that has many benefits; promoting flexibility, balance and endurance to name a few. Yoga is a mild, low-impact activity, therefore it is surprising that yoga injuries can occur, but they do. Like any form of exercise, if it is performed incorrectly or performed by persons with certain musculoskeletal conditions, injuries can result.

The most common yoga injuries occur as a result of repetitive strain on the wrists, shoulders, neck, knee, spine, hamstrings and the sacroiliac joint (which links the spinal column and the pelvis). The danger with yoga is that symptoms do not come on overnight and when they do appear it is usually too late. Also, beginners may try too hard and put a lot of strain on their joints. Pain, tenderness, difficulty with movements should alert that something is wrong and you should rest from the activity.

Some tips to avoid becoming injured while practicing Yoga:

- Find a qualified instructor: There are many books and tapes on the market and you may be tempted to learn from those, but you run the risk of performing the postures incorrectly and becoming injured.
- Perform warm up exercises before starting your Yoga session: Stretching cold muscles and tendons can lead to injury.
- Seek out the type of Yoga that best suits your needs: Not all forms of Yoga are created equal. Some are more strenuous and may be unsuitable for people with certain conditions.
    - Wear proper clothing that allows for ease of movement.
    - If you are a beginner, start slowly and do not try postures that you are not yet ready for.
    - Drink plenty of fluids, especially if participating in Bikram or 'hot' Yoga.
    - If you are not sure of a pose or movement, ask your instructor.
    - If you experience pain or exhaustion while performing Yoga, stop and rest.
    - Set personal goals: As with any project you should have a goal in mind. Work toward that goal consistently without allowing yourself to be swayed by what you see others doing. Everyone is different.

Yoga is a great addition to any fitness program, but you can become injured while performing Yoga if you do not know what you are doing, or if you have conditions for which Yoga may be contraindicated.

References

- Sport-Injury-Classification: physio-pedia.com, Retrieved 21 August, 2019
- The-physiology-of-sports-injuries-and-repair-processes, current-issues-in-sports-and-exercise-medicine: intechopen.com, Retrieved 20 July, 2019
- The-sprains-and-strains-of-sporting-injuries-article, sports-medicine-articles: nationwidechildrens.org, Retrieved 19 June, 2019
- Common-knee-injuries, diseases-conditions: orthoinfo.aaos.org, Retrieved 20 May, 2019
- Sports-hernia-athletic-pubalgia, diseases-conditions: orthoinfo.aaos.org, Retrieved 14 February, 2019
- Shin-splints, injuries-conditions-1: physioworks.com.au, Retrieved 21 August, 2019
- Sports-specific-injuries, patient-info: platinumphysio.co.uk, Retrieved 26 July, 2019
- Lateral-Epicondylitis: physio-pedia.com, Retrieved 16 April, 2019

Sports Injury: Treatment, Prevention and Rehabilitation

Cryotherapy, hydrotherapy, PRICE method, etc. are some methods that are widely used in sports injury preventions. Rehabilitation and physical therapy such as regenerative therapy seek to restore functional ability to those with physical impairments or disabilities. All these aspects related to sports injury treatment, prevention and rehabilitation have been carefully analyzed in this chapter.

Whether you play sports for competition or fitness, you don't want to be side-lined with an injury. Time away from the game or in forced inactivity is something we all want to avoid. While it is impossible to prevent every injury, research suggests that injury rates could be reduced by 25% if athletes took appropriate preventative action. Use these general rules for injury prevention no matter what sport you play.

Be in Proper Physical Condition to Play a Sport

Keep in mind the weekend warrior has a high rate of injury. If you play any sports, you should adequately train for that sport. It is a mistake to expect the sport itself to get you into shape. Many injuries can be prevented by following a regular conditioning program of exercises designed specifically for your sport.

Know and Abide by the Rules of the Sport

The rules are designed, in part, to keep things safe. This is extremely important for anyone who participates in a contact sport. You need to learn them and to play by the rules of conduct. Respect the rules on illegal procedures and insist on enforcement by referees, umpires, and judges. These rules are there to keep athletes healthy.

Wear Appropriate Protective Gear and Equipment

Protective pads, mouth guards, helmets, gloves, and other equipment are not for those you consider weak; they are for everyone. Protective equipment that fits you well can save your knees, hands, teeth, eyes, and head. Never play without your safety gear.

Rest

Athletes with a high number of consecutive days of training, have more injuries. While many athletes think the more they train, the better they'll play, this is a misconception. Rest is a critical component of proper training. Rest can make you stronger and prevent injuries of overuse, fatigue and poor judgment.

Always Warm-up Before Playing

Warm muscles are less susceptible to injuries. The proper warm-up is essential for injury prevention. Make sure your warm-up suits your sport. You may simply start your sport slowly, or practice specific stretching or mental rehearsal depending upon your activity.

Avoid Playing when Very Tired or in Pain

This is a set-up for a careless injury. Pain indicates a problem. You need to pay attention to warning signs your body provides.

Factors that Increase your Risk of Sport Injuries

Research provides us with helpful clues about the cause of sports injury. There are two factors that outweigh the rest when it comes to predicting a sports injury. They are:

- Having a history of injury. Previous injuries to a muscle or joint tend to develop into chronic problem areas for many athletes. It is extremely important to warm up, and stretch previously injured parts.
- A high number of consecutive days of training. Recovery days reduce injury rates by giving muscles and connective tissues an opportunity to repair between training sessions.

Sport Injury Prevention

Be in Proper Physical Condition

Before you engage in sports or training, always keep in mind that you should be in proper physical condition. Perform regular conditioning exercises that are designed specifically for your sport. Moreover, train slowly but surely. You do not learn any sports overnight. To condition your body, you need to undergo training.

Wear Protective Gear

You cannot tell if you will encounter accidents or emergencies in the middle of the game. You should be ready. Wear protective gears, equipment, and devices that will protect you from unexpected injuries. This includes mouth guards, helmets, gloves, protective pads and other equipment. Running shoes are also designed to improve your performance and decrease your risk to knee and foot injuries.

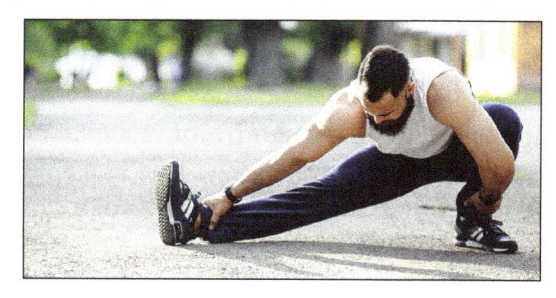

Warm up Before Playing

Warming up is a must before engaging into sports. It prepares your body, mind, and heart for the training or the sports. Warming-up gradually raises your heart rate, warms your muscles and connective tissues, improves your mobility and promotes functionality of all your body's movements. It also allows entry of oxygen to your muscles, tendons, ligaments and flexible joints, among others.

Have Enough Sleep

Sleep plays a vital part in your recovery which is vital in your overall training program and optimal performance. Sleep can make you stronger and will prevent you from fatigue, poor judgment, and certain injuries. Even famous athletes like Lebron James and Roger Federer gets 12 hours of sleep per night.

Do Not Over Work

It is extremely important that you always listen to your body. When you engage in sports, you have to begin slowly and steadily to avoid straining some of your muscles which may lead to injuries. Do not work beyond your limits.

Improve Technique

Based on the principles of biomechanics, the most effective way of improving your performance is by improving your techniques. Your physical built is just a small factor in your performance. The coordination of your body movements is important in performing well in different kinds of sports. For example, gymnasts are required to focus on improving their body techniques so they can perform well. Swimming, basketball and other sports require the application of biomechanics.

Keep Hydrated

Our body is composed of 60% of water. When we exercise or we do sports, we lose this water. Thus, we need to replace those water through proper hydration. According to sports dieticians, water is essential in maintaining blood volume, regulating body temperature and allowing muscle contractions. Apart from water, hydrating drinks that are rich in electrolytes are recommended for athletes.

Cool Down

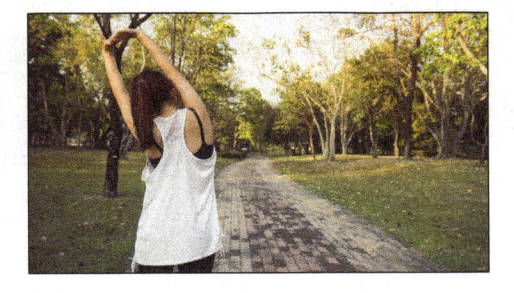

If warming up is important, cooling down is also essential. After working out or training, you have to spend at least 10 minutes of performing gentle exercises that will return your heart rate to a normal pace. By cooling down, you are allowing your body to remove excess wastes and allow the flow of oxygen and nutrients into your muscles.

Do Stretching

It is important that you maintain and develop flexibility in your body to prevent acquiring injuries. Poor flexibility is equivalent to short and tight muscles which cause muscle and tendon strains. Through stretching, you can improve or maintain your flexibility. After cooling down, make sure you spend time stretching.

Take Breaks

During a continuous training or a long play, remember to take a break so that your body and mind will have ample time to recover and gain energy. If you will not take a rest between sets or period, your mind will keep on pushing your body to work which will lead to injuries. It will also increase your risk to fatigue and decreased judgment. Thus, breaks are important for body recovery and mind refocusing.

Know the Rules of the Game

Basically, you have to be knowledgeable of the mechanics and rules of the sports. These rules are made to prevent athletes from acquiring injuries. For example, football restricts clipping, chop blocking and slapping a helmet to keep athletes safe. If you do not break the rules, then you do not endanger yourself to certain injuries.

Stop when Pain Occurs

Pain is the number one symptom of injury. If you experience a pain that is intolerable, stop playing or take a break. Pain is the earliest symptom of a possible injury. It will be followed by swelling, stiffness, instability, weakness, numbness, tingling and redness, among others. Pain can be felt in shoulders, elbows, wrists, fingers, spines, hips, knees, ankles and feet.

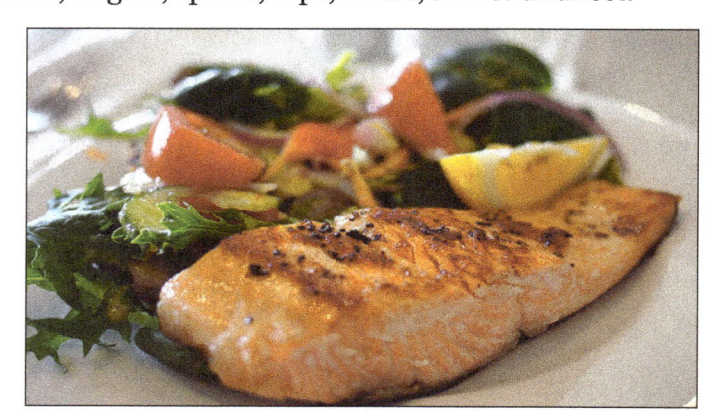

Eat Healthy

Diet and proper nutrition are important for athletes. A good nutrition plan is the foundation of an effective fitness program. The demands of sports and exercise on the body mean that you should replace all the energy and nutrients consumed by eating healthy food. For athletes, it is important that they eat regular, small meals to fuel their training or sport. They should also take protein to promote muscle health.

Price Method

Protection, Rest, Ice, Compression and Elevation, or P.R.I.C.E., adds the concept of "protection" to the traditional R.I.C.E. protocol formula. Protecting the injured area from further damage is crucial to the healing process.

Experts recommended acute injury patients use P.R.I.C.E. shortly after the injury occurs. It may be particularly helpful during the first 24 to 72 hours.

- P: Protection is meant to prevent further injury. For example, an injured leg or foot may be protected by limiting or avoiding weight-bearing through the use of crutches, a cane, or hiking poles. Partially immobilizing the injured area by using a sling, splint, or brace may also be a means of protection.

- R: Rest is important to allow for healing. However, many sports medicine specialists use the term "relative rest" meaning rest that allows for healing, but is not so restrictive that recovery is compromised or slowed. A person should avoid activities that stress the injured area to the point of pain or that may slow or prevent healing. Some movement, however, is beneficial. Gentle, pain-free, range-of-motion and basic isometric contractions of the joints and muscles surrounding an injury have been shown to speed recovery.

- I: Ice refers to the use of cold treatments, also known as cryotherapy, to treat acute injuries. Ice is recommended with the intent to minimize and reduce swelling as well as to decrease pain. There are many ways to employ cryotherapy at home. The most common and most convenient is a simple plastic bag of crushed ice placed over a paper towel on the affected area. It is important to protect the skin and limit the cold exposure to 10 to 15 minutes. Cycles of 10 to 15 minutes on and 1 to 2 hours off are generally agreed upon as effective as and safer than longer periods of continuous ice application.

    Skin sensitivity or allergy to cold exposure can occur. It may manifest as skin that becomes mottled, red and raised where the ice contacted the skin. If this is experienced, the ice treatments should be discontinued. Redness alone, however, is common and should resolve after a few minutes of re-warming.

- C: Compression is the use of a compression wrap, such as an elastic bandage, to apply an external force to the injured tissue. This compression minimizes swelling and provides mild support.

    Applying an elastic bandage does require some attention to detail. It should be applied directly to the skin by starting a few inches below the injury and wrapping in a figure eight or spiraling manner to a few inches above the injured area. A medium amount of tension should be applied to provide ample, but not too constrictive compression. The bandage should not cause numbness, tingling, or color change of the soft tissue. Loosening the bandage should quickly alleviate these should they occur. It is generally best to remove or significantly loosen the elastic bandage for sleeping and to re-apply it the next morning.

- E: Elevation is recommended to help reduce the pooling of fluid in the injured extremity or joint. Controlling swelling can help decrease pain and may limit the loss of range of motion, possibly speeding up recovery time.

- Elevation is accomplished by positioning the injured area above the level of the heart. Elevation during most of the waking hours, if possible, and positioning the injured limb on extra pillows for sleep is probably most effective in the initial 24 to 48 hours. If there is significant swelling which continues after 24 to 48 hours, or if swelling recurs during recovery, then continued periodic elevation is appropriate.

- For many sports and exercise injuries, ice can be secured over the affected area with an elastic bandage and the limb can then be elevated, achieving simultaneous Rest, Ice, Compression and Elevation—the optimum home treatment.

Cryotherapy

Cryotherapy literally means cold therapy. When you press a bag of frozen peas on a swollen ankle or knee, you are treating your pain with a modern (although basic) version of cryotherapy.

Cold therapy can be applied in various ways, including ice packs, coolant sprays, and ice massage, and whirlpools, or ice baths. When used to treat injuries at home, cold therapy refers to cold therapy with ice or gel packs that are usually kept in the freezer until needed. These remain one of the simplest, time-tested remedies for managing pain and swelling.

Using Cold Therapy

Cold therapy is the "I" component of R.I.C.E. (rest, ice, compression, and elevation). This is a treatment recommended for the home care of many injuries, particularly ones caused by sports.

Cold therapy for pain relief may be used for:

- Runner's knee.
- Tendonitis.
- Sprains.
- Arthritis pain.
- Pain and swelling after a hip or knee replacement.
- To treat pain or swelling under a cast or a splint.
- Lower back pain.

The benefits of applying ice include:

- It lowers your skin temperature.
- It reduces the nerve activity.
- It reduces pain and swelling.

Experts believe that cold therapy can reduce swelling, which is tied to pain. It may also reduce sensitivity to pain. Cold therapy may be particularly effective when you are managing pain with swelling, especially around a joint or tendon.

How to Apply Cold Therapy

Putting ice or frozen items directly on your skin can ease pain, but it also can damage your skin. It's best to wrap the cold object in a thin towel to protect your skin from the direct cold, especially if you are using gel packs from the freezer.

Apply the ice or gel pack for about 10 to 20 minutes several times a day. Check your skin often for sensation while using cold therapy. This will help make sure you aren't damaging the tissues.

You might need to combine cold therapy with other approaches to pain management:

- Rest: Take a break from activities that can make your pain worse.
- Compression: Applying pressure to the area can help control swelling and pain. This also stabilizes the area so that you do not further injure yourself.
- Elevation: Put your feet up, or elevate whatever body part is in pain.
- Pain medicine: Over-the-counter products can help ease discomfort.
- Rehabilitation exercises: Depending on where your injury is, you might want to try stretching and strengthening exercises that can support the area as recommended by your healthcare provider.

Stop applying ice if you lose feeling on the skin where you are applying it. If cold therapy doesn't help your pain go away, contact your healthcare provider. Also, you may want to avoid cold therapy if you have certain medical conditions, like diabetes, that affect how well you can sense tissue damage.

Cryotherapy can be delivered to just one area, or you can opt for whole-body cryotherapy. Localized cryotherapy can be administered in a number of ways, including through ice packs, ice massage, coolant sprays, ice baths, and even through probes administered into tissue.

The theory for whole-body cryotherapy (WBC) is that by immersing the body in extremely cold air for several minutes, you could receive a number of health benefits. The individual will stand in an enclosed chamber or a small enclosure that surrounds their body but has an opening for their head at the top. The enclosure will drop to between negative 200–300°F. They'll stay in the ultra-low temperature air for between two and four minutes.

You can get benefits from just one session of cryotherapy, but it's most effective when used regularly. Some athletes use cryotherapy twice a day. Others will go daily for 10 days and then once a month afterwards.

Benefits of Cryotherapy

Reduces Migraine Symptoms

Cryotherapy can help treat migraines by cooling and numbing nerves in the neck area. One study found that applying a neck wrap containing two frozen ice packs to the carotid arteries in the neck significantly reduced migraine pain in those tested. It's thought that this works by cooling the blood passing through intracranial vessels. The carotid arteries are close to the skin's surface and accessible.

Numbs Nerve Irritation

Many athletes have been using cryotherapy to treat injuries for years, and one of the reasons why is that it can numb pain. The cold can actually numb an irritated nerve. Doctors will treat the affected area with a small probe inserted into the nearby tissue. This can help treat pinched nerves or neuromas, chronic pain, or even acute injuries.

Helps Treat Mood Disorders

The ultra-cold temperatures in whole-body cryotherapy can cause physiological hormonal responses. This includes the release of adrenaline, noradrenaline, and endorphins. This can have a positive effect on those experiencing mood disorders like anxiety and depression. One study found that whole-body cryotherapy was actually effective in short-term treatment for both.

Reduces Arthritic Pain

Localized cryotherapy treatment isn't the only thing that's effective at treating serious conditions; one study found that whole-body cryotherapy significantly reduced pain in people with arthritis. They found that the treatment was well-tolerated. It also allowed for more aggressive physiotherapy and occupational therapy as a result. This ultimately made rehabilitation programs more effective.

May Help Treat Low-risk Tumors

Targeted, localized cryotherapy can be used as a cancer treatment. In this context, it's called "cryosurgery". It works by freezing cancer cells and surrounding them with ice crystals. It's currently being used to treat some low-risk tumors for certain types of cancer, including prostate cancer.

May Help Prevent Dementia and Alzheimer's Disease

While more research is needed to evaluate the effectiveness of this strategy, it's theorized that whole-body cryotherapy could help prevent Alzheimer's and other types of dementia. It's thought that may be an effective treatment because the anti-oxidative and anti-inflammatory effects of cryotherapy could help combat the inflammatory and oxidative stress responses that occur with Alzheimer's.

Treats Atopic Dermatitis and other Skin Conditions

Atopic dermatitis is a chronic inflammatory skin disease with signature symptoms of dry and itchy skin. Because cryotherapy can improve antioxidant levels in the blood and can simultaneously reduce inflammation, it makes sense that both localized and whole-body cryotherapy can help treat atopic dermatitis. Another study (in mice) examined its effect for acne, targeting the sebaceous glands.

Risks and Side Effects

The most common side effects of any type of cryotherapy are numbness, tingling, redness, and irritation of the skin. These side effects are almost always temporary. Make an appointment with your doctor if they don't resolve within 24 hours.

You should never use cryotherapy for longer than is recommended for the method of therapy you're using. For whole body cryotherapy, this would be more than four minutes. If you're using an ice pack or ice bath at home, you should never apply ice to the area for more than 20 minutes. Wrap ice packs in a towel so you don't damage your skin.

Those with diabetes or any conditions that affect their nerves should not use cryotherapy. They may be unable to fully feel its effect, which could lead to further nerve damage.

Tips and Guidelines for Cryotherapy

If you have any conditions you want to treat with cryotherapy, make sure you discuss them with the person assisting with or administering your treatment. It's always a good idea to consult your doctor before using any type of therapy.

If receiving whole body cryotherapy, wear dry, loose-fitting clothing. Bring socks and gloves to protect from frostbite. During therapy, move around if possible to keep your blood flowing.

If you're getting cryosurgery, your doctor will discuss specific preparations with you beforehand. This may include not eating or drinking for 12 hours beforehand.

Hydrotherapy

Hydrotherapy is the use of water to provide therapeutic effects for musculoskeletal and neural rehabilitation.

Hydrotherapy (sometimes called aquatic therapy) uses the principles of water to allow exercise and to alter exercise intensity. Increased buoyancy (opposite to gravity) allows for more exercise than is permitted on land. Increased temperature and hydrostatic pressure promote increases in circulation and flexibility and decrease in swelling. Increasing speed, turbulence and surface area can all be used to increase exercise difficulty.

A hydrotherapy pool is a swimming pool specifically designed for providing hydrotherapy treatments. The main difference is the increase in temperature. A hydrotherapy pool is heated to around 35 degrees Celsius. This allows for the patient to fully relax (and not tense up in cold water), promotes pain relief and encourages circulation.

Hydrotherapy pools should be rectangular in shape and may vary in depth to allow for walking as well as deepwater work. It should be easily accessible and have a hoist available to lower in those who are not able to enter the pool themselves.

Benefits of Hydrotherapy

Hydrotherapy can be very useful in treating many different types of soft tissue and bone injury as well as neuromuscular conditions such as muscular dystrophy. The benefits of hydrotherapy include:

- Pain relief.

- Reduction in muscle spasm.
- Increased joint range of motion.
- Strengthening of weak muscles.
- Increased circulation.
- Improvement of balance and coordination.
- Re-education of paralysed muscles.

Because of the buoyancy of the water, hydrotherapy allows many individuals to exercise, where they wouldn't be able to on land. The effect of this increased buoyancy and decreased gravitational force means that there is less stress on weight-bearing joints such as the knees and hips and many movements can be performed in water before they would be possible on land.

Uses of Hydrotherapy

Hydrotherapy may be useful in the following conditions:

- Arthritis – Both osteoarthritis and rheumatoid arthritis.
- Back pain.
- Musculoskeletal conditions – Such as frozen shoulder, ankle sprains and groin strains etc.
- Following surgery for conditions such as knee replacement, hip replacement, ACL reconstruction etc.
- Fibromyalgia.
- Neurological conditions including Muscular Dystrophy, Cerebral Palsy, Multiple Sclerosis, Parkinsons Disease etc.
- After strokes or head injuries.

Contraindications

In certain circumstances, hydrotherapy is not recommended.

- Inflammation – Acute injuries where redness and heat are still present are not recommended for hydrotherapy treatment.
- Fever – Whole body warming is not recommended if the temperature is present.
- Heart disease – Increased blood flow may place stress on the heart.
- Hypertension (high blood pressure).
- Vascular conditions – Increased circulation is not advised.
- Kidney problems.
- Cancer.
- Hemorrhage.

Exercises

There are many different types of exercise that can be undertaken in water and the form of exercise prescribed will vary to take into consideration the patient's injury or condition, ability and the facilities or equipment available.

Forms of Hydrotherapy

Hydrotherapy can include anything from floating in the water (Hot tubs) and simply benefiting from the increased temperature and relaxation properties, to full-on, intense exercise sessions. The form of hydrotherapy used will depend entirely on the individual in question and the facilities available.

Many land-based exercises can be adapted to use in the water. Walking in a pool is easier on the joints due to the buoyancy some state of the art facilities may even have underwater treadmills. Other exercises such as squats and lunges are easier too.

One method of hydrotherapy is known as the Bad Ragaz Ring Method. It is a method of muscle re-education where the patient is floated and specific patterns of resistance, endurance, elongation, relaxation, range of motion, and tonal reduction are used.

Exercise Difficulty

As mentioned above, all exercises can be progressed by increasing the speed of the movement or the turbulence of the water. Other methods of increasing difficulty include increasing surface area. This can be achieved for example by holding something wide in the hand (such as a racket or bat) when moving it through the water.

The buoyancy of the water can be used as either a tool to assist movement or to increase the difficulty of an exercise. For example, when exercising the shoulder, the water can be used to help in lifting the arm upwards from by the side. However, it will provide resistance against pushing the arm back down. This resistance can be increased further by attaching a float to the arm.

Treatment Options for Low Back Pain

Low back pain is one of the most common medical presentations in the general population. It is a common source of pain in athletes, leading to significant time missed and disability. The general categories of treatment for low back pain are medications and therapies.

The prevalence rates of low back pain in athletes range from 1% to 40%. Back injuries in the young athlete are a common phenomenon, occurring in 10% to 15% of participants. It is not clear if athletes experience low back pain more often than the general population. Comparisons of wrestlers, gymnasts, and adolescent athletes have found back pain more common versus age-matched controls. Other comparisons of athletes and nonathletes have found lower rates of low back pain in athletes than nonathletes.

Clinical examination and diagnostic skills are essential in the workup of low back pain. Athletes with neurologic compromise, fever, chills, or incontinence of bowel or bladder function or those with mechanism of action that could result in fracture or other serious injuries must first be evaluated for emergent causes. Workup and diagnosis must be individualized on the basis of differential diagnosis.

Because of the limited number of high-quality randomized controlled trials or systemic reviews involving athletes, most of the following recommendations are summaries of the current evidence for back pain in the general population.

Sports that have higher rates of back pain include gymnastics, diving, weight lifting, golf, football, and rowing. In gymnastics, the incidence of back injuries is 11%. In football linemen, it may be as high as 50%. Ninety percent of all injuries of professional golfers involve the neck or back. Injury rates for 15- and 16-year-old girls in gymnastics, dance, or gym training are higher than the general population, while cross-country skiing and aerobics are associated with a lower prevalence of low back pain. For boys, volleyball, gymnastics, weight lifting, downhill skiing, and snowboarding are associated with higher prevalence of low back pain, while cross-country skiing and aerobics show a lower prevalence.

Back pain is a symptom and has many causes. Muscle strains, ligament sprains, and soft tissue contusions account for as much as 97% of back pain in the general adult population. The majority of athletes with low back pain have a benign source of pain. Muscle strain may be the most common cause of low back pain in college athletes.

The clinical spectrum of spondylolysis, spondylolisthesis, and pars interarticularis stress fractures may be the most common cause of low back pain in adolescents. Repetitive hyperextension of the low back (gymnastics, figure skating, diving, and football linemen) is a risk factor for the development of spondylolysis.

Hyperlordosis (lordotic low back pain) is the second most common cause of adolescent low back pain. This condition is related to adolescent growth spurts when the axial skeleton grows faster than the surrounding soft tissue, resulting in muscular pain. Other causes of low back pain unique to children are vertebral endplate fractures and bacterial infection of the vertebral disk. Adolescents have weaker cartilage in the endplate of the outer annulus fibrosis, allowing avulsion and resulting in symptoms similar to a herniated vertebral disk. Additionally, the pediatric lumbar spine has blood vessels that traverse the vertebral bodies and supply the vertebral disk, increasing the chance of developing diskitis.

Treatment Options

Cold versus Heat

Cold can be applied to the low back with towels, gel packs, ice packs, and ice massage. Heat methods include water bottles and baths, soft packs, saunas, steam, wraps, and electric pads. There are few high-quality randomized controlled trials supporting superficial cold or heat therapy for the treatment of acute or subacute low back pain. A review cited moderate evidence supporting superficial heat therapy as reducing pain and disability in patients with acute and subacute low back pain, with the addition of exercise further reducing pain and improved function. The effects of superficial heat seem strongest for the first week following injury.

Ultrasound

There are no systemic reviews for ultrasound. One small nonrandomized trial for patients with acute sciatica found ultrasonography superior to sham ultrasonography or analgesics for relief of pain. All patients were prescribed bed rest. For patients with chronic back pain, the small trials were contradictory to whether ultrasonography was any better than sham ultrasonography.

Laser

Low-level laser therapy (LLLT) is a noninvasive light source treatment that generates a single wavelength of light without generating heat, sound, or vibration. Also called photobiology or biostimulation, LLLT may accelerate connective tissue repair and serve as an anti-inflammatory agent. Wavelengths from 632 to 904 nm are used in the treatment of musculoskeletal disorders. A review of 7 small studies with a total of 384 patients with nonspecific low back pain of varying durations found insufficient data to either support or refute the effectiveness of LLLT for the treatment of low back pain. Because of the varied length of treatment, LLLT dose, application techniques, and different populations, it was not possible to determine optimal administration of LLLT. No side effects were reported.

A recent double-blind randomized placebo-controlled study of 546 patients with acute low back pain (less than 4 weeks) with radiculopathy compared LLLT and nimesulide to nimesulide alone to sham LLLT. Treatment with LLLT and nimesulide improved movement, with more significant reduction in pain intensity and disability and with improvement in quality of life, compared with patients treated only with drugs or placebo LLLT.

Medications

Steroids

Three small higher quality trials found that systemic corticosteroids were not clinically beneficial compared with placebo when given parenterally or as a short oral taper for acute or chronic sciatica. With acute low back pain and a negative straight-leg raise test, no difference in pain relief through 1 month was found between a single intramuscular injection of methylprednisolone (160 mg) or placebo. Glucocorticosteroids are banned by the World Anti-doping Association.

Nonsteroidal Anti-inflammatory Drugs

A large review of 65 trials (11 237 patients) of nonsteroidal anti-inflammatory drugs (NSAIDs) and COX-2 inhibitors in the treatment of acute and chronic low back pain showed that NSAIDs had statistically better effects compared with placebo. The benefits included global improvement and less additional analgesia requirement. NSAIDs were associated with higher rate of side effects. There was no strong evidence that any one NSAID or COX-2-selective NSAID is clinically superior to the others. NSAIDs were not superior to acetaminophen, but NSAIDs had more side effects. NSAIDs were not more effective that physiotherapy or spinal manipulation for acute low back pain. COX-2-selective NSAIDs had fewer side effects than nonselective NSAIDs.

Muscle Relaxants

Several systemic reviews have found skeletal muscle relaxants effective for short-term symptomatic relief in acute and chronic low back pain. However, the incidence of drowsiness, dizziness, and other side effects is high. There is minimal evidence on the efficacy of the antispasticity drugs (dantrolene and baclofen) for low back pain.

Opioids

A 2007 review of opioids for chronic low back pain found that tramadol was more effective than placebo for pain relief and improving function. The 2 most common side effects of tramadol were headaches and nausea. One trial comparing opioids to naproxen found that opioids were significantly better for relieving pain but not improving function. Despite the frequent use of opioids for long-term management of chronic LBP, there are few high-quality trials assessing efficacy. The benefits of opioids for chronic LBP remain questionable. There is no evidence that sustained-release opioid formulations are superior to immediate-release formulations for low back pain. Long-acting opioids did not differ in head-to-head trials.[9] Opioids are banned by the World Anti-doping Association.

Antidepressants

A review of 10 antidepressant and placebo trials showed no difference in pain relief or depression severity. The qualitative analyses found conflicting evidence on the effect of antidepressants on pain intensity in chronic low back pain and no clear evidence that antidepressants reduce depression in chronic low-back-pain patients. Two pooled analyses showed no difference in pain relief between different types of antidepressants and placebo. Another systemic review found different results: Antidepressants were more effective than placebo, but the effects were not consistent with all antidepressants. Tricyclic antidepressants were moderately more effective than placebo, but paroxetine and trazodone were not. Antidepressants were associated with significantly higher risk for adverse events compared with placebo, with drowsiness, dry mouth, dizziness, and constipation the most commonly reported. Duloxetine has recently been approved by the Food and Drug Administration for treatment of chronic low back pain and osteoarthritis, and evidence suggests effectiveness in chronic low back pain.

Manipulation: Chiropractic, Osteopathic and Manual Physical Therapy

Three systemic reviews analyzed spinal manipulation therapy (SMT) for low back pain, including (1) high-velocity, low-amplitude manipulation of the spinal joints slightly beyond their passive range of motion; (2) high-velocity, low-amplitude technique rotating the thigh and leg; (3) mobilization within passive range of motion; and (4) instrument-based manipulations. There is moderate evidence of short-term pain relief with acute low back pain treated with SMT. Chronic low back pain showed moderate improvement with SMT, which is as effective as NSAIDs and more effective than physical therapy in the long term. Patients with mixed acute and chronic low back pain had better pain outcomes in the short and long terms compared with McKenzie therapy, medical care, management by physical therapists, soft tissue treatment, and back school. SMT was more effective in reducing pain and improving daily activities when compared with sham therapy. Dagenais found SMT effective in pain reduction in the short-, intermediate-, and long-term management of acute low back pain. However, a review in 2004 on SMT in acute and chronic low back pain concluded that there was no difference in pain reduction or ability to perform daily activities with SMT or standard treatments (medications, physical therapy, exercises, back school, or the care of a general practitioner).

Injections

A review of randomized controlled trials for subacute and chronic low back pain included 18 trials of 1179 participants. Studies that compared intradiscal injections, prolotherapy, ozone, sacroiliac joint injections, or epidural steroids for radicular pain were excluded unless injection therapy with another pharmaceutical agent was part of one of the treatment arms. Corticosteroids, local anesthetics, indomethacin, sodium hyaluronate, and B12 were used. Of 18 trials, 10 were rated for high methodological quality. Statistical pooling was not possible because of clinical heterogeneity in the trials yielding no strong evidence for or against the use of injection therapy.

Botulinum toxin was compared in a review that found significant study heterogeneity and low- to very-low-quality evidence for botulinum toxin in the treatment of nonspecific chronic low back pain. One new trial has shown no benefit with botulinum toxin injections for myofascial pain syndrome.

A small study on spinal injections in 32 athletes with acute, subacute, and chronic low back pain with sciatic nerve involvement showed that only 14% were able to return to participation.

Acupuncture

Thirty-five randomized controlled trials did not allow firm conclusions for the effectiveness of acupuncture for acute low back pain. For chronic low back pain, acupuncture is more effective for pain relief and functional improvement than no treatment or sham treatment in the short term only. Acupuncture is not more effective than other conventional or alternative treatments.

Massage

Massage might be beneficial for patients with subacute and chronic nonspecific low back pain, especially when combined with exercises and education. Acupressure or pressure point massage technique was more effective than classic massage. A second systemic review found insufficient evidence to determine efficacy of massage for acute low back pain. Evidence was insufficient to determine effects of the number or duration of massage sessions.

Traction

A meta-analysis found traction no more effective than placebo, sham, or no treatment for any outcome for low back pain with or without sciatica. The results consistently indicated that continuous or intermittent traction as a single treatment for low back pain is not effective. Side effects included worsening of signs and symptoms and increased subsequent surgery; however, the reports are inconsistent.

Transcutaneous Electrical Nerve Stimulation

Evidence from the small number of placebo-controlled trials does not support the use of transcutaneous electrical nerve stimulation in the routine management of chronic low back pain. Evidence from single lower quality trials is insufficient to accurately judge efficacy of transcutaneous electrical nerve stimulation versus other interventions for chronic low back pain or acute low back pain.

Bracing/Lumbar Supports

Braces are not effective in preventing back pain. However, there is conflicting evidence to whether braces are effective supplements to other preventive interventions. Bracing, in combination with activity restriction, is effective in the treatment of spondylolysis in adolescents. A meta-analysis of 15 observational spondylolysis and grade 1 spondylolisthesis treatment studies did not find a significant improvement in rates of healing with bracing when compared with conservative treatment without bracing. Most experts recommend surgical consultation for spondylolisthesis with 50% slippage or more (grade 3 and higher).

Back Schools

There is moderate evidence suggesting that back schools reduce pain and improve function and return-to-work status when compared with exercises, manipulation, myofascial therapy, advice, or placebo. The patients benefiting from back schools had chronic and recurrent nonspecific low back pain in an occupational setting.

Exercise

Exercise therapy appears to be slightly effective at decreasing pain and improving function in adults with chronic low back pain. In subacute low back pain, there is weak evidence that a graded activity program improves absenteeism. In acute low back pain, exercise therapy was no better than no treatment or conservative treatments. Exercise therapy using individualized regimens, supervision, stretching, and strengthening was associated with the best outcomes. The addition of exercise to other noninvasive therapies was associated with small improvements in pain and function.

A randomized single-blind controlled trial compared manual therapy and spinal stabilization rehabilitation to control (education booklet) for chronic back pain. Spinal stabilization rehabilitation was more effective than either manipulation or the education booklet in reducing pain, disability, medication intake, and improving the quality of life for chronic low back pain. A systemic review found segmental stabilizing exercises more effective in reducing the recurrence of pain in acute low back pain; however, exercises were no better than treatment by general practitioner in reducing short-term disability and pain. For chronic low back pain, segmental stabilizing exercises were more effective than treatment from general practitioners but no more effective than exercises using devices, massage, electrotherapy, or heat. In a trial of 30 hockey players, dynamic muscular stabilization techniques (an active approach to stabilization training) were more effective than a combination of ultrasound and short-wave diathermy and lumbar strengthening exercises.

The McKenzie method uses clinical examination to separate patients with low back pain into subgroups (postural, dysfunction, and derangement) to determine appropriate treatment. The goal is symptom relief through individualized treatment by the patient at home. The McKenzie method is not exclusively extension exercises; it emphasizes patient education to decrease pain quickly, restore function, minimize the number of visits to the clinic, and prevent recurrences. Two systemic reviews have compared the McKenzie method with different conclusions. Clare concluded that McKenzie therapy resulted in decreased short-term (less than 3 months) pain and disability when compared with NSAIDs, educational booklet, back massage with back care advice, strength training with therapist supervision, and spinal mobilization. Machado concluded that the McKenzie method does not produce clinically worthwhile changes in pain and disability when compared with passive therapy and advice to stay active for acute LBP.

A separate review evaluated bed rest versus activity in acute low back pain and sciatica. There were small benefits in pain relief and functional improvement from staying active compared with rest in bed.

Return-to-play

Return-to-play (RTP) guidelines are difficult to standardize for low back pain because of a lack of supporting evidence. A commonly encountered question is, can athletes play through pain? There is no simple answer to this question. For example, an athlete with suspected spondylolysis is generally advised that he or she should not play through pain, while athletes with chronic low back pain from muscular or ligamentous strain may continue to practice, exercise, and compete. However, there is little evidence to support either of these approaches. These athletes should always be monitored for their safety.

Expert opinion guidelines on RTP time frames have been published for lumbar spine conditions. Lumbar strains should achieve full range of motion before RTP. Patients with spondylolysis and spondylolisthesis (grade 1) should rest 4 to 6 weeks and then demonstrate full range of motion and pain-free extension before RTP. Athletes with herniated lumbar disks should rest 6 to 12 weeks following surgical treatment, while those with spinal fusion should wait 1 year to return to activity. Many surgeons advise against return to contact sports following spinal fusion. Iwamoto reviewed conservative and surgical treatments in athletes with lumbar disc herniation and time to return to previous level of sports activity. Seventy-nine percent of conservatively treated athletes returned in an average of 4.7 months, while 85% of those treated with microdiscectomy returned in 5.2 to 5.8 months. Sixty-nine percent of percutaneous discectomies returned in 7 weeks to 12 months.

Non-surgical Treatments

Bracing

Braces or splints are specifically designed devices that safely support an injured area in correct position to induce the healing process. Braces are comprised of specific material that provides warmth and compression to the affected joint and soft tissues. Bracing involves wrapping the specific brace or splint around the injured area as recommended by your physician.

How does Bracing Help

Braces are widely recommended for the management of injuries. Bracing plays an important role, both in prevention and therapeutic management. It helps to prevent further damage of the injured area, without affecting the daily activity of the person. Braces also are effective in healing muscular injuries, including damage to soft tissues such as tendons and ligaments.

The type of bracing depends upon the affected area (knee, wrist, and elbow etc.) and severity of the sports injury. Usually bracing will be more effective in treating mild to moderate injuries, rather than abrupt severe injuries.

For better recovery of injuries, bracing should be used along with physical therapy and strengthening exercises.

Cortisone Injection

Cortisone is a corticosteroid released by the adrenal gland in response to stress and is a potent anti-inflammatory agent.

Indications for Cortisone Injections

Cortisone injections are recommended in injuries that cause pain and inflammation, and those that don't require surgical treatment. One such condition is frozen shoulder.

Cortisone Injection Procedure

Artificial preparations containing cortisone are injected directly into the affected joint to relieve pain and reduce inflammation. The effects may last for several weeks and cortisone injections.

Risks and Complications of Cortisone Injections

Cortisone injections offer significant relief in pain and inflammation; however, is associated with certain adverse effects. The most common side effect is a "cortisone flare", a condition where cortisone crystallizes and cause severe pain for a brief period that lasts for a day or two. Cortisone flare can be minimized by applying ice to the injected area. Other adverse effects include whitening of the skin and infection at the injection site, a transient elevation in blood sugar if you are diabetic.

Shockwave Therapy

Shockwave therapy is a non-invasive method of treating soft tissue injuries. Shock wave is a short energy wave with high intensity, traveling faster than sound.

Indication for Shockwave Therapy

Shockwave therapy is used to treat many musculoskeletal conditions such as attachment points for ligaments and bones. A very common indication is heel spurs. It is also indicated for jumper's knee, Achilles tendon injury, connective tissue pain and degeneration, muscle pain and injuries. Shockwave therapy is also used for bone healing conditions like stress fractures, avascular necrosis (dead portion of bone), non-healing bone or slow healing bone.

Preparation for Shockwave Therapy

The shockwave treatment course involves two outpatient sessions. The duration between the sessions is 1 week. You should not consume heavy meals before the session and you will be asked to wear loose-fitting clothes.

Shockwave Therapy Procedure

During the session, you will sit comfortably on a table. A scanner will be used to guide the shockwave emitter exactly to the site of injury. Around 2000 shockwaves will be fired and a tapping sensation will be followed with each shockwave. Duration of each session is about 30 minutes.

Post-treatment Care for Shockwave Therapy

You can continue with your regular daily activities immediately after each session. In cases of heel spurs, running should be avoided for a week or more after the second session.

Advantages of Shockwave Therapy

The shockwave therapy does not disintegrate tissue; rather, it causes biological effects that help in tissue regeneration. It reduces pain and sensitivity immediately by over-stimulating pain transmission nerves. The therapy triggers the repair mechanism of the body by formation of new blood vessels. The shockwave stimulates osteoblasts (bone cells) in the body and promotes bone healing and new bone production.

Risks and Complications

Shockwave therapy is considered a safe and effective treatment option for soft tissue injuries. It has no major risks but may be associated with minor risks such as:

- Pain (energy levels of shock waves can be adjusted to your individual tolerance levels).
- It is not preferred if you have bone tumors, metabolic bone conditions, and nerve or circulation disorders.
- It is not recommended if you are pregnant, have areas of infection, locations where gas is present in the body and on locations where bone is still growing.

Viscosupplementation

Viscosupplementation refers to the injection of a hyaluronan preparation into the joint. Hyaluronan is a natural substance present in the joint fluid that assists in lubrication. It allows smooth movement of the cartilage covered articulating surfaces of the joint.

Indications of Viscosupplementation

Synvisc is one of the most commonly used hyaluronan preparations. It is indicated in the management of shoulder, knee, hip or ankle osteoarthritis that has not responded to non-surgical treatment options such as pain medications, physical therapy and corticosteroid injections.

Viscosupplementation Procedure

Synvisc provides symptomatic relief and delays the need for surgery. It is injected directly into the joint to replenish the diminished synovial fluid, thereby enhancing its lubricating properties. A single dose or a total of three separate doses of Synvisc, over several weeks, may be required for optimum benefit.

How does Viscosupplementation Work

Synvisc injection not only supplements the hyaluronan in the joint but also stimulates the production of hyaluronan in the treated knee. This provides gradual symptomatic relief over the course of the injections. This effect may last for several months.

Post-procedural Care Following Viscosupplementation

Ice packs and an analgesic may be used, if required, to ease the discomfort. Any strenuous activity such as jogging or tennis should be completely avoided for 48 hours to a week after the injection and should be resumed only after consultation with your doctor.

Risks of Viscosupplementation

You may experience mild pain, swelling, warmth and redness at the injection site for up to 48 hours following a Synvisc injection. Headache and joint stiffness may also occur in some cases.

Immediately consult your doctor if you develop fever or the pain and swelling fail to resolve after 48 hours following the injection.

Sports Injury Rehabilitation

Sports injury rehabilitation is a safe, therapeutic approach that helps athletes effectively treat pain and achieve optimal performance with targeted exercises to help you return to pre-injury function. Personalized exercise prescription to improve mobility restrictions reduced susceptibility to further sport-related injuries.

Musculoskeletal injuries are an inevitable result of sport participation. Football has the highest incidence of catastrophic injuries, with gymnastics and ice hockey close behind. Tissue injury from sports can be classified as macrotraumatic and microtraumatic.

- Macrotraumatic injuries are usually due to a strong force – such as a fall, accident, collision or laceration and are more common in contact sports such as football and rugby. These injuries can be primary (due to direct tissue damage) or secondary (due to transmission of forces or release of inflammatory mediators and other cytokinesis).
- Microtraumatic injuries are chronic injuries that result from overuse of a structure such as a muscle, joint, ligament, or tendon. This type of injury is more common in sports such as swimming, cycling and rowing.

The process of rehabilitation should start as early as possible after an injury and form a continuum with other therapeutic interventions. It can also start before or immediately after surgery when an injury requires a surgical intervention.

Rehabilitation Plan

The rehabilitation plan must take into account the fact that the objective of the patient (the athlete) is to return to the same activity and environment in which the injury occurred. Functional capacity after rehabilitation should be the same, if not better, than before injury.

The ultimate goal of the rehabilitation process is to limit the extent of the injury, reduce or reverse the impairment and functional loss, and prevent, correct or eliminate altogether the disability.

Multidisciplinary Approach

The rehabilitation of the injured athlete is managed by a multidisciplinary team with a physician functioning as the leader and coordinator of care. The team includes, but is not limited to, sports physicians, physiatrists (rehabilitation medicine practitioners), orthopaedists, physiotherapists, rehabilitation workers, physical educators, coaches, athletic trainers, psychologists, and nutritionists. The rehabilitation team works closely with the athlete and the coach to establish the rehabilitation goals, to discuss the progress resulting from the various interventions, and to establish the time frame for the return of the athletes to training and competition.

Communication is a vital factor. A lack of communication between medical providers, strength and conditioning specialists, and team coaches can slow or prevent athletes from returning to peak capability and increase the risk of new injuries and even more devastating reinjures.

Principles

Principles are the foundation upon which rehabilitation is based. Here are seven principles of rehabilitation, which can be remembered by the mnemonic: ATC IS IT.

A: Avoid Aggravation

It is important not to aggravate the injury during the rehabilitation process. Therapeutic exercise, if administered incorrectly or without good judgement, has the potential to exacerbate the injury, that is, makes it worse.

T: Timing

The therapeutic exercise portion of the rehabilitation program should begin as soon as possible—that is, as soon as it can occur without causing aggravation. The sooner patients can begin the exercise portion of the rehabilitation program, the sooner they can return to full activity. Following injury, rest is sometimes necessary, but too much rest can actually be detrimental to recovery.

C: Compliance

Without a compliant patient, the rehabilitation program will not be successful. To ensure compliance, it is important to inform the patient of the content of the program and the expected course of rehabilitation.

I: Individualization

Each person responds differently to an injury and to the subsequent rehabilitation program. Even though an injury may seem the same in type and severity as another, undetectable differences can change an individual's response to it. Individual physiological and chemical differences profoundly affect a patient's specific responses to an injury.

S: Specific Sequencing

A therapeutic exercise program should follow a specific sequence of events. This specific sequence is determined by the body's physiological healing response.

I: Intensity

The intensity level of the therapeutic exercise program must challenge the patient and the injured area but at the same time must not cause aggravation. Knowing when to increase intensity without overtaxing the injury requires observation of the patient's response and consideration of the healing process.

T: Total Patient

It must be considered the total patient in the rehabilitation process. It is important for the unaffected areas of the body to stay finely tuned. This means keeping the cardiovascular system at a preinjury level and maintaining range of motion, strength, coordination, and muscle endurance of the uninjured limbs and joints. The whole body must be the focus of the rehabilitation program, not just the injured area. Providing the patient with a program to keep the uninvolved areas in peak condition, rather than just rehabilitating the injured area, will help to better prepare the patient physically and psychologically for when the injured area is completely rehabilitated.

Components

Regardless of the specifics of the injury, however, here are fundamental components that need to be included in all successful rehabilitation programs.

Pain Management

Medications are a mainstay of treatment in the injured athlete - both for their pain relief and healing properties. It is recommended that they need to be used judiciously with a distinct regard for the risks and side effects as well as the potential benefits, which include pain relief and early return to play. Therapeutic modalities play a small, but important, part in the rehabilitation of sports injuries. They may help to decrease pain and enema to allow an exercise-based rehabilitation programme to proceed. By understanding the physiological basis of these modalities, a safe and appropriate treatment choice can be made, but its effectiveness will ultimately depend upon the patient's individualized and subjective response to treatment.

Flexibility and Joint ROM

Injury or surgery can result in decreased joint ROM mainly due to fibrosis and wound contraction. Besides that, it is common for post-injury flexibility to be diminished as a result of muscle spasm, inflammation, swelling and pain. In addition to impacting the injured area, this also affects the joints above and below the problem, and creates motor pattern issues. Flexibility training is an important component of rehabilitation in order to minimize the decrease in joint ROM. Also, a variety of stretching techniques can be used in improving range of motion, including PNF, ballistic stretching and static stretching.

Strength and Endurance

Injuries to the musculoskeletal system could result in skeletal muscle hypotrophy and weakness, loss of aerobic capacity and fatigability. During rehabilitation after a sports injury it is important to try to maintain cardiovascular endurance. Thus regular bicycling, one-legged bicycling or arm cycling, an exercise programme in a pool using a wet vest or general major muscle exercise programmes with relatively high intensity and short rest periods (circuit weight training) can be of major importance.

Proprioception and Coordination

Proprioception can be defined as 'a special type of sensitivity that informs about the sensations of the deep organs and of the relationship between muscles and joints'. Loss of proprioception occurs with injury to ligaments, tendons, or joints, and also with immobilization. Proprioceptive re-education has to get the muscular receptors working, in order to provide a rapid motor response (Scott 2000). Restoration of proprioception is an important part of rehabilitation. The treatment has to be adapted to each individual, considering the type of injury and the stress to which the athlete will be exposed when practicing his or her sport.

Coordination can be defined as 'the capacity to perform movements in a smooth, precise and controlled manner'. Rehabilitation techniques increasingly refer to neuromuscular re-education. Improving coordination depends on repeating the positions and movements associated with different sports and correct training. It has to begin with simple activities, performed slowly and perfectly executed, gradually increasing in speed and complexity. The technician should make sure that the athlete performs these movements unconsciously, until they finally become automatic.

Functional Rehabilitation

All rehabilitation programs must take into account, and reproduce, the activities and movements required when the athlete returns to the field post-injury. The goal of function-based rehabilitation programmes is the return of the athlete to optimum athletic function. Optimal athletic function is the result of physiological motor activations creating specific biomechanical motions and positions using intact anatomical structures to generate forces and actions.

The use of Orthotics

The use of orthotic devices to support musculoskeletal function and the correction of muscle imbalances and inflexibility in uninjured areas should receive the attention of the rehabilitation team. Appropriate orthotic application will result in restraint forces that oppose an undesired motion. A complete orthotic prescription should include the patient's diagnosis, consider the type of footwear to be used, include the joints it encompasses and specify the desired biomechanical alignment, as well as the materials for fabrication. Communication with the orthotist, who will fabricate or fit the brace, is of utmost importance in order to obtain a good clinical result.

Psychology of Injury

Injury is more than physical; that is, the athlete must be psychologically ready for the demands of his or her sport. The most immediate emotional response at the point of injury is shock. Its degree may range from minor to significant, depending upon the severity of the injury. It is important to note that denial itself is an adaptive response that allows an individual to manage extreme emotional responses to situational stress. Many individuals assist athletes through the recovery process and can foster psychological readiness, but they can also identify those who are physically recovered but require more time or intervention to be fully prepared to return to competition. Thus, rehabilitation and recovery are not purely physical but also psychological.

Mental skills in sports are often viewed as part of an individual's personality and something that cannot be taught. Many physicians feel that injured athletes either have or do not have the mental toughness to progress through rehabilitation. Mental skills, however, can be learned. One example for this is to provide proper goal setting, which has very important role in sports rehabilitation, because they can enhance recovery from injury. Goal setting needs to be measurable and stated in behavioral terms. The research indicates that goals should be challenging and difficult, yet attainable. It is important for physicians to help them focus on short-term goals as a means to attain long-term goals. For example, to set daily and weekly goals in rehabilitation process which will end in long-term goal like returning to play after an injury? It is important for sports medicine physicians to assist patients in setting goals related to performance process rather than outcomes, such as returning to play.

Stages of Rehabilitation

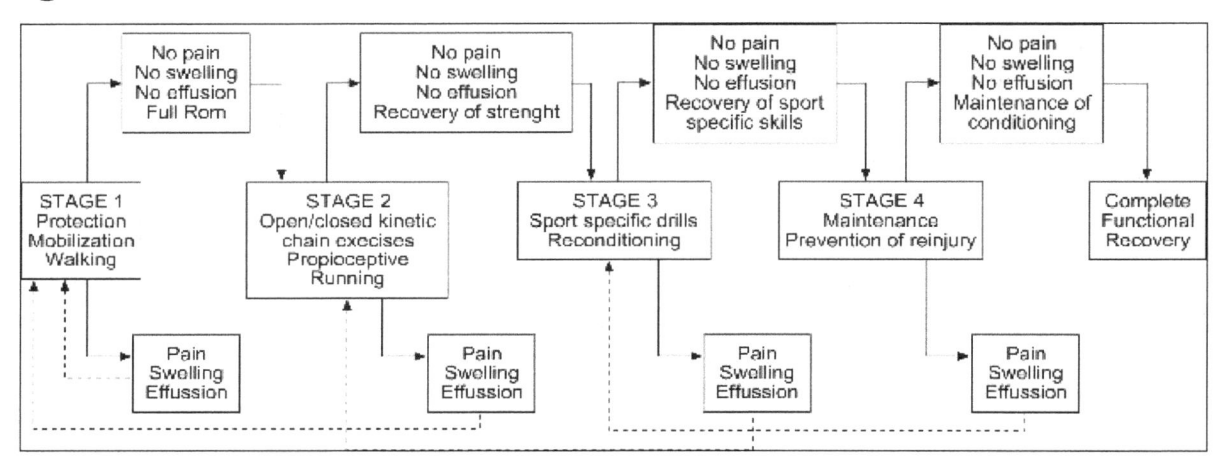

Stage	Criteria	Focus
STAGE 1	No pain, No swelling, No effusion, Full Rom	Protection, Mobilization, Walking
STAGE 2	No pain, No swelling, No effusion, Recovery of strenght	Open/closed kinetic chain excises, Propioceptive, Running
STAGE 3	No pain, No swelling, No effusion, Recovery of sport specific skills	Sport specific drills, Reconditioning
STAGE 4	No pain, No swelling, No effusion, Maintenance of conditioning	Maintenance, Prevention of reinjury
Complete Functional Recovery		

(If Pain, Swelling, Effussion occur at any stage, return to previous stage.)

Initial Stage of Rehabilitation

This phase lasts approximately 4-6 days. The body's first response to an injury is inflammation. It's main function is to defend the body against harmful substances, dispose of dead or dying tissue and to promote the renewal of normal tissue. The goals during the initial phase of the rehabilitation process include limitation of tissue damage, pain relief, control of the inflammatory response to injury, and protection of the affected anatomical area. The pathological events that take place immediately after the injury could lead to impairments such as muscle atrophy and weakness and limitation in the joint range of motion. These impairments result in functional losses, for example, inability to jump or lift an object. The extent of the functional loss may be influenced by the nature and timing of the therapeutic and rehabilitative intervention during the initial phase of the injury. If functional losses are severe or become permanent, the athlete now with a disability may be unable to participate in his/her sport.

The physiotherapist is usually the professional in charge of this phase although the process may be started by a medical doctor.

Intermediate Stage of Rehabilitation

This phase lasts from day 5 to 8-10 weeks. After the inflammatory phase, the body begins to repair the damaged tissue with similar tissue, but the resiliency of the new tissue is low. Repair of the weakened injury site can take up to eight weeks if the proper amount of restorative stress is applied, or longer if too much or too little stress is applied.

Joint ROM and Muscle Conditioning

The goals during the second phase of rehabilitation include the limitation of the impairment and the recovery from the functional losses. Early protected motion hastens the optimal alignment of collagen fibers and promotes improved tissue mobility. A number of physical modalities are used to enhance tissue healing. Exercise to regain flexibility, strength, endurance, balance, and coordination become the central component of the intervention. To the extent that these impairments and functional losses were minimized by early intervention, progress in this phase can be accelerated. Again, the maintenance of muscular and cardiorespiratory function remains essential for the uninjured areas of the body. The strength and conditioning professional has considerable expertise to offer the other members of the sports medicine team regarding selection of the appropriate activities.

Possible exercise forms during this phase include strengthening of the uninjured extremities and areas proximal and distal to the injury, aerobic and anaerobic exercise, and improving strength and neuromuscular control of the involved areas:

- Isometric exercise may be performed provided that it is pain free and otherwise indicated. Submaximal isometric exercise allows the athlete to maintain neuromuscular function and improve strength with movements performed at an intensity low enough that the newly formed collagen fibers are not disrupted.

- Isokinetic exercise can be an important aspect of strengthening following injury. This type of exercise uses equipment that provides resistance to movement at a given speed (e.g., 60°/s or 120°/s).

- Isotonic exercise involves movements with constant external resistance and the amount of force required moving the resistance varies, depending primarily on joint angle and the length of each agonist muscle. Isotonic exercise uses several different forms of resistance, including gravity (i.e., exercises performed without equipment, with gravitational effects as the only source of resistance), dumbbells, barbells, and weight-stack machines. The speed at which the movement occurs is controlled by the athlete; movement speed can be a program design variable, with more acute injuries calling for slower movement and the later phases of healing amenable to faster, more sport-specific movement.

- Specific types of exercises exist to improve neuromuscular control following injury and can be manipulated through alterations in surface stability, vision, and speed. Mini-trampolines, balance boards, and stability balls can be used to create unstable surfaces for upper and lower extremity training. Athletes can perform common activities such as squats and push-ups on uneven surfaces to improve neuromuscular control.

- Exercises may also be performed with eyes closed, thus removing visual input, to further challenge balance.

Finally, increasing the speed at which exercises are performed provides additional challenges to the system. Specifically controlling these variables within a controlled environment will allow the athlete to progress to more challenging exercises in the next stage of healing.

Advanced Stage of Rehabilitation

This phase begins at around 21 days and can continue for 6-12 months. The outcome of the previous phase is the replacement of damaged tissue with collagen fibers. After those fibers are laid down, the body can begin to remodel and strengthen the new tissue, allowing the athlete to gradually return to full activity. This phase of rehabilitation represents the start of the conditioning process needed to return to sports training and competition. Understanding the demands of the particular sport becomes essential as well as communication with the coach. This phase also represents an opportunity to identify and correct risk factors, thus reducing the possibility of re-injury.

Functional Training

The combination of clinic-based and sport-specific functional techniques will provide an individualized, sport-specific rehabilitation protocol for the athlete. Rehabilitation and reconditioning exercises must be functional to facilitate a return to competition. Examples of functional training include joint angle-specific strengthening, velocity-specific muscle activity, closed kinetic chain exercises, and exercises designed to further enhance neuromuscular control. Strengthening should transition from general exercises to sport-specific exercises designed to replicate movements common in given sports. Cross-training is encouraged, especially with activities that do not produce any symptoms from the injury.

It is essential that the rehabilitation and training be sufficiently vigorous to prepare the injured tissue for the demands of the game. With each increase in activity, signs of recurring pain or weakness should trigger a slowdown or a reversal to a tolerable level of activity. The player will have returned to game during this phase and will have ceased physiotherapy or individual rehabilitation while this process is still continuing. Unrestricted sports activity is not allowed until all of these steps have been completed and full-effort sports-specific activity is tolerated without symptoms.

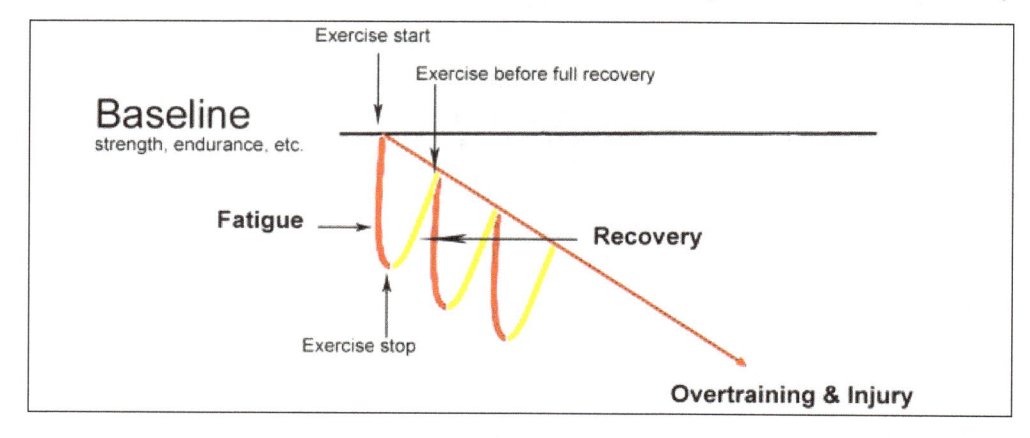

Return to Sport

At some point in the recovery process, athletes return to strength and conditioning programs and resume sport-specific activities in preparation for return to play. The transition is important for several reasons. First, although the athlete may have recovered in medical terms (ie, improvements in flexibility, range of motion, functional strength, pain, neuromuscular control, inflammation), preparation for competition requires the restoration of strength, power, speed, agility, and endurance at levels exhibited in sport.

Return to play is defined as the process of deciding when an injured or ill athlete may safely return to practice or competition. Early return to training and sport are considered sensible goals if the rate of return is based on the affected muscle, the severity of the injury and the position of the athlete.

Criteria for return to play must emphasize gradual return to sport-specific functional progressions. Sport-specific function occurs when the activations, motions and resultant forces are specific and efficient for the needs of that sport. Sport-specific functional rehabilitation should focus on restoration of the injured athlete's ability to have sport-specific physiology and biomechanics to interact optimally with the sport-specific demands. That means that they need to be replicated at the same speed, on the same surface and with the same level of fatigue to be truly effective.

Once an athlete has been medically cleared to return-to-play there are some fundamental steps that need to be followed:

- The athlete has to fulfill the fitness standards of the team he is returning to.
- The athlete needs to pass some skill specific tests applicable to his playing position.
- The player may then begin practicing with the team.
- Exposure to the match situation should be gradual, with the match time gradually increasing.

There are simple guidelines which need to be developed by each team with contributions and support from each member of the medical team.

Monitoring

Regarding these aspects from the text above, there are several problems: are all the mechanic parameters of the performance (force, velocity, power) regained at that time? Are there any ways to conduct the rehabilitation program in order to obtain better parameters and so the return to the sports activity to be safely done? Which could be the most suitable evaluation methods in order to be sure about the athletes well-training?

Monitoring athlete well-being is essential to guide training and to detect any progression towards negative health outcomes and associated poor performance. Objective (performance, physiological, biochemical) and subjective measures (mood disturbance, perceived stress and recovery and symptoms of stress) are all options for athlete monitoring. Appropriate load monitoring can aid in determining whether an athlete is adapting to a training program and in minimizing the risk of developing non-functional overreaching, illness, and injury.

In order to gain an understanding of the training load and its effect on the athlete, a number of potential markers are available for use. There are a number of external load quantifying and monitoring tools, such as power output measuring devices, time-motion analysis, as well as internal load unit measures, including perception of effort, heart rate, blood lactate, and training impulse. Other monitoring tools used by high-performance programs include heart rate recovery, neuromuscular function, biochemical/hormonal/immunological assessments, questionnaires and diaries, psychomotor speed, and sleep quality and quantity. Coaching staffs and administrative personnel must work to ensure that care can be provided at all points of the rehabilitation process, especially when funding dictates the need to hire personnel capable of addressing injuries at multiple levels. A clear understanding of the injury and of the interventions from each provider is vital to an efficient and successful return to play.

Appropriate monitoring of training load can provide important information to athletes and coaches; however, monitoring systems should be intuitive, provide efficient data analysis and interpretation, and enable efficient reporting of simple, yet scientifically valid, feedback. If accurate and easy-to-interpret feedback is provided to the athlete and coach, load monitoring can result in enhanced knowledge of training responses, aid in the design of training programs, provide a further avenue for communication between support staff and athletes and coaches and ultimately enhance an athlete's performance.

Injury Recovery and Rehabilitation Exercises

Below are some of the types of injury recovery exercises for specific types of injuries and what to expect as you return to exercise after your injury. These are exercises you can repeat multiple times daily to promote strength and rehabilitation.

Back Injury Recovery

Properly recovering from a back injury is critical to your spinal health. It ensures you maintain your mobility, posture and muscle strength so you can protect your spine. The key to recovering from a back injury is your core.

After having suffered a back injury, it's important to focus on strengthening your core—a powerhouse muscle group consisting of over 30 muscles in your abdomen and low back. Having a strong core will reduce the risk of developing chronic pain from your injury and will mitigate the chance of reinjuring your back.

If you're returning to exercise after an injury to your back, try these core strengthening moves:

- Pelvic Tilts: Lie with your back flat on the floor, knees bent. Place your hands on your hip bones and slowly tilt your pelvis toward and then away from your rib cage. You'll feel your low back lift. Continue this movement for one minute.
- Bird Dogs: Begin on hands and knees with a tight core. Slowly extend one arm straight forward and the opposite leg straight behind, holding for 3-5 seconds. Bring your arm and leg back to center and switch sides. Repeat 6 times per side.

Shoulder Injury

Shoulder injuries such as bursitis or tendonitis can be chronic and take a long time to heal. They can cause severe pain and impact your quality of life, making it difficult to perform movements such as reaching, pulling or pushing.

Because shoulder injuries often occur due to overuse, such as from repetitive motions, it's difficult to perform shoulder injury rehab right away. Your shoulder needs time to rest so it can actually get stronger before you start exercising again.

Once you've been cleared to begin using it again, shoulder injury rehab is the next step. You can rehabilitate and strengthen your shoulder muscle with the following exercises:

- Pendulum: In a standing position bend forward at the waist and support yourself on a counter or chair with one arm. Let your injured arm hang down. Gently swing your arm back and forth, side to side, then in circles. Repeat on the other side. Perform this exercise 3 times daily.
- Crossover Arm Stretch: Stand with shoulders straight and relaxed. Gently pull one arm straight across your chest. Hold the stretch for 30 seconds and repeat on the other side.

Hamstring Injury

Hamstring strains can be incredibly painful and debilitating. Like shoulder injuries, if a hamstring injury isn't properly rehabilitated, it can become a chronic or recurring problem. To properly rehabilitate your hamstring, it's important to find ways way to continue to use it without straining it even more.

You can perform isometric hamstring exercises which flex the muscles without stretching them. Additionally, as part of hamstring injury rehab, you'll want to strengthen your glutes. Because your hamstrings and glutes work together, having strong glute muscles can prevent future hamstring injuries.

To start your rehabilitation, try these two hamstring exercises after injury:

- Single Leg Bridge: Lie on the ground, back flat and knees bent. Activate your glute muscles and raise one leg up. Keeping your leg raised, push into your heel and raise your hips off the floor. Keep your shoulders flat to the ground, and your core, glutes and hamstring engaged. Repeat 10 times on each side.
- Hamstring Curl: Lie on your front with your legs straight. Place a pillow under your stomach if it's more comfortable. Slowly bend the knee of your affected leg toward your buttock, stopping when you feel resistance. Continue this motion 8-12 times per side.

Groin Injury

Groin injuries can be caused by pulled or strained groin muscles (adductors). These injuries typically affect athletes and can recur if not properly treated.

After resting and icing a groin injury, you may decide to return to physical activity with some groin injury rehab exercises:

- Adductor Squeeze: Lie down with your back flat on the ground. Raise bent legs so your shins are parallel with the floor. Place a soccer ball between your knees and squeeze them together until you feel your groin muscles activate. Hold the squeeze for 2 seconds. Release and repeat 10 times.

- Side-Lying Leg Lift with Crossover: Lie down on the side of your injury. Bend your top leg and place your foot flat on the ground in front on your bottom leg. Keeping your bottom leg straight, slowly raise it up as far as it will go. Hold for 5 seconds and repeat 15 times. Switch sides and repeat for 2 sets.

Knee Injury

Knee injuries are very common as it's one of the most used joints in the body—and the most susceptible to wear and tear. Initially following a knee injury, you'll want to work on getting your range of motion back, and it's advisable to work with a physiotherapist for this.

Chronic knee injuries can be rehabilitated by strengthening the muscles around the knee joint, which provide stability and mobility. Additionally, having strong hips takes pressure off the knee so it can continue to function properly.

To help rehabilitate, try the following knee strengthening exercises after injury:

- Straight Leg Raises: Lie with your back flat on the ground, one knee bent and foot flat to the floor. Extend your other leg long and raise it slowly up to the height of your bent knee. Repeat 15 times per leg, 3 times daily.

- Step-Ups: Standing on the bottom stair of a staircase, bend one knee and lightly touch the other foot to the floor behind you. Raise it back up. Repeat 15 times then switch legs. You can increase the height of the step-up as your knee feels stronger.

Tips for Safe Injury Recovery and Rehabilitation

It's important to be cautious before diving into any injury recovery exercises. Achieving safe, sustainable rehabilitation should be the ultimate goal of any injury recovery program. Suffering an injury drastically increases your risk of developing a recurrence or even a new injury. We can mitigate these risks by being safe and smart about how we hard we push ourselves.

Come Back Slow

One of the biggest mistakes that you can make when recovering from an injury is to get back to a full exercise routine too quickly. It's wise to start off slowly—even slower than you feel is necessary—and gradually increase your exercise intensity. Coming back slowly helps you build confidence and prevent a recurring injury. It also gives you the opportunity to notice any changes and build better body awareness.

Undergo Therapy

If you've suffered a particularly bad injury or you're experiencing chronic pain, it's important to seek professional therapy to help you better understand what's happening. Depending on your injury, you may wish to see a chiropractor or a physiotherapist or both. Chiropractors can help you alleviate chronic musculoskeletal pain, while physiotherapists can put together a rehabilitation plan for you. Getting an expert opinion can give you the reassurance to return to exercising safely.

Listen to your Body

Not only is it important to listen to your physical symptoms (don't ignore your pain), it's also essential to listen to any emotional symptoms you may be experiencing. Injuries, and the chronic pain that accompanies them, can take a toll on your emotional wellbeing. You may feel frustrated and helpless that you're not able to perform tasks like you used to. You may also feel anxious about returning to exercise for the fear of re-injuring yourself. Remember to practice self-compassion and get support as you need it.

Exercises to Recover from Sports Hernia

A sports hernia typically takes about 4 to 6 weeks to fully heal before you can return to your sport. Treatment begins with about two weeks of rest before physical therapy, which according to Stevens will:

- Develop pelvic stability so your pelvis is less reliant on support tissues to maintain stability.
- Learn to properly activate your hip flexors so the muscles that are intended to flex your hips are actually doing their job.
- Increase core strength so your core muscles are strong enough to lock down your trunk during explosive lower-body movements.

Stevens has his clients perform three exercises that help achieve these goals to fully recover from a sports hernia. You can also use these as general prehab exercises to improve your hip and core function, and decrease your chance of sustaining a sports hernia.

Banded Hip Flexion

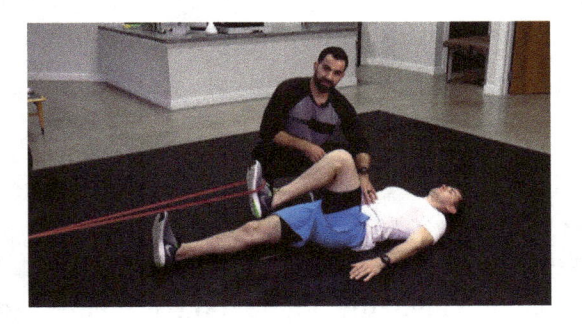

- How to: Attach a resistance band to a fixed object, lie down on the ground and wrap it around your left foot. Position yourself so there's tension in the band. With your core tight and feet dorsiflexed, bend your left knee and hip until both joints are at a 90-degree angle. Slowly straighten your leg to return to the starting position.
- Sets/Reps: 2-3 × 6-8 each leg.

Physioball Dead Bug

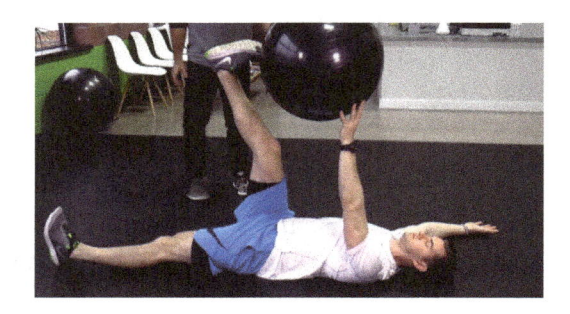

- How to: Lie on your back with your arms and legs straight over your shoulders and hips, respectively, and hold a physioball between your hands and feet. Keeping your core tight, simultaneously extend your left arm and right leg. Return your arm and leg to the physioball, and repeat with your opposite arm and leg. Continue alternating back and forth.
- Sets/Reps: 2-3 × 6-8 each leg.

Glute Bridge Leg Lifts

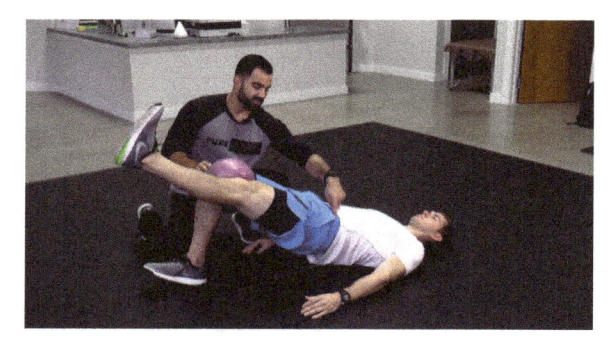

- How to: Lie on the ground with your knees bent and feet flat on the ground positioned about hip-width apart. Place a med ball between your knees and squeeze it with your legs. Drive your hips up as if performing a Glute Bridge. Tighten your core and glutes to create stability in this position. Without moving your hips, slowly straighten your left leg before returning it to the starting position. Repeat with your opposite leg and continue alternating back and forth.
- Sets/Reps: 2-3 × 6-8 each leg.

Recovery Techniques for Athletes

Professionalism in sport has provided the foundation for elite athletes to focus purely on training and competition. Furthermore, high-performance sport and the importance of successful performances have led athletes and coaches to continually seek any advantage that may improve performance. It follows that the rate and quality of recovery are extremely important for the high-performance athlete and that optimal recovery may provide numerous benefits during repetitive high-level training and competition. Therefore, investigating different recovery interventions and their effects on fatigue, muscle injury, recovery and performance is important.

Adequate recovery has been shown to result in the restoration of physiological and psychological processes, so that the athlete can compete or train again at an appropriate level. Recovery from training and competition is complex and typically dependent on the nature of the exercise performed and any other outside stressors. Athletic performance is affected by numerous aspects and therefore, adequate recovery should also consider such factors.

Table: Factors affecting athletic performance.

Training competition	Volume: intensity duration type of training/sport degree of fatigue recovery from previous training/competition.
Nutrition	Carbohydrate protein and other nutrient intake, fluid and electrolyte balance.
Psychological stress	Stress and anxiety from competition.
Lifestyle	Quality and amount of sleep; schedule housing situation leisure/social activities relationship with team member : coach; friends and family, job or schooling situation.
Health	Illnesses; infection injury, iii muscle soreness and damage.
Environment	Temperature, humidity: altitude.

Methods to Enhance Recovery

There are a number of popular methods used by athletes to enhance recovery. Their use will depend on the type of activity performed, the time until the next training session or event and equipment and personnel available. Some of the most popular recovery techniques for athletes include hydrotherapy, active recovery, stretching, compression garments, massage, sleep and nutrition.

Endurance Exercise

Various forms of water immersion recovery techniques are becoming increasingly popular with elite athletes. While athletes have been using hydrotherapy for a number of years, research into the potential recovery effects of water immersion, recovery and performance are now appearing. The most common forms of water immersion are cold water immersion (CWI), hot water immersion (HWI) and contrast water therapy (CWT), where the athlete alternates between hot and cold water immersion.

Coffey investigated the effects of three recovery interventions (active, low-intensity exercise; passive, seated rest; and CWT) on repeated treadmill running performance separated by 4 h. Contrast water therapy was associated with a perception of improved recovery. However, performance during the high-intensity treadmill running task returned to baseline levels 4 h after the initial exercise task regardless of the recovery intervention performed. Hamlin also found CWT to have no beneficial effect on performance during repeated sprinting. Twenty rugby players performed two repeated sprint tests separated by 1 h and completed either CWT or active recovery between trials. An active recovery generally consists of aerobic exercise that can be performed using different modes such as cycling, jogging, aqua jogging or swimming. Active recovery is often thought to be better for recovery than passive recovery due to enhanced blood flow to the exercised area and clearance of lactate and other metabolic waste products via increased oxygen delivery and oxidation.

Even though substantial decreases in blood lactate concentration and heart rate were observed following CWT when compared to active recovery, performance in the second exercise bout was decreased compared with the first exercise bout regardless of the intervention.

In a study investigating the dose-response effect of CWT, the authors reported substantially improved cycling time trial and sprint performance following 6 min of CWT (hot water: 38.4 °C; cold water: 14.6 °C; 1 min rotations) when compared to control (passive rest). The time between cycling bouts was 2 h and the duration of each cycling bout was 75 min. However, there was no improvement in repeat performance with 18 min of CWT, indicating that a dose-response relationship does not exist under these conditions. Twelve minutes of CWI also improved sprint total work and peak power. The same research group repeated the above study with trained runners using identical water immersion times and temperatures and the same time between exercise bouts (2 h). However, in this instance, the first bout consisted of a 3,000 m time trial and 8 x 400 m intervals. The second bout of exercise was a 3,000 m time trial. The results of this study again demonstrated that CWT for 6 min improved performance, whereas 12 and 18 min did not, indicating the lack of a dose-response relationship between running performance and CWT. Importantly, this study was performed outdoors at an environmental temperature of 14.9°C and the increased duration of cold water exposure may have reduced the potential benefits of longer water immersion durations.

The effectiveness of CWI and CWT on recovery from simulated team sport performance (running) was assessed across a 48 h period. Each subject completed three testing trials lasting 3 d with CWI, CWT or passive recovery completed immediately after the initial exercise bout and again at 24 h after exercise. Performance (time taken to complete 10 x 20 m sprints and leg extension/flexion isometric force) was assessed before exercise and 48 h after exercise. Cold water immersion (2 x 5 min in 10°C) was significantly better than both CWT (2 min cold in 10°C, 2 min in 40°C x 3) and passive recovery in reducing ratings of muscle soreness, and reducing decrements in isometric leg extension, flexion force and sprint performance from baseline value. Contrast water therapy also improved muscle soreness at 24 h when compared with passive recovery.

The effects of three hydrotherapy interventions on next day performance recovery following strenuous training was investigated on 12 male cyclists, who completed four experimental trials differing only in recovery intervention: CWI, HWI, CWT or passive recovery. Each trial consisted of five consecutive exercise days (105 min duration, including 66 maximal effort sprints) followed by recovery on each day. After completing each exercise session, participants performed one of the four recovery interventions in a randomised crossover design. Sprint (0.1–2.2%) and time trial (0.0– 1.7%) performance were enhanced across the 5 d trial following both CWI and CWT when compared to HWI and passive recovery.

Vaile also examined different water immersion temperatures (15 min of intermittent immersion in 10 °C, 15 °C, 20° C, continuous immersion in 20 °C water, and active recovery). Two 30 min cycling bouts performed in the heat were separated by 60 min, with one of the five recovery strategies performed immediately after the first exercise bout. Each trial was separated by seven days. All water immersion protocols significantly improved subsequent cycling performance when compared to active recovery.

Team Sports

Rowsell conducted a study in high-performance junior soccer players, with four matches played over 4 d and recovery completed after each match. No effect of cold water immersion was observed when compared to thermoneutral water immersion (control condition) on indicators of soccer performance. However, the perception of fatigue and muscle soreness was lower in the cold water immersion group.

In rugby players, researchers have reported that CWT had no beneficial effect on performance during repeated sprinting (Hamlin, 2007). Twenty participants performed two repeated sprint tests separated by 1 h. They completed either CWT or active recovery between trials. While substantial decreases in blood lactate concentration and heart rate were observed following CWT compared to the first exercise bout, performance in the second exercise bout was decreased similarly regardless of the intervention.

When examining the effect of various recovery strategies (passive, active, CWI, CWT), King and Duffield reported no significant effects of any of the strategies on performance during a simulated netball circuit (vertical jump, 20-m sprint, 10-m sprint and total circuit time). However, effect sizes showed trends for a smaller decline in sprint performance and vertical jumps with both CWT and CWI. The time frame between testing sessions was 24 h, suggesting that complete recovery may have occurred prior to repeat testing. It is possible that the water immersion protocols were not substantial enough to have an effect, with immersion to the iliac crest only and showers used for the hot water exposure in the CWT. This finding may suggest that muscle temperature is a key factor when considering the timing of recovery strategies.

The effectiveness of three recovery strategies (carbohydrate intake and stretching, CWI and full leg compression garments) was examined before and after a 3 d basketball tournament in state-level athletes. Recovery was performed each day and the athletes played one full 48 min game per day. Sprint, vertical jump, line-drill performance and agility performance and 20 m acceleration decreased across the 3 d tournament, indicating accumulated fatigue. CWI was substantially better than other strategies in maintaining 20 m acceleration. CWI and compression showed similar benefits in maintaining line-drill performance when compared to carbohydrate and stretching.

It should be noted that in well-controlled laboratory studies that have examined the effects of recovery on performance, positive effects of various forms of hydrotherapy have been demonstrated. However, limited studies utilising team sports scenarios combined with large differences in methodology have resulted in less clear findings in team sport athletes when compared to previous laboratory research.

Active Recovery

It is not clear whether there are benefits of an active recovery between training sessions or following competition in various sports. No detrimental effects on performance have been reported following an active recovery (when compared to a passive recovery) between training sessions, along with a small amount of literature reporting enhanced performance. Many researchers, however, use the removal of lactate as their primary indicator of recovery and this may not be a valid indicator of enhanced recovery and the ability to repeat performance at a previous level.

A recent study investigated the effects of a swim recovery session on subsequent running performance and reported an increase in performance when compared to passive recovery. Well-trained triathletes completed a high-intensity running session followed 10 h later by either a swim session (20 x 100 m at 90% of 1 km time trial speed) or passive recovery. Twenty-four hours following the initial running session, a time to fatigue run test was performed. The swim trial resulted in subjects running for 830 + 98 s, compared to the passive trial in which subjects ran for 728 + 183 s. This improvement may have been due to the hydrostatic benefits of water (thought to increase venous return and blood flow) and the active recovery per sec.

The influence of the intensity of active recovery on the clearance of blood lactate has also been investigated. Different running intensities during active recovery were compared to passive recovery and it was reported that lactate was lower following higher intensities (60-100% of lactate threshold) than lower intensities (0-40% of lactate threshold). Maximum lactate clearance occurred during active recovery at intensities close to lactate threshold. It should be noted that maximal lactate concentrations were low (3.9 mm) in this study and subjects were only moderately trained. Carter investigated the effects of mode of exercise recovery on thermoregulatory and cardiovascular responses, with the data suggesting that mild active recovery may play an important role for post-exertional heat dissipation. However, the mechanism(s) behind these altered responses during active recovery is unknown.

The role of active recovery in reducing lactate concentrations after exercise may be an important factor for athletes, although the research in this area is incomplete. This is anecdotally reported to be one of the most common forms of recovery and utilised by the majority of athletes for these reasons.

Stretching

Although stretching is anecdotally one of the most used recovery strategies, the literature examining the effects of stretching as a recovery method is sparse. In team sport athletes, Kinugasa and Kilding, assessed the effects of 7 min of static stretching following a football game. Stretching was not as effective as CWT or a combined recovery (CWT and active recovery) for improving the subject's perceived recovery. Similarly, Montgomery reported that a combined recovery strategy (stretching and carbohydrate intake) performed immediately after three basketball games over 3 d was not as effective as CWI for restoring physical performance (20 m sprint, basketball specific running drill, sit and reach test).

In contrast, Dawson and colleagues reported that stretching following an Australian football match significantly improved power output during a 6 s cycle sprint 15 h after the match, compared to a control. Additionally, Miladi and colleagues reported that dynamic stretching was significantly superior to active or passive recovery for maintaining a second bout of cycling to exhaustion. Finally, following a muscle damaging protocol, stretching was found to improve range of motion and reduce muscle soreness compared to a control.

As can be concluded from the above findings, there have been mixed reports regarding the benefit of stretching as a recovery strategy. However, two separate reviews of recovery methods concluded that there was no benefit for stretching as a recovery modality. It is important to note that to date, there have not been any detrimental effects on performance associated with post-exercise stretching.

Compression Garments

Many recovery strategies for elite athletes are based on medical equipment or therapies used in patient populations. Compression clothing is one of these strategies that have been traditionally used to treat various lymphatic and circulatory conditions. Compression garments are thought to improve venous return through application of graduated compression to the limbs from proximal to distal. The external pressure created may reduce the intramuscular space available for swelling and promote stable alignment of muscle fibres, attenuating the inflammatory response and reducing muscle soreness.

Recreational runners wearing compression garments have been examined during and after intermittent and continuous running. The authors found that there was a reduction in delayed onset muscle soreness 24 h after wearing compression garments during a continuous exercise task (10 km). While not statistically significant, there was a trend for participants in the compression trial to perform the 10 km in a faster time than when not wearing the compression garments. Subjects wore commercially available graduated compression stockings, with the compression highest at the ankle (18-22 mmHg) and reduced by 70% to the top of the stocking, which ended below the knee. Recently, a reduction in the perception of muscle soreness after wearing compression garments during sprinting and bounding exercise and for 24 h after exercise was reported. While perceptions of soreness were reduced, there was no change in sprint performance while wearing the garments.

While there is currently minimal research into compression garments and recovery for endurance athletes, the small amount of data suggests that there may be some small benefits and there is no indication that they impede the recovery process.

Massage

Massage is a widely used recovery strategy among athletes. However, apart from perceived benefits of massage on muscle soreness, few reports have demonstrated positive effects on repeated exercise performance. Furthermore, increased blood flow is one of the main mechanisms proposed to improve recovery (thus improving clearance of metabolic waste products). However, many studies reported no increase in blood flow or lactate removal during massage. Indeed, in a recent study, Wiltshire and colleagues reported that massage actually impaired blood flow and lactate removal.

Lane and Wenger reported that massage was superior to passive recovery in maintaining cycle performance separated by 24 h. However, active recovery and cold water immersion provided greater (non-significant) benefits compared to massage. Monedero and Donne reported that massage was no more effective than passive recovery performed between two simulated 5 km cycle time trials separated by 20 min. However, a combined recovery consisting of active cycling and massage was significantly superior at maintaining performance than active cycling or massage in isolation, or passive recovery. In contrast, in high-intensity cycle sprints (8 x 5 sec sprints repeated twice), Ogai and colleagues reported that when massage was performed between the two bouts, total power output of the second bout was enhanced compared to the control. It should be noted that no other recovery strategies were performed, and as such, it is difficult to make recommendations for massage over other forms of recovery.

Several reviews of the effects of massage have concluded that while massage is beneficial in improving psychological aspects of recovery, most evidence does not support massage as a modality to improve recovery of functional performance. However, as massage may have potential benefits for injury prevention and management; massage should still be incorporated in an athlete's training program for reasons other than recovery.

Practical Applications

While there are not a large number of scientific studies investigating recovery strategies in athletes, current evidence as well as anecdotal evidence from athletes suggests that completing appropriate recovery can aid in enhancing performance. At present, the following general recommendations can be made:

- Consideration should be given to the amount of time until the next training session or competition. Is a recovery procedure necessary? What can be practically performed in the time frame? What strategies have scientific evidence to support their use in the given time?

- Use appropriate temperatures and duration for water immersion. Research has found positive effects of water immersion at temperatures of 10–15 °C for cold water and 38–40 °C for hot water.

- Cold water immersion or contrast water therapy for duration of 14–15 min has been shown to improve performance in selected studies.

- The ratio of hot-cold water immersion during contrast-water therapy should be 1:1. Research that has reported positive performance effects used seven rotations of 1 min hot and 1 min cold.

- Compression garments and active recovery may be beneficial for recovery in endurance-trained athletes. While the positive evidence is minimal at present, there does not appear to be harmful effects relating to their use, and anecdotal evidence for their support is high. Further well-controlled research is needed.

Regenerative Therapy

Regenerative Therapy is becoming popular for treating sports injuries, not only for professional athletes but also local competitors. Stem cell injections, platelet-rich plasma (PRP), and prolotherapy are examples of regenerative medicine treatments available to treat sports injuries.

Depending on the injury, regenerative therapy may be the sole treatment, or it may be used in conjunction with other conventional treatments. For example, PRP can be used alone as a therapeutic injection or applied during cartilage regeneration surgery.

As the field of regenerative medicine advances, more people are turning to therapies that utilize biological substances, such as stem cells, to heal sports-related injuries faster.

Regenerative therapy takes advantage of the body's natural ability to heal itself by using healthy regenerative cells found throughout the body. The treatment has the potential to accelerate the body's natural healing process, repair damaged tissues, reduce pain, and improve function.

Regenerative therapy is the process of taking the body's own cells and injecting them into an area of the body that has been injured or otherwise needs to heal. This treatment has given birth to the term orthobiologics, which is the use of high concentrations of biological substances, such as platelet-rich plasma (PRP) or stem cells, to help speed the healing process for musculoskeletal injuries.

Laboratory and clinical research have found it is possible to use platelet-rich plasma (PRP) and adult stem cells to heal (and even regenerate) lost, damaged, or aging tissue. In many cases, the therapy provides patients an alternative to surgery. In sports medicine, regenerative therapies are beneficial for treating both acute, chronic, and common conditions that result from overuse.

Stem cell therapy and PRP have benefits over cortisone injections. Administering a cortisone injection basically shuts down all cellular activity, which causes inflammation to decrease. Cortisone, except for isolated circumstances, is a stop-gap measure that can also affect the body's ability to sense pain which can lead to further injury.

Who has used Regenerative Therapy for Sports & Athletic Injuries?

Many prominent sports personalities have made the headlines for using Stem Cell Therapy or Platelet-Rich Plasma (PRP) treatments.

Athletes of all skill levels can benefit from regenerative medicine therapies and treatments, from younger adults, active seniors, and baby boomers, to amateur and professional athletes.

Types of Regenerative Therapy Treatments are Available for Sports and Athletic Injuries

All regenerative therapy treatments are outpatient procedures; however, it may take more than one treatment to achieve optimal results. As with any medical treatment, results are not guaranteed.

Stem Cell Treatments

A stem cell does not serve a specific bodily function, but it can develop into a cell that does, such as a cartilage cell or a tendon cell. Medical professionals theorize stem cells can transform to meet a medical need when placed in a specific environment. For example, stem cells that are injected into a damaged Achilles tendon develop into healthy Achilles tendon cells. Furthermore, the collection of the stem cells for treatment come from the patient's fat, blood, or bone marrow.

Platelet-rich Plasma (PRP)

The patient's blood is processed, often in a centrifuge, to create a concentrated solution of platelets and plasma to make PRP. The natural healing properties found in the blood's platelets and plasma help facilitate healing and repair of the injury. PRP can also be injected or applied to an injured area during surgery.

PRP therapies vary, depending on factors such as differences in patients' blood, the method of blood processing, and the addition of other substances, such as an anesthetic.

Prolotherapy

Inflammation increases blood flow and attracts other cells that can repair and heal damaged tissues; therefore, sports injuries usually cause inflammation. In some cases, the inflammation subsides before the injury is completely healed. When this occurs, a physician may use prolotherapy to increase inflammation to allow the body time to heal.

Prolotherapy includes an injection of an irritant into the injured area temporarily increases inflammation, which facilitates further healing. However, prolotherapy treatments are not considered regenerative therapy unless they include platelet-rich plasma (PRP) and stem cells.

How are Regenerative Therapies used?

Stem cell therapy is used to treat shoulder, knee, hip, and spine degeneration, in addition to soft tissue (muscle, tendon, ligament) and other bone-related injuries. Adult stem cells can treat many types of chronic pain and degeneration. Under the right conditions, stem cells hold the potential to regenerate damaged tissue.

The application of stem cells to an injured area may be by:

- Injection: A physician may inject stem cells directly into the affected area, often using ultrasound or other medical imaging to help deliver the cells directly to the damaged tissue.
- Direct surgical application: A surgeon may apply stem cells directly to the torn ligament, tendon, or bone for repair.
- Stem-cell bearing sutures: A surgeon may stitch together a torn muscle, ligament, or tendon using a thread-like material coated with stem cells. (The sutures dissolve over time, and the body absorbs the stem cells).

Soft tissue injuries are most responsive to PRP treatment. Some examples of these injuries include:

- Joint pain resulting from inflammation after an acute injury.
- Chronic degenerative joint disease.
- Ligament and muscle injuries.
- Tendonitis, such as tennis elbow and golfer's elbow.
- Partial tendon tears when caught early.

Tendonitis, such as Achilles tendonitis, patellar tendonitis in the knee, or tennis elbow are common overuse conditions that plague many athletes. Many of these injuries involve microscopic tearing and formation of scar tissue. It is often difficult for these tendon injuries to heal due to inadequate blood supply to the area. With PRP treatment, however, the concentrated platelet injection enhances the nutrients and growth factors in the injury which allow the body to heal itself.

Both research studies and clinical practice have shown PRP therapy to be very effective at relieving pain and returning patients to their normal lives. Ultrasound and MRI imaging show definitive tissue repair and healing following PRP therapy. Treating injured tissues before damage progresses and making the condition irreversible, can significantly reduce the need for surgery.

PRP therapy alone can be effective for acute sports injuries, but it is often not sufficient for treating chronic arthritic joint injuries and degenerative disc disease that cause lower back pain. Much more profound results (tissue regeneration and pain relief) are often seen when PRP is utilized in combination with the injection of stem cells. In many cases, both stem cells and PRP are used to treat an injury.

Is Regenerative Therapy an Alternative to Surgery?

Treatment for patients suffering from chronic musculoskeletal injuries traditionally involves arthroscopic surgery or joint replacement. These treatment options can often require months of rehabilitation to regain strength and mobility. There are also the typical surgical risks including complications from the anesthesia, blood transfusions, blood clots (deep vein thrombosis), slow healing, and even paralysis (possible with spinal surgery).

Most cases of stem cell and PRP treatments are successful and avoid the pain, disability, downtime, and the risks associated with major surgery. Regenerative Therapy does involve some soreness and bruising in the treated area; even so, there is minimal recovery from a stem cell or PRP treatment.

Stem cell treatment can be repeated in a joint, if necessary, to obtain optimal results where a second surgery may not always be possible. Additionally, undergoing regenerative therapy does not preclude a patient from future surgery in the area.

Finally, there have been no reports of serious adverse effects in the scientific literature when adult mesenchymal stem cells are used in these procedures.

Guidelines for Who Can Receive Stem Cell Therapy

Right now, there are no formal medical guidelines regarding who can receive stem cell therapy for sports injuries. The use of stem cells for treatment is up to patients and their doctor. Some physicians have specific criteria for recommending stem cell therapy or PRP treatments. The suitability of regenerative therapy is decided on a case-by-case basis after a thorough examination and medical history.

For professional athletes, the World Anti-Doping Agency (WADA) regulations for regenerative therapy may or may not prohibit the use of stem cell therapy or PRP, depending on how the cellular material is manipulated or modified for use. Stem cell injections are prohibited if the product is modified in a way that can offer performance-enhancing benefits. WADA further clarifies that athletes are not permitted to use both normal and genetically modified cells in any way, if the process causes performance enhancement. Athletes should be aware that the use of stem cell products cannot justify a positive doping test, if any prohibited substances are identified in a sample.

References

- How-to-prevent-sports-injuries-3119270: verywellfit.com, Retrieved 19 March, 2019
- 14-effective-ways-to-prevent-sports-injury: isbglasgow.com, Retrieved 23 May, 2019
- Cryotherapy-benefits: healthline.com, Retrieved 10 July, 2019

- Hydrotherapy, treatments-therapies: sportsinjuryclinic.net, Retrieved 15 August, 2019
- Price-protocol-principles: sports-health.com, Retrieved 20 April, 2019
- Rehabilitation-in-Sport: physio-pedia.com, Retrieved 25 July, 2019
- Injury-recovery-and-rehabilitation-exercises: relaxtheback.com, Retrieved 30 April, 2019
- 120-recovery-techniques-for-athletes, sports-science-exchange: gssiweb.org, Retrieved 02 May, 2019
- Regenerative-therapy-for-sports-athletic-injuries, pain-treatments: novusspinecenter.com, Retrieved 05 January, 2019

Sports Nutrition and Supplements

Sports nutrition is defined as the study and practice of implementing appropriate diet and nutrition to improve the athletic performance of a person. It studies the nutrition and quantity of fluids and food taken by an athlete. This chapter closely examines the different dietary supplements under sports nutrition to provide an extensive understanding of the subject.

Sports nutrition is a topic of constant change and has grown as a dynamic field of clinical study. Research continues to advise improved nutritional guidelines and support for both active adults and competitive athletes. Science recognizes sports nutrition and energy intake as the "cornerstone of the athlete's diet".

Sports nutrition is the foundation of athletic success. It is a well-designed nutrition plan that allows active adults and athletes to perform at their best. It supplies the right food type, energy, nutrients, and fluids to keep the body well hydrated and functioning at peak levels. A sports nutrition diet may vary day to day, depending on specific energy demands.

Sports Nutrition Basics: Macronutrients

The energy required for living and physical activity comes from the food we eat and fluid intake. Macronutrients in the following food groups supply the energy essential to optimal body function:

- Carbohydrates are either simple or complex, and the most important energy source for the human body. Simple carbs include sugars naturally occurring in foods like fruits, vegetables, and milk. Whole grain bread, potatoes, most vegetables, and oats are examples of healthy complex carbs. Your digestive system breaks own carbohydrates into glucose or blood sugar which feeds energy to your cells, tissues, and organs.

- Proteins are made up of a chain of amino acids and are essential to every cell of the human body. Protein can either be complete or incomplete. A complete protein contains all the amino acids needed by the body, and includes animal sources like meat, fish, poultry, and milk. Incomplete protein sources (typically plant-based proteins) often lack one or more of the essential amino acids. Essential amino acids can't be made by the body and must be supplied by food. Protein plays an important role in muscle recovery and growth.

- Fats can be saturated or unsaturated, and they play a vital role in the human body. Unsaturated fats are considered healthy and come from plant sources like olive oil and nuts. Saturated fats are found in animal products like red meats and high-fat dairy, which are indicated to increase the risk of disease. Healthy fats provide energy, help with body development, protect our organs, and maintain cell membranes.

The Goal of Sports Nutrition

Active adults and competitive athletes turn to sports nutrition to help them achieve their goals.

Examples of individual goals could include gaining lean mass, improving body composition, or enhancing athletic performance. These sport-specific scenarios require differing nutritional programs. Research findings indicate the right food type, caloric intake, nutrient timing, fluids, and supplementation are essential and specific to each individual. The following are different states of training and competitive sport benefiting from sports nutrition:

Eating for Exercise/Athletic Performance

Training programs require a well-designed diet for active adults and competitive athletes. Research shows a balanced nutrition plan should include sufficient calories and healthy macronutrients to optimize athletic performance. The body will use carbohydrates or fats as the main energy source, depending on exercise intensity and duration. Inadequate caloric intake can impede athletic training and performance.

For example, and according to research, energy expenditure for extreme cyclists competing in the Tour de France is approximately 12,000 calories per day.

- Carbohydrates are the main fuel source for an active adult or competitive athlete. General guidelines for carbohydrate intake are based on body size and training characteristics. Carbohydrate needs in a daily diet can range from 45 to 65 percent of total food intake depending on physical demands.

- Proteins are responsible for muscle growth and recovery in the active adult or athlete. Sufficient amounts of protein per individual help maintain a positive nitrogen balance in the body, which is vital to muscle tissue. Protein requirements can vary significantly ranging from .8g to 2g per kilogram of body weight per day.

- Fats help maintain energy balance, regulate hormones, and restore muscle tissue. Omega-3 and omega-6 are essential fatty acids that are especially important to a sports nutrition diet. Research findings recommend an athlete consume approximately 30 percent of their total daily caloric intake as a healthy fat.

Eating for Endurance

Endurance programs are defined as one to three hours per day of moderate to high-intensity exercise. High-energy intake in the form of carbohydrates is essential. According to research, target carbohydrate consumption for endurance athletes ranges from 6g to 10g per kilogram of body weight per day. Fat is a secondary source of energy used during long-duration training sessions. Endurance athletes are more at risk for dehydration. Replacing fluids and electrolytes lost through sweat are necessary for peak performance.

Eating for Strength

Resistance training programs are designed to gradually build the strength of skeletal muscle. Strength training is high-intensity work. It requires sufficient amounts of all macronutrients for muscle development. Protein intake is especially vital to increase and maintain lean body mass. Research indicates protein requirements can vary from 1.2g to 3.1g per kilogram of body weight per day.

Eating for Competition

Preparing for a competitive sport will vary in sports nutrition requirements. For example, strength athletes strive to increase lean mass and body size for their sport. Endurance runners focus on reduced body weight/fat for peak body function during their event. Athletic goals will determine the best sports nutrition strategy. Pre and post-workout meal planning are unique for each athlete and essential for optimal performance.

Hydration and Sports Performance

Adequate hydration and electrolytes are essential for health and athletic performance. We all lose water throughout the day, but active adults and athletes lose additional body water (and a significant amount of sodium) sweating during intense workouts.

Dehydration is the process of losing body water, and fluid deficits greater than 2 percent of body weight can compromise athletic performance and cognitive function. Athletes are recommended to use fluid replacement strategies as part of their sports nutrition to maintain optimal body functioning. Rehydration with water and sports drinks containing sodium are often consumed depending on the athlete and sporting event. Lack of sufficient hydration for athletes may lead to the following:

- Hypohydration (dehydration).
- Hypovolemia (decreased plasma/blood volume).
- Hyponatremia (low blood sodium levels/water intoxication).

Supplements in Sports Nutrition

Sports supplements and foods are unregulated products marketed to enhance athletic performance. According to the Academy of Sports Medicine, "the ethical use of sports supplements is a personal choice and remains controversial". There are limited supplements backed by clinical research. The Australian Institute of Sport has provided a general guide ranking sports performance supplements and foods according to the significance of scientific evidence:

- Sports food: Sports drinks, bars, and gels, electrolyte supplements, protein supplements, liquid meal supplements.
- Medical supplements: Iron, calcium, vitamin D, multi-vitamin/mineral, omega-3 fatty acids.
- Performance supplements: Creatine, caffeine, sodium bicarbonate, beta-alanine, nitrate.

Sports Nutrition for Special Populations and Environments

Sports nutrition covers a wide spectrum of needs for athletes. Certain populations and environments require additional guidelines and information to enhance athletic performance.

- Vegetarian athlete: A vegetarian diet contains high intakes of plant proteins, fruits, vegetables, whole grains, and nuts. It can be nutritionally adequate, but insufficient evidence exists on long-term vegetarianism and athletic performance. Dietary assessments are recommended to avoid deficiencies and to ensure adequate nutrients to support athletic demands.

- High altitude: Specialized training and nutrition are required for athletes training at high altitude. Increasing red blood cells to carry more oxygen is essential. Iron-rich foods are an important component for this athlete as well. Increased risk of illness is indicated with chronic high altitude exposure. Foods high in antioxidants and protein are essential. Fluid requirements will vary per athlete, and hydration status should be individually monitored.

- Hot environments: Athletes competing in hot conditions are at greater risk of heat illness. Heat illness can have adverse health complications. Fluid and electrolyte balance is crucial for these athletes. Hydration strategies are required to maintain peak performance while exercising in the heat.

- Cold environments: Primary concerns for athletes exercising in the cold are adequate hydration and body temperature. Leaner athletes are at higher risk of hypothermia. Modifying caloric and carbohydrate intake are important for this athlete. Appropriate foods and fluids that withstand cold temperatures will promote optimal athletic performance.

Special Topics in Sports Nutrition

Eating disorders in athletes are not uncommon. Many athletes are required to maintain lean bodies and low body weight and exhibit muscular development. Chronic competitive pressure can create psychological and physical stress of the athlete leading to disordered eating habits. Without proper counseling, adverse health effects may eventually develop. The most common eating disorders among athletes may include:

- Anorexia nervosa.

- Bulimia.

- Compulsive exercise disorder.

- Orthorexia.

Obviously, the nutritional needs of these individuals greatly differ from that of other active adults or athletes. Until someone with an eating disorder is considered well again, the primary focus should be put on treating and managing the eating disorder and consuming the nutrition needed to achieve and maintain good health, rather than athletic performance.

Micronutrient deficiencies are a concern for active adults and athletes. Exercise stresses important body functions where micronutrients are required. Additionally, athletes often restrict calories and certain food groups, which may potentially lead to deficiencies of essential micronutrients. Research indicates the most common micronutrient deficiencies include:

- Iron deficiency: Can impair muscle function and compromise athletic performance.

- Vitamin D deficiency: Can result in decreased bone strength and reduced muscle metabolic function.

- Calcium deficiency: Can impair the repair of bone tissue, decrease regulation of muscle contraction, and reduce nerve conduction.

Roles of a Sports Dietitian

Athletes and active adults are seeking guidance from sports professionals to enhance their athletic performance. Sports dietitians are increasingly hired to develop nutrition and fluid programs catered to the individual athlete or teams. A unique credential has been created for sports nutrition professionals: Board Certified Specialist in Sports Dietetics (CSSD). Sports dietitians should have knowledge in the following areas:

- Clinical nutrition.
- Nutrition science.
- Exercise physiology.
- Evidence-based research.
- Safe and effective nutrition assessments.
- Sports nutrition guidance.
- Counseling for health and athletic performance.
- Medical nutrition therapy.
- Design and management of effective nutrition strategies.
- Effective nutrition programming for health, fitness, and optimal physical performance.

Sports Supplements

Sports supplements represent a multi-million dollar industry. Active adults and athletes are often enticed by effective supplement marketing. The promises of enhanced performance among other claims are motivating factors to purchase alternative nutrition to achieve results. Lack of supplement regulation and quality control may mean unreliable and ineffective products are being used. It's estimated between 39 and 89 percent of the international supplement market are athletes with the highest frequency among older and elite athletes.

Supplements are considered an addition to an already healthy diet. Active adults or athletes may include supplements to help meet nutritional needs, improve nutrient deficiencies, enhance athletic performance or achieve personal fitness goals. Without a well-designed nutrition plan in place, supplementation is said to be rarely effective.

Supplement Regulation and Standards

Dietary supplements have been placed in a special food category and not considered drugs. Supplements aren't required to be submitted to the *Food and Drug Administration* (FDA) for regulation. Although the FDA has the ability to review ingredients and health claims of supplements, very few are investigated.

Sport supplement manufacturers are allowed to make health claims with FDA approval as long as the product statements are true and based on scientific evidence. Unfortunately, very few supplements claiming ergogenic benefits are supported by clinical research. This leaves the active adult or athlete without a guarantee of safety, effectiveness, potency or purity of supplements for dietary or ergogenic purposes.

- Dietary supplements include vitamins, minerals, amino acids, herbs, botanicals, and extracts or concentrates from plants or foods. They are typically sold as capsules, tablets, liquids, powders or bars and required to be clearly labeled as a dietary supplement.
- Ergogenic aids include substances, drugs or techniques used to enhance athletic performance. They can range from acceptable practices of carbohydrate loading to "illegal and unsafe approaches such as anabolic-androgenic steroid use".

Evaluating the Benefit of Supplements

Supplement use remains controversial and is a personal choice. Common questions asked by active adults, athletes, and sports nutritionists relate to manufacturing and supplement quality. Locating evidence-based research information is highly advised before considering sports foods and supplements. The *International Society of Sports Nutrition* (ISSN) recommends evaluating the validity and scientific merit behind supplement claims for enhanced athletic performance. The following questions are suggested:

- Does the supplement claim make sense?
- Is there scientific evidence available?
- Is the supplement legal or safe?

Supplements are marketed for health and exercise performance based on hypothetical applications gathered from preliminary research. The claims sound promising but often don't agree with clinical findings.

If working with a sports dietitian or specialist, they can be a valuable resource in supplement research interpretation. The information gathered will enable you to make the best decision about taking sports supplements for health and athletic goals.

How Science Classifies Supplements

Dietary supplements and ergogenic aids are marketed and claim to enhance the diet and athletic performance of an active adult or athlete. Clinical research continues to uncover flaws in these supplement health claims. The International Society of Sports Nutrition (ISSN) has provided a classification for supplements based on clinical research:

- Apparently effective: The majority of supplement research studies show safe and effective.
- Possibly effective: Initial supplement findings are good, but more research is required to examine the effects on training and athletic performance.
- Too early to tell: Supplement theory makes sense but lacks sufficient research to support using it.

- Apparently ineffective: Supplements lack sound scientific evidence and research has shown the supplement to be clearly ineffective and unsafe.

The International Society of Sports Nutrition (ISSN) indicates the foundation of a good training program is a sound energy balanced, nutrient-dense diet. If supplements are being considered, the ISSN suggests supplements only from category one (apparently effective). Any other supplements would be considered experimental. They further discourage supplements in category three (too early to tell) and don't support athletes taking supplements in category four (apparently ineffective).

Supplement Value of Vitamins and Exercise Performance

Vitamins are organic compounds essential to regulating metabolic processes, energy production, neurological functioning and protection of our cells. Dietary analysis on active adults or athletes has reported vitamin deficiencies. Although research shows a possible benefit of taking vitamins for general health, there has been minimal to no ergogenic benefits reported. The following vitamins common to athletes have been researched as proposed nutritional ergogenic aids:

Nutrient	Ergogenic Claim	Research Findings
Vitamin A	may improve sports vision.	no improvement in athletic performance.
Vitamin D	may help prevent bone loss.	may help with calcium co-supplement.
Vitamin E	may prevent free radicals.	Decrease in oxidative stress found/more research required.
Vitamin K	may help bone metabolism.	elite female athletes show improved balance of bone formation and resorption.
Thiamin (B1)	may improve anaerobic threshold.	doesn't appear to enhance exercise capacity at normal intake.
Riboflavin (B2)	may enhance energy availability during exercise.	doesn't appear to enhance exercise capacity at normal intake.
Niacin (B3)	may enhance energy metabolism, improve cholesterol and blunt fat stores.	shown to decrease cholesterol but decrease exercise capacity.
Pyridoxine (B6)	may improve lean mass, strength, aerobic capacity and mental focus.	well-nourished athletes show no improvement in athletic performance. Some improved fine motor skills when combined with Vitamins B1 and B12.
Cyano-cobalamin (B12)	may increase muscle mass and decrease anxiety.	no ergogenic effect reported, however, when combined with vitamins B1 and B6 may reduce anxiety.
Folic acid (folate)	may increase red blood cells for better oxygen to muscle and decrease birth defects.	found to decrease birth defects in pregnant women, but shown not to enhance athletic performance.
Pantothenic acid	may benefit aerobic energy.	research reports no enhanced aerobic performance.
Beta-carotene	may help exercise-induced muscle damage.	may help decrease exercise-induced muscle damage, but more research is required for improved athletic performance.
Vitamin C	may improve metabolism during exercise.	well-nourished athletes indicate no enhanced performance.

Supplement Value of Minerals for Athletes

Minerals are inorganic elements essential for metabolic processes, tissue structure and repair, hormone regulation and neurological function. Research indicates active adults or athletes have been deficient in these important elements. Mineral deficiency may negatively affect athletic performance and therefore supplementation may be helpful. The following mineral supplements common to athletes have been researched as proposed nutritional ergogenic aids:

Nutrient	Ergogenic Claim	Research Findings
Boron	May promote muscle growth during resistance training.	No evidence currently exists to support this theory.
Calcium	May promote bone growth and fat metabolism.	Shown to stimulate bone growth taken with vitamin D and may promote fat metabolism. No ergogenic benefit for athletic performance.
Chromium	Sold as chromium picolinate and claims to increase lean mass and reduce body fat.	Recent studies show no improvement in lean mass or reduced body fat.
Iron	May help improve aerobic performance.	Shown to only improve aerobic performance in athletes suffering from iron deficiency or anemia.
Magnesium	May improve energy metabolism/ATP availability.	Shown to only improve exercise performance in athletes suffering from magnesium deficiency.
Phosphorus (phosphate salts)	May improve energy systems in the body.	Shown to enhance the aerobic energy system during endurance training. More research is required.
Potassium	May help with muscle cramping.	No ergogenic benefits reported and research remains unclear if it helps with muscle cramping.
Selenium	May improve aerobic exercise performance.	Improvements in aerobic exercise performance have not been demonstrated
Sodium	May help with muscle cramping and reduce risk of hyponatremia.	Shown to maintain fluid balance during heavy training and prevent hyponatremia.
Vanadyl sulfate (vanadium)	May stimulate muscle growth, enhance strength and power.	Not shown to have any effect on muscle mass, strength or power.
Zinc	May reduce upper respiratory tract infections during heavy training.	Shown to minimize exercise-induced changes to immune function during training.

Water as an Ergogenic Aid for Athletes

Water is considered the most important nutritional ergogenic aid for active adults and athletes. If 2 percent or more of body weight is lost through sweat, athletic performance may be significantly impaired. Weight loss of 4 percent or more during exercise may lead to heat illness, heat exhaustion, or more severe adverse health effects. It is critical for active adults and athletes to implement hydration management during training and competitive events. The International Society of Sports Nutrition(ISSN) recommends:

- Consuming a sufficient amount of water and sports drinks to maintain fluid balance and hydration.

- Athletes should drink 0.5 to 2 liters per hour of fluid in order to offset weight loss.

- Don't depend on thirst as an indicator to drink water or sports drinks.
- Athletes should weigh themselves prior to and following exercise.
- Consume three cups of water for every pound lost during athletic training.
- Avoid excessive weight loss techniques including sauna sweats, wearing rubber suits, using diuretics, vomiting, or severe dieting.

The takeaway is to become well educated on proper hydration methods during athletic training. This will help you maintain proper fluid balance and provide a positive exercise experience.

The Role of Dietary Supplements for Athletes

Dietary supplements can play an important role in an athletic diet. However, they should be viewed as supplements to the diet, not replacements for a good diet. While there are very few supplements backed by scientific evidence to enhance athletic performance, there are some shown to be helpful for exercise and recovery. Whether you're an active adult, athlete working alone, or have hired a sports nutrition specialist, it's important to stay current on supplement research. The following common nutritional supplements have been researched and classified as either: apparently effective, possibly effective, too early to tell, or apparently ineffective.

Apparently Effective and Generally Safe

- Muscle building supplements:
  - Weight gain powders.
  - Creatine.
  - protein.
  - Essential amino acids (EAA).
- Weight loss supplements:
  - Low-calorie foods, meal replacement powders (mrps), ready-to-drink shakes (rtds).
  - Ephedra, caffeine, and salicin containing thermogenic supplements taken in recommended doses for appropriate populations (ephedra is banned by the FDA).
- Performance-enhancing supplements:
  - Water and sports drinks.
  - Carbohydrates.
  - Creatine.
  - Sodium phosphate.
  - Sodium bicarbonate.
  - Caffeine.
  - B-alanine.

Possibly Effective but more Research Required

- Muscle building supplements:
  - HMB in untrained individuals, start-up training programs.
  - BCAA (branched chain amino acids).
- Weight loss supplements:
  - High-fiber diets.
  - Calcium.
  - Green tea extract.
  - conjugated linoleic acids (CLA).
- Performance-enhancing supplements:
  - Post-exercise carbohydrate and protein.
  - Essential amino acids (EAA).
  - Branched chain amino acids (BCAA).
  - HMB.
  - Glycerol.

Too Early to tell and Lacks Sufficient Research

- Muscle building supplements:
  - α-Ketoglutarate.
  - α-Ketoisocaproate.
  - Ecdysterones.
  - Growth hormone releasing peptides and secretogues.
  - Ornithine α-ketoglutarate.
  - Zinc/magnesium aspartate.
- Weight loss supplements:
  - Gymnema sylvestre, chitosan.
  - Phosphatidl choline.
  - Betaine.
  - Coleus forskolin.
  - DHEA.
  - Psychotropic Nutrients/Herbs.

- Performance-enhancing supplements:
    - Medium chain triglycerides.

Apparently not Effective and Unsafe

- Muscle building supplements:
    - Glutamine.
    - Smilax.
    - Isoflavones.
    - Sulfo-polysaccharides (myostatin inhibitors).
    - Boron.
    - Chromium.
    - Conjugated linoleic acids.
    - Gamma oryzanol.
    - Prohormones.
    - Tribulus terrestris.
    - Vanadyl sulfate (vanadium).
- Weight loss supplements:
    - Calcium Pyruvate.
    - Chitosan.
    - Chromium (for people who don't have diabetes).
    - HCA.
    - L-Carnitine.
    - Phosphates.
    - Herbal diuretics.
- Performance-enhancing supplements:
    - Glutamine.
    - Ribose.
    - Inosine.

General Health Supplements Suggested for Athletes

Maintaining good health for active adults and athletes is essential. It is suggested athletes supplement with a few additional nutrients to stay healthy during intense exercise. The American

Medical Association (AMA) recommends all Americans "ingest a daily low-dose multivitamin" to ensure proper amounts of nutrients in the diet. Although not recommended to enhance athletic performance, a multi-vitamin may be helpful for general health. Other research recommends the following additional nutrients for active adults and athletes:

- Glucosamine and chondroitin (preventative for joint pain and slowed cartilage degeneration).
- Vitamin C, glutamine, echinacea, and zinc (may enhance immune function).
- Omega-3 fatty acids (heart healthy fats endorsed by the *American Heart Association* (AHA)).

Dietary Supplements

Dietary supplements to enhance exercise and athletic performance come in a variety of forms, including tablets, capsules, liquids, powders, and bars. Many of these products contain numerous ingredients in varied combinations and amounts. Among the more common ingredients are amino acids, protein, creatine, and caffeine. According to one estimate, retail sales of the category of "sports nutrition supplements" totaled $5.67 billion in 2016, or 13.8% of $41.16 billion total sales for dietary supplements and related nutrition products for that year.

Several surveys have indicated the extent of dietary supplement use for bodybuilding and to enhance exercise and athletic performance:

- International surveys found that two-thirds of 3,887 adult and adolescent elite track and field athletes participating in world-championship competitions took one or more dietary supplements containing such ingredients as vitamins, minerals, creatine, caffeine, and amino acids. Supplement use increased with age and was significantly more common among women than men.

- A survey of 1,248 students aged 16 years or older in five U.S. colleges and universities in 2009–2010 found that 66% reported use of any dietary supplement. The reasons for use included enhanced muscle strength (20% of users), performance enhancement (19% of users), and increased endurance (7% of users). Products taken for these purposes included protein, amino acids, herbal supplements, caffeine, creatine, and combination products.

- In a national survey of about 21,000 U.S. college athletes, respondents reported taking protein products (41.7%), energy drinks and shots (28.6%), creatine (14.0%), amino acids (12.1%), multivitamins with caffeine (5.7%), beta-hydroxy-beta-methylbutyrate (HMB; 0.2%), dehydroepiandrosterone (DHEA; 0.1%), and an unspecified mix of "testosterone boosters" (1.6%). Men were much more likely to take performance-enhancing products than women, except for energy drinks and shots. Among the sports with the highest percentage of users of performance-enhancing products were ice hockey, wrestling, and baseball among the men and volleyball, swimming, and ice hockey among the women.

- In a review of studies on adolescent use of performance-enhancing substances, the American Academy of Pediatrics concluded that protein, creatine, and caffeine were the most commonly used ingredients and that use increased with age. Although athletes used these ingredients more than nonathletes, teenagers not involved in organized athletic activities often took them to enhance their appearance.

- A survey of 106,698 U.S. military personnel in 2007–2008 found that 22.8% of the men and 5.3% of the women reported using bodybuilding supplements, such as creatine and amino acids, and 40.5% of the men and 35.5% of the women reported using energy supplements that might contain caffeine and energy-enhancing herbs. Use of these products was positively associated with deployment to combat situations, being younger than 29 years, being physically active, and reporting 5 or fewer hours of sleep a night.

It is difficult to make generalizations about the extent of dietary supplement use by athletes because the studies on this topic are heterogeneous. But the data suggest that:

- A larger proportion of athletes than the general U.S. population take dietary supplements.
- Elite athletes (e.g., professional athletes and those who compete on a national or international level) use dietary supplements more often than their non-elite counterparts.
- The supplements used by male and female athletes are similar, except that a larger proportion of women use iron and a larger proportion of men take vitamin E, protein, and creatine.

For any individual to physically perform at his or her best, a nutritionally adequate diet and sufficient hydration are critical. Athletes require adequate daily amounts of calories, fluids, carbohydrates (to maintain blood glucose levels and replace muscle glycogen; typically 1.4 to 4.5 g/lb body weight [3 to 10 g/kg body weight]), protein (0.55 to 0.9 g/lb body weight [1.2 to 2.0 g/kg body weight]), fat (20% to 35% of total calories), and vitamins and minerals.

A few dietary supplements might enhance performance only when they add to, but do not substitute for, this dietary foundation. Athletes engaging in endurance activities lasting more than an hour or performed in extreme environments (e.g., hot temperatures or high altitudes) might need to replace lost fluids and electrolytes and consume additional carbohydrates for energy. Even with proper nutritional preparation, the results of taking any dietary supplement(s) for exercise and athletic performance vary by level of training; the nature, intensity, and duration of the activity; and the environmental conditions.

Sellers claim that dozens of ingredients in dietary supplements can enhance exercise and athletic performance. Well-trained elite and recreational athletes might use products containing one or more of these ingredients to train harder, improve performance, and achieve a competitive edge. However, the National Athletic Trainers' Association acknowledges in a position statement that because the outcomes of studies of various performance-enhancing substances are often equivocal, using these substances can be controversial and confusing.

Most studies to assess the potential value and safety of supplements to enhance exercise and athletic performance include only conditioned athletes. Therefore, it is often not clear whether the supplements may be of value to recreational exercisers or individuals who engage in athletic activity only occasionally. In addition, much of the research on these supplements involves young adults (more often male than female), and not adolescents who may also use them against the advice of paediatric and high-school professional associations. The quality of many studies is limited by their small samples and short durations, use of performance tests that do not simulate real-world conditions or are unreliable or irrelevant, and poor control of confounding variables. Furthermore, the benefits and risks shown for the supplements might not apply to the supplement's use to enhance types of physical performance not assessed in the studies. In most cases, additional research is needed to fully understand the efficacy and safety of particular ingredients.

Selected Ingredients in Dietary Supplements for Exercise and Athletic Performance

Many exercise and athletic-performance dietary supplements in the marketplace contain multiple ingredients (especially those marketed for muscle growth and strength). However, much of the research has focused only on single ingredients. One therefore cannot know or predict the effects and safety of combinations in these multi-ingredient products unless clinical trials have investigated that particular combination. Furthermore, the amounts of these ingredients vary widely among products. In some cases, the products contain proprietary blends of ingredients listed in order by weight, but labels do not provide the amount of each ingredient in the blend. Manufacturers and sellers of dietary supplements for exercise and athletic performance rarely fund or conduct scientific research on their proprietary products of a caliber that reputable biomedical journals require for publication.

Antioxidants (Vitamin C, Vitamin E and Coenzyme Q)

Exercise increases the body's consumption of oxygen and induces oxidative stress, leading to the production of reactive oxygen and nitrogen species (i.e., free radicals) and the creation of more oxidized molecules in various tissues, including muscle. In theory, free radicals could impair exercise performance by impeding muscles' ability to produce force, thereby accelerating muscle damage and fatigue and producing inflammation and soreness. Some researchers have suggested that supplements containing antioxidants, such as vitamins C and E and coenzyme Q (CoQ), could reduce this free-radical formation, thereby minimizing skeletal muscle damage and fatigue and promoting recovery.

Efficacy: Studies suggest that the use of large doses of antioxidant supplements, especially vitamins C and E, may actually reduce rather than promote some of the beneficial effects of exercise. One study, for example, randomly assigned 54 healthy Norwegian men and women aged 20–30 years, most of whom were recreational exercisers, to receive 1,000 mg vitamin C and 235 mg (about 520 IU) vitamin E as DL-alpha-tocopherol or a placebo daily for 11 weeks while engaging in an endurance training program consisting mostly of running. Compared with placebo, the supplements had no effect on maximal oxygen consumption (VO_2max, a measure of aerobic fitness and endurance capacity) or running performance. However, they significantly lowered levels of biochemical markers related to mitochondrial creation and exercise-induced cell signaling, thereby diminishing the desirable training-induced adaptations within skeletal muscle. The same research group conducted another trial using the same doses of vitamins C and E in 32 young men and women who followed a strength-training program for 10 weeks. Compared with placebo, the supplements did not affect muscle growth, but they significantly reduced the gain in arm strength as measured by biceps curls and blunted cellular signaling pathways linked to muscle hypertrophy. Another study randomly assigned 18 young men aged 20 to 34 years to receive 120 mg/day CoQ for 22 days or a placebo. After 7 days of high-intensity cycling sprints, the CoQ group had, on average, a significantly smaller improvement in mean power output than the placebo group, suggesting a poorer adaptation to training.

The preponderance of research to date suggests that exercise-induced reactive oxygen species and nitric oxide are beneficial. These free radicals induce adaptive changes in muscle that lead to greater production of mitochondria and hypertrophy of myofibers. Exposure of cells to high concentrations of various antioxidant supplements (of which vitamins C and E have the most evidence) appears to blunt or block cell signaling and thereby inhibit some favorable physiological and physical adaptations to exercise. However, these adaptations might not prevent improvements in VOmax or endurance performance.

Safety: Studies on the safety of vitamins C, E, and other antioxidant supplements taken during exercise show no evidence of adverse effects, aside from potentially reducing some of the benefits of exercise, but such studies have only lasted a few weeks or months. The Tolerable Upper Intake Level (UL) of vitamin C that the Food and Nutrition Board established as the maximum amount associated with little or no risk of adverse health effects is 1,800 mg/day for adolescents and 2,000 mg/day for adults. These amounts are substantially higher than the doses that studies have typically used for exercise and athletic performance. The UL of vitamin E, at 800 mg/day for adolescents and 1,000 mg/day (1,100–1,500 IU) for adults, is likewise higher than the dose that these studies typically used.

Among the potential adverse effects of excess vitamin C are diarrhea, nausea, abdominal cramps, and other gastrointestinal disturbances. The intake of excessive amounts of vitamin E increases the risks of hemorrhagic effects. Moreover, results from a large clinical trial show that vitamin E supplements, even at doses below the UL (400 IU/day taken for several years), might increase men's risk of prostate cancer. The side effects of CoQ_{10} are mild and can include fatigue, insomnia, rashes, nausea, upper abdominal pain, heartburn, sensitivity to light, irritability, dizziness, and headaches.

Implications for use: Little research supports the use as ergogenic aids of antioxidant supplements containing greater amounts than those available from a nutritionally adequate diet. In fact, they can adversely affect some measures of exercise and athletic performance. The Australian Institute of Sport, part of the government of Australia, does not recommend supplementation with vitamins C and E by athletes, except when they use these products as part of a research protocol or with proper monitoring.

Arginine

L-arginine is an amino acid found in many protein-containing foods, especially animal products and nuts. The typical dietary intake is 4–5 grams/day. The body also synthesizes arginine (from citrulline), mainly in the kidneys.

Some experts suggest that taking arginine in supplement form enhances exercise and athletic performance in several ways. First, some arginine is converted to nitric oxide, a potent vasodilator that can increase blood flow and the delivery of oxygen and nutrients to skeletal muscle. Second, increased vasodilation can speed up the removal of metabolic waste products related to muscle fatigue, such as lactate and ammonia that the body produces during exercise. Third, arginine serves as a precursor for the synthesis of creatine, which helps supply muscle with energy for short-term, intense activity. Fourth, arginine may increase the secretion of human growth hormone (HGH), which in turn increases insulin-like growth factor-1 (IGF-1) levels, both of which stimulate muscle growth.

Efficacy: The research to support supplemental arginine as a performance enhancer is limited and conflicting. Overall, it suggests that doses of 2–20 g/day arginine have little to no effect on performance in either anaerobic or aerobic exercise. Furthermore, arginine typically had no effect on nitric oxide concentration, blood flow, or exercise metabolites (e.g., lactate and ammonia), especially when well-trained athletes—including cyclists, tennis players, and judo practitioners—took the supplement for 1–28 days. A recent review assessed 54 clinical studies examining the effects of arginine supplementation on strength performance, endurance, muscle blood volume and flow, cardiorespiratory measures, and nitric oxide production in healthy, active adults. The authors concluded that supplemental arginine (either alone or, more commonly, in combination with other ingredients, such as branched-chain amino acids [BCAAs] and lysine) provided little or no enhancement of athletic performance and did not improve recovery from exhaustion. Most of the studies included few participants, primarily young men aged 18–25 years (only four studies included women), and lasted only 4–8 weeks (with none lasting 3 months or longer). In the 18 studies that compared arginine alone with a placebo, the most common doses were 2–10 g/day as a single dose and up to 20 g/day divided into three doses.

Research on the ability of supplemental arginine to raise HGH and IGF-1 serum concentrations also has had conflicting findings. Depending on the study (and therefore participants' age, fitness level, and use of other supplements as well as the nature and duration of the exercise), extra arginine might either reduce HGH secretion or raise HGH and IGF-1 secretion. Even raised HGH secretion, however, might not translate into more blood flow into muscle or greater protein synthesis. Little evidence shows supplemental arginine by itself increases muscle creatine concentrations or is superior or complementary to direct consumption of creatine.

Safety: Most study results suggest that up to 9 g/day arginine for several days or weeks is safe and well tolerated. At doses of 9–30 g/day, the most commonly reported adverse reactions are gastrointestinal discomfort, such as diarrhea and nausea, and slightly reduced blood pressure. The safety of taking high-dose arginine supplements for more than 3 months is not known.

Implications for use: Arginine supplementation's ability to enhance strength, improve exercise or athletic performance, or promote muscular recovery after exercise has little scientific support.

Beetroot or Beet juice

Beets are one of the richest food sources of inorganic nitrate. Ingested nitrate might enhance exercise and athletic performance in several ways, primarily through its conversion into nitric oxide in the body. Nitric acid is a potent vasodilator that can increase blood flow and the delivery of oxygen and nutrients to skeletal muscle. Ingested nitrate might also enhance performance by dilating blood vessels in exercising muscle when oxygen levels decline, thereby increasing oxygen and nutrient delivery, reducing the oxygen cost of submaximal exercise, attenuating the adenosine triphosphate (ATP)-creatine phosphate energy system's cost associated with skeletal muscle force production, and improving oxidative phosphorylation in mitochondria. Beetroot is available as a juice or juice concentrate and in powdered form; the amount of nitrate can vary considerably among products.

Efficacy: A growing number of clinical trials investigating beetroot juice or concentrate as an ergogenic aid have been published since 2007. Beetroot has generally improved performance and endurance to different extents compared with placebo among runners, swimmers, rowers, and cyclists in time trials and time-to-exhaustion tests, but not in all studies. Performance benefits are more likely in recreationally active non-athletes than elite athletes. One study in 10 recreationally active, young male cyclists suggested a dose-response relationship. Although consuming beetroot juice concentrate on each of 4 days to supply 4.2 mmol nitrate (70 ml) provided no performance benefits compared with placebo, larger amounts of juice supplying 8.4 mmol nitrate (140 ml) did. However, consumption of even more beetroot juice supplying 16.8 mmol nitrate (280 ml) produced no further performance benefits. There has been little study of the effects of beetroot on anaerobic performance, such as high-volume resistance exercise with many repetitions.

More research is needed to clarify the potential benefits of nitrate supplementation from beetroot juice on exercise and athletic performance and to determine the best doses and dosing protocols. No research has assessed longer-term supplementation with beetroot-derived nitrate beyond several weeks as an ergogenic aid.

Safety: Studies have not identified any safety concerns with the consumption of beetroot juice in moderate amounts (about 2 cups/day) for several weeks. The amount of nitrate that this amount of juice provides is less than half the total nitrate consumption from a diet rich in vegetables and fruits. Although not a safety concern, beetroot consumption can color the urine pink or red due to the excretion of red pigments in the beets.

Implications for use: In a position statement, the Academy of Nutrition and Dietetics (AND), the Dietitians of Canada (DoC), and the American College of Sports Medicine (ACSM) state that nitrate sources, such as beetroot juice, enhance exercise tolerance and economy and they improve endurance exercise performance in recreational athletes. researchers support the use of beetroot juice for improving sports performance in suitable athletic competitions under the direction of an expert in sports medicine, but it notes that more research might be required to understand how the supplement should be used for best results.

Most studies have used 500 ml/day (about 2 cups) of beetroot juice taken once (about 2.5 to 3 hours before exercise) or daily for up to 15 days. This amount of juice provides about 5–11 mmol (or 310–682 mg) nitrate, depending on the product. Potential benefits persist for up to 24 hours after ingestion. The labels on beetroot juice and concentrate usually indicate that these products are foods and not dietary supplements. Some dietary supplements contain beetroot powder in varying amounts, but studies have not assessed whether these are viable alternatives to beetroot juice or beetroot-juice concentrate.

Beta-alanine

Beta-alanine, a type of amino acid that the body does not incorporate into proteins, is the rate-limiting precursor to the synthesis of carnosine—a dipeptide of histidine and beta-alanine—in skeletal muscle. Carnosine helps buffer changes in muscle pH from the anaerobic glycolysis that provides energy during high-intensity exercise but results in the buildup of hydrogen ions as lactic acid accumulates and dissociates to form lactate, leading to reduced force and to fatigue. More carnosine in muscle leads to greater potential attenuation of exercise- induced reductions in pH, which could enhance performance of intense activities of short to moderate duration, such as rowing and swimming.

Beta-alanine is produced in the liver, and relatively small amounts are present in animal-based foods such as meat, poultry, and fish. Estimated dietary intakes range from none in vegans to about 1 g/day in heavy meat eaters. Carnosine is present in animal-based foods, such as beef and pork. However, oral consumption of carnosine is an inefficient method of increasing muscle carnosine concentrations because the dipeptide is digested into its constituent amino acids. Consumption of beta-alanine, in contrast, reliably increases the amount of carnosine in the body. Four to six grams of beta-alanine for 10 weeks, for example, can increase muscle carnosine levels by up to 80%, especially in trained athletes, although the magnitude of response differs widely. For example, in one study of young, physically active but untrained adult men who took 4.8 g/day beta-alanine for 5–6 weeks, the percent increase in muscle carnosine content after 9 weeks of follow-up ranged from 2% to 69%. Among the "low responders," the duration of the washout period when beta alanine concentrations returned to baseline values was less than half that for the "high responders" (6 weeks vs. 15 weeks).

Efficacy: Studies have evaluated beta-alanine as a potential ergogenic aid with a variety of participants, exercise and activity protocols, and dosing regimens. Some studies suggest that beta-alanine consumption could provide small performance benefits in competitive events requiring high-intensity effort over a short period, such as rowing, swimming, and team sports (e.g., hockey and football) that involve repeated sprints and intermittent activity. Other studies have found no such benefits. Evidence is conflicting on whether beta-alanine consumption improves performance in endurance activities, such as cycling. Experts have not reached consensus on whether beta-alanine consumption primarily benefits trained athletes or recreationally active individuals. Studies provide little consistent evidence of a relationship between the dose of beta-alanine and performance effect.

The authors of a Department of Defense-sponsored review concluded that the limited evidence from 20 human trials did not support consumption of beta-alanine (alone or in combination products) by active adults to enhance athletic performance or improve recovery from exercise-related exhaustion. Most of the studies in this review included young men aged 18–25 years who took 1.6–6.4 g/day beta-alanine supplements (in two to four separate servings) over 4–8 weeks. In contrast, the International Society of Sports Nutrition (ISSN) concluded from its literature review that beta- alanine supplements (4–6 g/day consumed for at least 2–4 weeks) can improve high-intensity exercise performance that lasts over 60 seconds, especially in time-to-exhaustion tasks. However, performance benefits are more modest in exercise tests lasting more than 4 minutes because aerobic metabolic pathways increasingly meet energy demands. The ISSN called for more research to determine whether beta-alanine increases the strength and muscle mass that regular resistance exercise, such as weightlifting, can produce.

The authors of the most recent review of studies on beta-alanine's effects on exercise concluded that supplementation has a statistically significant and positive effect on performance (including in both isolated-limb and whole-body exercises), especially in protocols lasting 30 seconds to 10 minutes. However, this review also highlighted the fact that small studies of short duration using varied exercise and supplement protocols dominate this scientific literature. The 40 placebo-controlled studies reviewed, for example, employed 65 exercise protocols and 70 exercise measures in a total of 1,461 participants. Furthermore, the total dose of beta-alanine that participants consumed ranged from 84 to 414 g in studies lasting 28–90 days.

Safety: Beta-alanine supplementation appears to be safe at 1.6–6.4 g/day for up to 8 weeks. Some evidence does show, however, that consuming a conventional dose of beta-alanine of at least 800 mg or exceeding 10 mg/kg body mass can provoke moderate to severe paresthesia. This tingling, prickling, or burning sensation is common in the face, neck, back of the hands, and upper trunk and typically lasts 60–90 minutes but is not a painful, serious, or harmful reaction. Use of divided doses or a sustained-release form of the supplement can attenuate paresthesia resulting from beta-alanine consumption. Some research has also found that beta-alanine supplements can produce pruritus (itchy skin), but the authors do not indicate the severity of this effect. There are no safety data on use of the supplement for more than 1 year.

Implications for use: There is insufficient expert consensus on the value of taking beta-alanine to enhance performance in intense, short-term activities or its safety, particularly when users take it regularly for at least several months. In a position statement, AND, DoC, and ACSM advise that beta-alanine supplementation might improve training capacity and does enhance performance, especially of high-intensity exercise lasting 60-240 seconds, that acid-base disturbances resulting from increased anaerobic glycolysis would otherwise impair. In its position statement, ISSN concludes that beta-alanine supplementation improves exercise performance and attenuates neuromuscular fatigue. Researchers support the use of beta- alanine for improving sports performance in suitable athletic competitions under the direction of an expert in sports medicine, but it notes that more research might be required to understand how the supplement should be used for best results.

For healthy individuals willing to use beta-alanine supplements, ISSN recommends a daily loading dose of 4 to 6 g/day in divided doses of 2 g or less for at least 2 weeks. The society states that bepnfits increase after 4 weeks, when muscle carnosine concentrations rise by 40–60%. It advises users to take beta-alanine supplements with meals to augment muscle carnosine levels and to use divided lower doses or take a sustained-release form if paresthesia occurs.

Beta-hydroxy-beta-methylbutyrate

Beta-hydroxy-beta-methylbutyrate (HMB) is a metabolite of the branched-chain amino acid leucine. About 5% of the body's leucine is converted into HMB, which is then converted in the liver to a precursor (known as beta-hydroxy-beta-methylglutaryl coenzyme A) needed for cholesterol biosynthesis. Some experts hypothesize that skeletal muscle cells that become stressed and damaged from exercise require an exogenous source of the coenzyme for synthesis of cholesterol in their cellular membranes to restore structure and function. Experts also believe that the conversion of leucine to HMB activates muscle protein synthesis and reduces protein breakdown. Supplementation is the only practical way to obtain 3 g/day HMB because one would otherwise need to consume over 600 g/day of high-quality protein (from 5 lb of beef tenderloin, for example) to obtain enough leucine (60 g) for conversion into HMB.

Efficacy: Although studies have investigated HMB for two decades, they have used substantially different periods of supplementation (1 day to 6 weeks) and daily doses (1.5 to 6 g; most commonly 3 g based on evidence that this dose provides equivalent results to 6 g and better results than 1.5 g). Studies also used participants of different ages (19 to 50 years), training status (e.g., untrained or trained athletes), training protocols (e.g., with machines or free weights), training duration (10 days to 12 weeks), consumption of other supplements (such as creatine), and other factors. It is therefore difficult to predict what, if any, benefits an exercising individual might experience from consuming HMB.

There is general agreement that HMB helps speed up recovery from exercise of sufficient amount and intensity to induce skeletal muscle damage. Therefore, trained athletes must exert themselves more than untrained individuals to potentially benefit from using the supplement. Some studies suggest that HMB use has additional benefits, including an ability to enhance strength, power, skeletal muscle hypertrophy, and aerobic performance in both trained and untrained people.

Safety: A review of safety data from nine studies found that users tolerate HMB well, and it is safe at daily intakes of 3 g for 3 to 8 weeks in younger (ages 18–47 years) and older (ages 62–81) adults of both sexes who do or do not exercise. Assessments of blood chemistry, hematology, and emotional affect found no adverse effects. Another study randomized 37 untrained males aged 18–29 years participating in a resistance training program to take either no HMB or about 3–6 g/day HMB. Use of HMB did not alter or adversely affect any measured hematologic, hepatic, or renal-function parameters in these young men. Although 3 g/day HMB appears to be safe for short-term use in adults, its safety profile (and efficacy) has not been studied in adolescents.

Implications for use: There is no expert consensus on the value of taking HMB for several months or longer or its safety. HMB is not on a list of evidence-based ergogenic aids issued by the AND, DoC, and the ACSM. The researchers support not recommends HMB supplementation by athletes, except as part of a research protocol or with proper monitoring. However, ISSN notes that HMB can enhance recovery by reducing exercise-induced skeletal muscle damage in both trained and untrained individuals.

HMB is available in two forms: as a mono-hydrated calcium salt (HMB-Ca) and a calcium-free form (HMB-free acid [HMB-FA]). HMB-Ca is approximately 13% calcium by weight, and a daily dose of 3 g/day adds about 400 mg calcium to the diet. Those who wish to limit their calcium intake can use HMB-FA. Although the latter form appears to have a faster and greater effect based on its ability to raise HMB plasma levels, more studies are needed to compare the effects of HMB-Ca with those of HMB-FA.

The ISSN recommends that healthy adults interested in using HMB supplements take 1–2 g HMB-Ca 60 to 120 minutes before exercise or 1–2 g HMB-FA 30 to 60 minutes before exercise. It also suggests that supplement users ideally consume 3 g/day HMB (in three equal servings of 1 g) for at least 2 weeks before high-intensity exercise to optimize HMB's protective effects on muscle.

Betaine

Betaine, also known as trimethylglycine, is found in foods such as beets, spinach, and whole-grain breads. Average daily intakes of betaine range from 100 to 300 mg/day. The mechanisms by which betaine might enhance exercise and athletic performance are not known, but many are hypothesized. For example, betaine might increase the biosynthesis of creatine, levels of blood nitric acid, and the water retention of cells.

Efficacy: A limited number of small studies in men have assessed betaine in supplemental form as a potential ergogenic aid. These studies, which typically examined strength- and power-based performance in bodybuilders and, occasionally, cyclists, provided conflicting results, and performance improvements tended to be modest. The typical dose of betaine that studies used ranged from 2 to 5 g/day for up to 15 days.

Safety: The several small studies of athletes described in the previous paragraph who took betaine supplements for up to several weeks found no side effects or safety concerns. However, research has not adequately evaluated the safety of betaine.

Implications for use: More research on betaine supplementation to enhance various types of performance, training protocols, and exercise during specific sports is needed before any recommendations for its use can be made.

Branched-chain Amino Acids

Three essential amino acids—leucine, isoleucine, and valine—are the branched-chain amino acids (BCAAs), whose name reflects their chemical structure. BCAAs make up approximately 25% of the amino acids in foods containing complete proteins (including all essential amino acids); most of these foods are animal products, such as meat, poultry, fish, eggs, and milk. BCAAs comprise about 14%–18% of the amino acids in human skeletal muscle proteins. Unlike other essential amino acids, the BCAAs can be metabolized by mitochondria in skeletal muscle to provide energy during exercise. The BCAAs, especially leucine, might also stimulate protein synthesis in exercised muscle.

Efficacy: The limited research on the potential ergogenic effects of the BCAAs has found little evidence to date that supplements of these amino acids improve performance in endurance-related aerobic events. The BCAAs might delay feelings of fatigue or help maintain mental focus by competing with the amino acid tryptophan (a precursor of the neurotransmitter serotonin that regulates mood and sleep) for entry into the brain, but this effect has not been well studied. The results of several short-term studies lasting about 3 to 6 weeks suggest that about 10–14 g/day supplemental BCAAs might enhance gains in muscle mass and strength during training. Overall, however, studies to date provide inconsistent evidence of the ability of BCAAs to stimulate muscle protein synthesis beyond the capacity of sufficient dietary amounts of any high-quality protein to perform this function. Furthermore, it is not clear from existing research whether consumption of protein and BCAAs before versus after a workout affects their ability to maximize muscle protein synthesis and reduce protein catabolism.

Safety: Up to 20 g/day BCAA supplements in divided doses appear to be safe. For leucine alone, studies suggest an upper safe limit of intake of 500 mg/kg per day in healthy young and elderly men, or about 38 g/day for a man weighing 75 kg (165 lb).

Implications for use: Studies have not consistently shown that taking supplements of BCAAs or any of their three constituent amino acids singly enhances exercise and athletic performance, builds muscle mass, or aids in recovery from exercise. Consuming animal foods containing complete proteins—or a combination of plant-based foods with complementary proteins that together provide all essential amino acids—automatically increases consumption of BCAAs. This is also true of consuming protein powders made from complete proteins, especially whey, which has more leucine than either casein or soy.

Caffeine

Caffeine is a methylated xanthine naturally found in variable amounts in coffee; tea; cacao pods (the source of chocolate); and other herbal/botanical sources, such as guarana, kola (or cola) nut, and yerba mate. Caffeine stimulates the central nervous system, muscles, and other organs, such as the heart, by binding to adenosine receptors on cells, thereby blocking the activity of adenosine, a neuromodulator with sedative-like properties. In this way, caffeine enhances arousal, increases vigor, and reduces fatigue. Caffeine also appears to reduce perceived pain and exertion. During the early stages of endurance exercise, caffeine might mobilize free fatty acids as a source of energy and spare muscle glycogen.

Caffeine is commonly used in energy drinks and "shots" touted for their performance-enhancement effects. It is also found in energy gels containing carbohydrates and electrolytes as well as in anhydrous caffeine-only pills.

Efficacy: Many studies have shown that caffeine might enhance performance in athletes when they ingest about 2–6 mg/kg body weight before exercise by improving endurance, strength, and power in high-intensity team sports activities. For an individual weighing 154 pounds (70 kg), this dose is equivalent to 210–420 mg caffeine. Taking more, however, is unlikely to improve performance further and increases the risk of side effects.

A review of the literature found that caffeine intake affected sport-specific performance (e.g., running, cycling, swimming, and rowing), as measured in time trials. Although 30 of the 33 trials showed positive improvements in performance, the improvements were not statistically significant in half of them. In these studies, performance improvement ranged from a decrease of 0.7% to an increase of 17.3%, suggesting that the caffeine was very helpful to some participants but slightly impaired performance in others. Factors such as the timing of ingestion, caffeine intake mode or form, and habituation to caffeine could also have accounted for the varied effects on performance.

Caffeine supplementation is more likely to help with endurance-type activities (such as running) and activities of long duration with intermittent activity (such as soccer) than more anaerobic, short-term bouts of intense exercise (such as sprinting or lifting weights). Some evidence suggests that caffeine is more likely to improve performance in people who are not habituated to it. Limiting caffeine intake to 50 mg/day or abstaining from caffeine for 2–7 days before taking it for an athletic event might maximize any ergogenic effect. However, other evidence shows no habituation effect of caffeine consumption on performance.

Safety: Heavy caffeine use (500 mg/day or more) might diminish rather than enhance physical performance and could also disturb sleep and cause irritability and anxiety. Other adverse effects of caffeine include insomnia, restlessness, nausea, vomiting, tachycardia, and arrhythmia. Caffeine does not induce diuresis or increase sweat loss during exercise and therefore does not reduce fluid balance in the body that would adversely affect performance.

For healthy adults, the U.S. Food and Drug Administration (FDA) states that 400 mg/day caffeine does not usually have dangerous adverse effects. The American Medical Association recommends that adults limit their intake of caffeine to 500 mg/day and that adolescents consume no more than 100 mg/day. The American Academy of Pediatrics warns that caffeine-containing energy drinks in particular "have no place in the diets of children or adolescents" and are not suitable for use during routine physical activity.

Pure powdered caffeine is available as a dietary supplement and is very potent. A single tablespoon contains 10 g caffeine, and an acute oral dose of 10 to 14 g caffeine (approximately 150–200 mg/kg) can be fatal. Furthermore, combining caffeine with other stimulants could increase the potential for adverse effects. At least two young men have died as a result of taking an unknown amount of pure powdered caffeine.

Implications for use: Caffeine is easily and rapidly absorbed, even from the buccal membranes in the mouth, and is distributed throughout the body and brain. It reaches peak concentrations in the blood within 45 minutes of consumption and has a half-life of about 4–5 hours. For a potential benefit to athletic performance, users should consume caffeine 15 to 60 minutes before exercise. Consumption of caffeine with fluid during exercise of long duration might extend any performance improvements.

In a position statement, AND, DoC, and ACSM state that caffeine supplementation reduces perceived fatigue and enables users to sustain exercise at the desired intensity longer. The U.S. Department of Defense states that caffeine supplementation at 2–6 mg/kg body weight is linked to enhanced physical performance and the effects of smaller doses usually last longer and are greater in people who do not usually consume caffeine. It adds that caffeine could reduce perceived exertion when exercise lasts longer. In a position statement, ISSN describes caffeine as effective in trained athletes for improving sports performance and notes that supplementation with about 3–6 mg/kg has an ergogenic effect on "sustained maximal endurance exercise" but not necessarily on "strength-power performance. Researchers support the use of caffeine for improving sports performance in suitable athletic competitions under the direction of an expert in sports medicine, but it notes that more research might be required to understand how caffeine should be used for best results.

The International Olympic Committee considers caffeine to be a "controlled or restricted substance;" Olympic athletes may consume it until urinary concentrations exceed 12 mcg/ml. The National Collegiate Athletic Association prohibits use of caffeine from any source in amounts that would lead to urine concentrations exceeding 15 mcg/ml. (Consuming about 500 mg caffeine produces a urinary caffeine concentration of 15 mcg/ml within 2–3 hours). The World Anti-Doping Agency does not prohibit or limit caffeine use.

Citrulline

L-citrulline is a nonessential amino acid produced in the body, mainly from glutamine, and obtained from the diet. Watermelon is the best-known source; 1 cup diced seedless watermelon has about 365 mg citrulline. About 80% of the body's citrulline is converted in the kidneys into arginine, another amino acid. The subsequent conversion of arginine to nitric oxide, a potent dilator of blood vessels, might be the mechanism by which citrulline could serve as an ergogenic aid. In fact, consumption of citrulline might be a more efficient way to raise blood arginine levels than consumption of arginine because more citrulline is absorbed from the gut than arginine.

Most studies have used citrulline malate, a combination of citrulline with malic acid (a constituent in many fruits that is also produced endogenously), because malate, an intermediate in the Krebs cycle, might enhance energy production.

Efficacy: The research to support supplemental citrulline as an ergogenic aid is limited and conflicting at best. The few published studies have had heterogeneous designs and ranged in duration from 1 to 16 days. As an example, in one randomized controlled study with a crossover design, 41 healthy male weight lifters aged 22–37 years consumed 8 g citrulline malate or a placebo 1 hour before completing barbell bench presses to exhaustion. Overall, participants could complete significantly more repetitions when taking the supplement and reported significantly less muscle soreness 1 and 2 days after the test. Another study that randomized 17 young healthy men and women to take citrulline without malate (either 3 g before testing or 9 g over 24 hours) or a placebo found that participants using the citrulline did not perform as well as those taking the placebo on an incremental treadmill test to exhaustion. Although citrulline supplementation might increase plasma levels of nitric oxide metabolites, such a response has not been directly related to any improvement in athletic performance.

Safety: Studies have not adequately assessed the safety of citrulline, particularly when users take it in supplemental form for months at a time. In the study of weight lifters described above, 6 of the 41 participants reported "stomach discomfort" after taking the supplement. Additional short-term studies in which supplemental citrulline was provided to non-athletes at up to 6 g/day for 4 weeks and 1.35 g/day for 6 weeks found no adverse effects.

Implications for use: The research to date does not provide strong support for taking citrulline or citrulline malate to enhance exercise or athletic performance. Whether athletes in specific sports or activities might benefit from taking supplemental citrulline remains to be determined.

Dietary supplements that contain citrulline provide either citrulline or citrulline malate. Citrulline malate is 56.64% citrulline by weight so, for example, 1 g citrulline malate provides 566 mg of citrulline. Sellers of some citrulline malate dietary supplements claim that they provide a higher percentage of citrulline (with labels listing, for example, citrulline malate 2:1 or tri-citrulline malate), but studies have not determined whether these supplements are superior to standard citrulline or citrulline malate supplements.

Creatine

Creatine is one of the most thoroughly studied and widely used dietary supplements to enhance exercise and sports performance. Creatine is produced endogenously and obtained from the diet in small amounts. It helps generate ATP and thereby supplies the muscles with energy, particularly for short-term events. Creatine might improve muscle performance in four ways: by increasing stores of phosphocreatine used to generate ATP at the beginning of intense exercise, accelerating the re-synthesis of phosphocreatine after exercise, depressing the degradation of adenine nucleotides and the accumulation of lactate, and enhancing glycogen storage in skeletal muscles.

The liver and kidneys synthesize about 1 g/day creatine from the amino acids glycine, arginine, and methionine. Animal-based foods, such as beef (2 g/lb), pork (2.3 g/lb), and salmon (2 g/lb), also contain creatine. A person weighing 154 pounds has about 120 g creatine and phosphocreatine in his or her body, almost all in the skeletal and cardiac muscles. However, it is only when users consume much greater amounts of creatine over time as a dietary supplement that it could have ergogenic effects. Metabolized creatine is converted into the waste product creatinine, which is eliminated from the body through the kidneys.

Efficacy: Studies in both laboratory and sports settings have found that short-term creatine supplementation (for 5 to 7 days) in both men and women often significantly increases strength (e.g., for bench presses) and power (e.g., for cycling), work involving multiple sets of maximal effort muscle contractions, and sprinting and soccer performance. In one example, a study randomized 14 healthy, resistance-trained men (aged 19–29 years) to receive 25 g creatine monohydrate or a placebo for 6–7 days. Participants taking the supplement had significant improvements in peak power output during all five sets of jump squats and in repetitions during all five sets of bench presses on three occasions. In another study, 18 well-trained male sprinters aged 18–24 years received either 20 g/day creatine or a placebo for 5 days. Compared with those taking the placebo, participants taking the creatine improved their performance in both 100- meter sprints and six intermittent 60 m sprints.

Supplementation with creatine over weeks or months helps training adaptations to structured, increased workloads over time. For example, in a randomized study of 14 female collegiate soccer players during the off-season, those who received creatine (15 g/day for 1 week and then 5 g/day for 12 weeks) had significantly greater increases in muscle strength, as measured by bench press and full-squat maximal strength testing, but not lean tissue compared with participants who took a placebo.

Individuals have varied responses to creatine supplementation, based on factors such as diet and the relative percentages of various muscle fiber types. Vegetarians, for example, with their lower muscle creatine content, might have greater responses to supplementation than meat eaters. Overall, creatine enhances performance during repeated short bursts of high-intensity, intermittent activity, such as sprinting and weight lifting, where energy for this predominantly anaerobic exercise comes mainly from the ATP-creatine phosphate energy system.

Creatine supplementation seems to be of little value for endurance sports, such as distance running or swimming, that do not depend on the short-term ATP-creatine phosphate system to provide short-term energy, and it leads to weight gain that might impede performance in such sports. Furthermore, in predominantly aerobic exercise lasting more than 150 seconds, the body relies on oxidative phosphorylation as the primary energy source, a metabolic pathway that does not require creatine.

Safety: Studies have found no consistent set of side effects from creatine use, except that it often leads to weight gain, because it increases water retention and possibly stimulates muscle protein synthesis. Several studies have found that supplemental creatine monohydrate, when used for a strength-training program, can lead to a 1–2 kg increase in total body weight in a month.

Creatine is considered safe for short-term use by healthy adults. In addition, evidence shows that use of the product for several years is safe. Anecdotal reactions to creatine use include nausea, diarrhea and related gastrointestinal distress, muscle cramps, and heat intolerance. Creatine supplementation may reduce the range of motion of various parts of the body (such as the shoulders, ankles, and lower legs) and lead to muscle stiffness and resistance to stretching. Adequate hydration while taking creatine might minimize these uncommon risks.

Implications for use: In a position statement, AND, DoC, and ACSM advise that creatine enhances performance of cycles of high-intensity exercise followed by short recovery periods and improves training capacity. In its position statement, ISSN states that creatine monohydrate is the most effective nutritional supplement currently available for enhancing capacity for high- intensity exercise and lean body mass during exercise. The ISSN contends that athletes who supplement with creatine have a lower incidence of injuries and exercise-related side effects compared to those who do not take creatine. Researchers support the use of creatine for improving sports performance in suitable athletic competitions under the direction of an expert in sports medicine, but it notes that more research might be required to understand how the supplement should be used for best results.

A typical protocol for creatine supplementation in adults, regardless of sex or body size, consists of a loading phase for 5–7 days, when users consume 20 g/day creatine monohydrate in four portions of 5 g, followed by a maintenance phase of 3–5 g/day. In some studies, the loading dose is based on body weight (e.g., 0.3 g/kg). Another creatine supplementation protocol consists of taking single doses of about 3–6 g/day (0.03–0.1 g/kg body weight) for 3 to 4 weeks, without a loading phase, to produce ergogenic effects.

Creatine monohydrate, which is 88% creatine by weight, is the most widely used and studied form. Other, usually more expensive, forms of creatine (e.g., creatine ethyl ester, creatine alpha-ketoglutarate, and buffered forms of creatine) have not been proven to have superior ability to creatine monohydrate for enhancing muscle creatine levels, digestibility, product stability, or safety.

Deer Antler Velvet

Deer antler velvet consists of cartilage and epidermis from growing deer or elk antlers before ossification. It is used as a general health aid in traditional Chinese medicine. Several growth factors have been detected in deer antler velvet, such as IGF-1, that could promote muscle tissue growth in a similar way to the quick growth of deer antlers.

Efficacy: Three randomized controlled trials in a total of 95 young and middle-aged men and 21 young females provide virtually no evidence that deer antler velvet supplements improve aerobic or anaerobic performance, muscular strength, or endurance. One of the trials randomized 38 active men aged 19–24 years to take 300 mg/d of a deer-antler-velvet extract, 1.5 g/d of a deer-antler-velvet powder, or a placebo and begin a strength- and endurance-training program. The supplements provided no significant ergogenic effects compared with placebo.

Safety: Studies have not adequately assessed the safety of deer antler velvet. The studies cited above found no side effects in participants taking deer-antler-velvet supplements. IGF-1 is available as a prescription medication, and its reported side effects include hypoglycemia, headache, edema, and joint pain. An evaluation of six deer-antler-velvet dietary supplements that were commercially available in 2013 found that five of them contained no deer IGF-1, and four were adulterated with human IGF-1. Only one of the six supplements contained a low level of deer IGF-1.

Implications for use: The research to date does not support taking deer-antler-velvet supplements to enhance exercise or athletic performance. The National Collegiate Athletic Association and the World Anti-Doping Agency ban the use of IGF-1 and its analogues in athletic competition.

Dehydroepiandrosterone

Dehydroepiandrosterone (DHEA) is a steroid hormone secreted by the adrenal cortex. The body can convert DHEA to the male hormone testosterone; testosterone's intermediary, androstenedione; and the female hormone estradiol. Testosterone is an anabolic steroid that promotes gains in muscle mass and strength when combined with resistance training.

Efficacy: The minimal research on DHEA's use to enhance exercise and athletic performance provides no evidence of benefit. One study, for example, randomly assigned 40 male weight lifters (average age 48 years) to receive DHEA (100 mg/day), androstenedione (100 mg/day), or a placebo for 12 weeks while continuing their training programs. Compared to placebo, the DHEA and androstenedione produced no statistically significant increase in strength, aerobic capacity, lean body mass, or testosterone levels. Another study randomly assigned 20 sedentary men 19–29 years of age to receive either 150 mg/day DHEA or a placebo for 6 of 8 weeks in combination with a resistance-training program. The supplement provided no benefits compared with placebo in increasing muscle strength, lean body mass, or testosterone concentrations.

Safety: Studies have not adequately assessed the safety of DHEA. The two short-term studies in men described above found no side effects from the DHEA; blood lipid levels and liver function remained normal. Other studies have found that in women, use of DHEA for months significantly raises serum testosterone but not estrogen levels, which can cause acne and growth of facial hair.

Implications for use: The research to date does not support taking DHEA supplements to enhance exercise or athletic performance. The National Collegiate Athletic Association and the World Anti-Doping Agency ban the use of DHEA.

Ginseng

Ginseng is a generic term for botanicals from the genus *Panax*. Some popular varieties are known as Chinese, Korean, American, and Japanese ginseng. Preparations made from ginseng roots have been used in traditional Chinese medicine for millennia as a tonic to improve stamina and vitality. So-called Siberian or Russian ginseng (*Eleutherococcus senticosus*), although unrelated to *Panax* ginseng, has also been used in traditional Chinese medicine to combat fatigue and strengthen the immune system.

Efficacy: Numerous small studies, with and without placebo controls, have investigated *Panax* ginseng's potential to improve the physical performance of athletes, regular and occasional exercisers, and largely sedentary individuals. In almost all cases, the studies found that *Panax ginseng* in various doses and preparations had no ergogenic effect on such measures as peak power output, time to exhaustion, perceived exertion, recovery from intense activity, oxygen consumption, or heart rate.

One review of studies of the effects of Siberian ginseng on endurance performance found that the five studies with the most rigorous research protocols (with a total of 55 men and 24 women) showed no effect of supplementation for up to 6 weeks on exercise performed for up to 120 minutes. A subsequent randomized controlled trial using a crossover design with nine male college tennis players found that 800 mg/day Siberian ginseng (prepared from the root and rhizome) for 8 weeks significantly improved endurance in a cycling trial, elevated VO_2max and heart rate, and increased fat oxidation.

Safety: Short-term *Panax* ginseng use appears to be safe; the most commonly reported adverse effects include headache, sleep disturbances, and gastrointestinal disorders. Short-term Siberian ginseng use also appears to be safe. The studies cited above reported no adverse effects, although other reports of clinical trials have listed insomnia as a rare side effect.

Implications for use: The research to date provides little support for taking ginseng to enhance exercise or athletic performance.

Glutamine

Glutamine is the most abundant amino acid in muscle, blood, and the body's free-amino-acid pool. It is synthesized in the body primarily from the BCAAs, and an adult consumes about 3–6 g/day in protein-containing foods. Glutamine is a key molecule in metabolism and energy production, and it contributes nitrogen for many critical biochemical reactions. It is an essential amino acid for critically ill patients when the body's need for glutamine exceeds its capacity to produce sufficient amounts.

Efficacy: Few studies have examined the effect of glutamine supplementation alone as an ergogenic aid. One study randomized 31 male and female weight lifters to receive either glutamine (0.9 g/kg lean body mass, or almost 45 g/day) or placebo while completing a 6-week strength-training program. There were no significant differences between the two groups in measures of strength, torque, or lean tissue mass, demonstrating that glutamine had no effect on muscle performance, body composition, or muscle-protein degradation. Another study compared the effect of glutamine (four doses of 0.3 g/kg body weight over 3 days) or placebo in 16 young adult men and women on recovery from eccentric exercise consisting of unilateral knee extensions. Supplementation with glutamine reduced the magnitude of strength loss, accelerated strength recovery, and diminished muscle soreness more quickly than placebo; these effects were more pronounced in the men. Some athletes use glutamine supplements in the hope that they will attenuate exercise-induced immune impairment and reduce their risk of developing upper respiratory tract infections. However, there is little research-based support for this benefit.

Safety: In the studies described above, the glutamine had no reported side effects. Many patients with serious catabolic illnesses, such as infections, intestinal diseases, and burns, take glutamine safely as part of their medical care. Daily oral doses ranging from 0.21 to 0.42 g/kg body weight glutamine (equivalent to 15–30 g/day in a person weighing 154 pounds) have provided no biochemical or clinical evidence of toxicity.

Implications for use: The research to date does not support taking glutamine alone to improve exercise and athletic performance.

Iron

Iron is an essential mineral and a structural component of hemoglobin, an erythrocyte protein that transfers oxygen from the lungs to the tissues, and myoglobin, a protein in muscles that provides them with oxygen. Iron is also necessary to metabolize substrates for energy as a component of cytochromes and to dehydrogenase enzymes involved in substrate oxidation. Iron deficiency impairs oxygen-carrying capacity and muscle function, and it limits people's ability to exercise and be active. Its detrimental effects can include fatigue and lethargy, lower aerobic capacity, and slower times in performance trials.

Iron balance is an important consideration for athletes who must pay attention to both iron intakes and iron losses. Teenage girls and premenopausal women are at increased risk of obtaining insufficient amounts of iron from their diets. They require more iron than teenage boys and men because they lose considerable iron due to menstruation, and they might not eat sufficient amounts of iron-containing foods.

Athletes of both sexes lose additional iron for several reasons. Physical activity produces acute inflammation that reduces iron absorption from the gut and iron use via a peptide, hepcidin, that regulates iron homeostasis. Iron is also lost in sweat. The destruction of erythrocytes in the feet because of frequent striking on hard surfaces leads to foot-strike hemolysis. Also, use of antiinflammatories and pain medications can lead to some blood loss from the gastrointestinal tract, thereby decreasing iron stores.

The richest dietary sources of heme iron (which is highly bioavailable) include lean meats and seafood. Plant-based foods—such as nuts, beans, vegetables, and fortified grain products—contain non-heme iron, which is less bioavailable than heme iron.

Efficacy: Although iron deficiency anemia decreases work capacity, there is conflicting evidence on whether milder iron deficiency without anemia impairs sport and exercise performance. One systematic review and meta-analysis to determine whether iron treatments (provided orally or by injection) improved iron status and aerobic capacity in iron-deficient but non- anemic endurance athletes identified 19 studies involving 80 men and 363 women with a mean age of 22 years. Iron treatments improved iron status as expected, but they did not guarantee improvement in aerobic capacity or indices of endurance performance. Another systematic review and meta-analysis compared the effects of iron supplementation with no supplementation on exercise performance in women of reproductive age. Most of the 24 studies identified were small (i.e., they randomly assigned fewer than 20 women to a treatment or control group) and had a risk of bias. Based on the limited data and heterogenicity of results, the study authors suggested that preventing and treating iron deficiency could improve the performance of female athletes in sports that require endurance, maximal power output, and strength.

Safety: Athletes can safely obtain recommended intakes of iron by consuming a healthy diet containing iron-rich foods and by taking an iron-containing dietary supplement as needed. High doses of iron may be prescribed for several weeks or months to treat iron deficiency, especially if anemia is present.

The UL for iron is 45 mg/day for men and women aged 14 and older and 40 mg/day for younger children. Acute intakes of more than 20 mg/kg iron from supplements or medicines can lead to gastric upset, constipation, nausea, abdominal pain, vomiting, and fainting, especially if users do not consume food at the same time. Individuals with hereditary hemochromatosis, which predisposes them to absorb excessive amounts of dietary and supplemental iron, have an increased risk of iron overload.

Implications for use: Correcting iron deficiency anemia improves work capacity, but there is conflicting evidence on whether milder iron deficiency without anemia impairs athletic performance. In a position statement, AND, DoC, and ACSM do not recommend routine supplementation of iron except in response to a healthcare provider's instruction, and note that such supplementation is only ergogenic if the individual has iron depletion. Furthermore, they warn that iron supplementation can cause gastrointestinal side effects.

The recommended dietary allowance (RDA) for iron is 11 mg for teenaged boys and 15 mg for teenaged girls. The RDA is 8 mg for men and 18 mg for women aged 50 and younger, and 8 mg for older adults of both sexes. Individuals who engage in intense exercise might require 30% to 70% more iron than moderately active and sedentary people. Recommended intakes of iron for vegetarians and vegans are 1.8 times higher than for people who eat meat.

Protein

Protein is necessary to build, maintain, and repair muscle. Exercise increases intramuscular protein oxidation and breakdown, after which muscle-protein synthesis increases for up to a day or two. Regular resistance exercise results in the accretion of myofibrillar protein (the predominant proteins in skeletal muscle) and an increase in skeletal muscle fiber size. Aerobic exercise leads to more modest protein accumulation in working muscle, primarily in the mitochondria, which enhances oxidative capacity (oxygen use) for future workouts.

Athletes must consider both protein quality and quantity to meet their needs for the nutrient. They must obtain essential amino acids (EAAs) from the diet or from supplementation to support muscle growth, maintenance, and repair. The nine EAAs are histidine, isoleucine, leucine, lysine, methionine, phenylalanine, threonine, tryptophan, and valine. Most complete proteins (those that contain all EAAs) are composed of about 40% EAAs, so a meal or snack with 25 g total protein provides about 10 g EAAs.

The potential of these amino acids to enhance exercise and athletic performance is not related to their incorporation into proteins.

Efficacy: Adequate protein in the diet is required to provide the EAAs necessary for muscle-protein synthesis and to minimize muscle-protein breakdown. Dietary protein consumption increases the concentration of amino acids in the blood, which muscle cells then take up. Sufficient protein is necessary primarily to optimize the training response to, and the recovery period after, exercise.

Muscle protein synthesis leading to increases in strength and muscle mass appears to be optimal with the consumption of high-quality protein (providing about 10 g EAAs) within 0–2 hours after exercise, in the early recovery phase. However, a meta-analysis of randomized clinical trials found that ingesting protein within an hour before or after exercise does not significantly increase muscle strength or size or facilitate muscle repair or remodeling. The period after exercise when protein intake reduces muscle protein breakdown, builds muscle, and increases mitochondrial proteins to enhance oxygen use by working muscles (the so-called "window of anabolic opportunity") can last for up to 24 hours.

Several studies in people engaged in resistance training show that consuming some protein before sleep can increase the rate of protein synthesis during the night and augment muscle mass and strength. Participants in these studies consumed a bedtime drink containing 27.5 or 40 g of the milk protein casein, which increased circulating amino acid levels throughout the night. Some studies show increased muscle protein synthesis when plasma levels of amino acids are raised.

Safety: The Food and Nutrition Board has not set a UL for protein, noting that the risk of adverse effects from excess protein from food is "very low". However, it advises caution for those obtaining high protein intakes from foods and supplements because of the limited data on their potential adverse effects. High-protein diets (e.g., those providing two to three times the RDA of 0.8 g/kg/day for healthy adults and 0.85 g/kg/day for adolescents) do not appear to increase the risk of renal stones or dehydration; compromise renal function; reduce bone health; or, when consumed for several months, alter glomerular filtration rate or blood levels of lipids, glucose, creatine, or blood urea nitrogen. Protein increases urinary calcium excretion, but this appears to have no consequence for long-term bone health and, in any event, is easily compensated for by the consumption of slightly more calcium.

Implications for use: Many foods—including meats, poultry, seafood, eggs, dairy products, beans, and nuts—contain protein. Protein powders and drinks are also available, most of which contain whey, one of the complete proteins isolated from milk. Digestion of casein, the main complete protein in milk, is slower than that of whey, so the release of amino acids from casein into the blood is slower. Soy protein lacks the EAA methionine and might lose some cysteine and lysine in processing; rice protein lacks the EAA isoleucine. Many protein supplements consist of a combination of these protein sources. All EAAs are necessary to stimulate muscle protein synthesis, so users should select singular or complementary protein sources accordingly. To maximize muscle adaptations to training, AND, DoC, and ACSM recommend that athletes consume 0.3 g/kg body weight of high-quality protein (e.g., about 20 g for a person weighing 150 lb) 0 to 2 hours after exercise and then every 3 to 5 hours.

Since the Food and Nutrition Board developed the RDA for protein, more recent data have suggested that athletes require a daily protein intake of 1.2 to 2.0 g/kg to support metabolic adaptations, muscle repair and remodeling, and protein turnover. Athletes might benefit from even greater amounts for short periods of intense training or when they reduce their energy intake to improve physique or achieve a competition weight. The 2007–2008 National Health and Nutrition Examination Survey showed that the average daily intake of protein by adult men is 100 g and by women is 69 g. Athletes who require additional protein can obtain it by consuming more protein-containing foods and, if needed, protein supplements and protein-fortified food and beverage products.

Quercetin

Quercetin is a polyphenolic flavonol that is naturally present in a variety of fruits (such as apples), vegetables (such as onions), and beverages (such as wine and, especially, tea). An analysis of National Health and Nutrition Examination Survey 1999–2002 data found that estimated daily total flavonol (including quercetin) consumption by adults averaged about 13 mg/day. The mechanisms by which quercetin might enhance exercise and athletic performance when taken in much larger amounts are not known, but many have been hypothesized. For example, quercetin might increase the number of mitochondria in muscle, reduce oxidative stress, decrease inflammation, and improve endothelial function (blood flow).

Efficacy: Numerous small studies have assessed quercetin in supplemental form as a potential ergogenic aid in young adult, mostly male, participants. These studies typically examined the endurance performance and VO_2max of participants engaged in aerobic activities, such as running or cycling trials, who received either quercetin (most often 1,000 mg/day) or placebo for 1 to 8 weeks. The effects of quercetin supplementation were inconsistent and varied by study, but they generally ranged from no ergogenic benefit to only a trivial or small improvement that might not be meaningful in real-world (in contrast to laboratory) exercise conditions.

Safety: The studies of trained athletes and untrained participants cited in the previous paragraph who took as much as 1,000 mg/day quercetin for up to 2 months found no side effects or safety concerns. The safety of longer-term use of that amount of quercetin or more has not been studied. FDA considers up to 500 mg/serving quercetin to be generally recognized as safe (GRAS) as an ingredient in foods such as beverages, processed fruits and fruit juices, grain products, pastas, and soft candies.

Implications for use: More research, including larger clinical trials, on quercetin supplementation to improve aerobic capacity in trained athletes during specific sports and competitions is needed before any recommendations can be made.

Ribose

Ribose, a naturally occurring 5-carbon sugar synthesized by cells and found in some foods, is involved in the production of ATP. The amount of ATP in muscle is limited, and it must continually be resynthesized. Therefore, theoretically, the more ribose in the body, the more potential ATP production.

Efficacy: The limited amount of research on ribose shows little if any benefit of doses ranging from 625 to 10,000 mg/day for up to 8 weeks for exercise capacity in both trained and untrained healthy adults.

Safety: The authors of the short-term studies investigating ribose as a potential ergogenic aid have not reported any safety concerns. No studies have assessed the safety of long-term ribose use as a dietary supplement.

Implications for use: Supplemental ribose does not appear to improve aerobic or anaerobic performance.

Sodium Bicarbonate

Sodium bicarbonate is commonly known as baking soda. The consumption of several teaspoons of sodium bicarbonate over a short time temporarily increases blood pH by acting as a buffering agent. The precise mechanism by which this induced alkalosis leads to an ergogenic response to exercise is unclear. It is thought that "bicarbonate loading" enhances disposal of hydrogen ions that accumulate and efflux from working muscles as they generate energy in the form of ATP via anaerobic glycolysis from high-intensity exercise, thereby reducing the metabolic acidosis that contributes to fatigue. As a result, supplementation with sodium bicarbonate might improve performance in short-term, intense exercises (e.g., sprinting and swimming) and in intermittently intense sports (e.g., boxing and tennis).

Efficacy: Many studies have assessed sodium bicarbonate as an ergogenic aid in swimmers, cyclists, rowers, boxers, tennis and rugby players, judo practitioners, and others. These studies usually included a small number of participants who underwent one or more trials in a laboratory over several days.

Because the research results are conflicting, the activities and individuals most likely to benefit from sodium bicarbonate supplementation in real-world conditions is not clear. Reviewers of these studies generally agree that taking about 300 mg/kg body weight sodium bicarbonate might provide a minor to moderate performance benefit in strenuous exercise over several minutes and in sports that involve intermittent, high-intensity activity. However, individuals have varied responses to bicarbonate loading; the practice does not benefit some users, and it can worsen rather than enhance performance in others. Recreationally active individuals, in particular, might find the supplements to be ergogenic for one exercise session but not another. Many study findings suggest that supplementation with sodium bicarbonate is most likely to improve the performance of trained athletes.

Safety: The main side effect of sodium bicarbonate supplementation in gram quantities is gastrointestinal distress, including nausea, stomach pain, diarrhea, and vomiting. Supplement users can reduce or minimize this distress by consuming the total dose in smaller amounts multiple times over an hour with fluid and a snack of carbohydrate-rich food. Sodium bicarbonate is 27.4% sodium by weight; 1 teaspoon (4.6 g) contains 1,259 mg sodium. A 70-kg individual ingesting a recommended dose of 300 mg/kg body weight would consume approximately 5,750 mg sodium. Such a large intake of sodium with fluid can lead to temporary hyperhydration, which could be useful in activities where large sweat losses might otherwise lead to significant fluid deficits. However, the slight increase in body weight from fluid retention might hinder performance in other sports. Studies have not evaluated the safety (and effectiveness) of long-term use of sodium bicarbonate as an ergogenic aid over months or longer.

Implications for use: The amount of sodium bicarbonate in recommended servings of dietary supplements—about 300 mg/kg body weight, or the equivalent of 4–5 teaspoons of baking soda for most individuals taken 1–2 hours before exercise in one or multiple doses as a pill or as a powder mixed with a flavored fluid—is generally much less than the quantity that could enhance exercise and athletic performance. Many athletes find this amount of sodium bicarbonate powder dissolved in fluid to be unpalatably salty. Researchers support the use of bicarbonate for improving sports performance in suitable athletic competitions under the direction of an expert in sports medicine, but it notes that more research might be required to understand how the supplement should be used for best results.

Tart or Sour Cherry

The Montmorency variety of tart or sour cherry (*Prunus cerasus*) contains anthocyanins and other polyphenolic phytochemicals, such as quercetin. Researchers hypothesize that these compounds have antiinflammatory and antioxidant effects that might facilitate exercise recovery by reducing pain and inflammation, strength loss and muscle damage from intense activity, and hyperventilation trauma from endurance activities. The labels on tart-cherry juice and concentrate products do not usually indicate that they are dietary supplements, although the labels on products containing encapsulated tart-cherry powder do.

Efficacy: Much of the limited research on use of tart cherry to enhance exercise and athletic performance involves short-term use of a tart-cherry product or placebo by young resistance- trained men for about a week before a test of strength (such as single-leg extensions or back squats); participants continue taking the supplements for about 2 days after the test. Study results vary, but the benefits appear to include more rapid recovery of strength and lower perceived muscle soreness. One pilot study investigated the use of tart-cherry juice (472 ml/day; the equivalent of 100–120 whole cherries) or a placebo for a week before a marathon and 2 days afterward in 13 male and 7 female runners (age range 24–50 years). None of the participants who drank the juice experienced airway inflammation causing upper respiratory tract symptoms after the marathon (a common complaint in many marathon runners), but half of those drinking the placebo did. Another study compared a supplement containing 480 mg freeze-dried Montmorency tart-cherry-skin powder (CherryPURE) with a placebo in 18 male and 9 female endurance-trained runners and triathletes (age range 18–26 years). Participants took the supplements once a day for 10 days, including the day they ran a half-marathon, then for 2 days after the run. Participants taking the tart-cherry supplement averaged a statistically significant 13% shorter race finish time and had lower levels of blood markers of inflammation and muscle catabolism than the placebo takers, but perceptions of soreness of the quadriceps muscles did not differ significantly between the groups.

Further research is needed to determine the value of tart-cherry products for enhancing performance and recovery from intense exercise or participation in sports—especially when used on a regular basis—and the amounts of supplement, juice, or concentrate needed to provide any benefits.

Safety: Studies have not identified any side effects of the fresh tart-cherry juice or concentrate or of supplements of dried tart-cherry-skin powder. However, they have not adequately assessed the safety of tart-cherry dietary supplements.

Implications for use: There is no expert consensus on the value of taking tart-cherry products to enhance exercise and athletic performance.

Tribulus Terrestris

Tribulus terrestris (common names include bindii, goat's-head, bullhead, and tackweed), is a fruit-bearing plant that is most common in Africa, Asia, Australia, and Europe. It has been used since ancient times in Greece, China, and Asia to treat low libido and infertility. *Tribulus terrestris* extracts contain many compounds, including steroidal saponins. Some marketers claim that *Tribulus terrestris* enhances exercise and athletic performance by increasing serum concentrations of testosterone and luteinizing hormone, but studies have not adequately determined its potential mechanisms of action.

Efficacy: Only a few small, short-term clinical trials have investigated *Tribulus terrestris* as an ergogenic aid, and none since 2007. In one study, 10 mg/kg or 20 mg/kg *Tribulus terrestris* or a placebo taken for 4 weeks by men aged 20–36 years did not raise levels of either hormone. A study in 15 resistance-trained men found no differences among those taking 3.21 mg/kg *Tribulus terrestris* or placebo for 8 weeks in improvements in bench and leg press scores or in muscle mass. In 22 elite male rugby players aged 19.8 years, on average, who were randomly assigned to take 450 mg/day *Tribulus terrestris* or a placebo for 5 weeks, the supplement did not have a superior effect on strength or lean body mass.

Safety: The only toxicity studies of *Tribulus terrestris* were conducted in animals, where unspecified high intakes led to severe heart, liver, and kidney damage. The clinical studies described above found no side effects of *Tribulus terrestris*. One case report involved a morbidly obese Iranian man, age 28, who consumed 2 L/day *Tribulus terrestris* water for 2 days before being hospitalized with seizures, severe weakness in the legs, malaise, and poor appetite. Subsequent tests indicated hepatotoxicity, nephrotoxicity, and neurotoxicity. The man's condition improved after he discontinued the water, but the water was not tested to determine the presence or amount of *Tribulus terrestris* or any other potential toxin or contaminant.

Implications for use: The Australian Institute of Sport advises against the use of *Tribulus terrestris* by athletes, noting that this supplement and other claimed testosterone boosters are banned from athletic competitions or have a high risk of being contaminated with substances that, if ingested, could lead to positive drug-screening results.

Ingredients Banned from Dietary Supplements

Androstenedione

Androstenedione is an anabolic steroid precursor, or prohormone, that the body converts to testosterone (which induces muscle growth) and estrogen. Major League Baseball slugger Mark McGwire popularized androstenedione as an ergogenic aid in 1998. However, two randomized clinical trials found no performance benefits from androstenedione supplements. In one study, 10 healthy young men (ages 19–29 years) took a single 100-mg dose of androstenedione. Another 20 were randomized to receive either 300 mg/day androstenedione or a placebo for 6 of 8 weeks while undergoing resistance-training and muscle-strengthening exercises. The short-term or longer-term use of the supplement did not affect serum testosterone concentrations, nor did it produce any significantly greater gains in resistance-training performance, muscle strength, or lean body mass. However, participants who took androstenedione for the 6 weeks experienced significant declines in their high-density lipoprotein (HDL) cholesterol levels and significant increases in serum estrogens. A similar study randomized 50 men (ages 35–65 years) to take 200 mg/day androstenedione, 200 mg/day of the related androstenediol, or a placebo for 12 weeks while participating in a high-intensity resistance training program. The supplements did not improve participants' muscular strength or lean body mass compared with placebo, but they significantly decreased HDL cholesterol levels and raised levels of serum estrogens. Among participants taking the androstenedione, testosterone levels increased significantly by 16% after 1 month of use but declined to pre-treatment levels by 12 weeks, in part due to downregulation of endogenous testosterone synthesis.

In March 2004, FDA warned companies to cease distributing androstenedione-containing dietary supplements. The rationale was the lack of sufficient information to establish that such products could reasonably be expected to be safe and that FDA had never approved androstenedione as a new dietary ingredient permitted in supplements. The U.S. Department of Justice classified androstenedione as a Schedule III controlled substance (defined as a drug with a moderate to low potential for physical and psychological dependence) in 2004. The National Collegiate Athletic Association, International Olympic Committee, and World Anti-Doping Agency ban the use of androstenedione.

Dimethylamylamine

Dimethylamylamine (DMAA) is a stimulant formerly included in some pre-workout and other dietary supplements claimed to enhance exercise performance and build muscle. Studies have not evaluated DMAA in humans as a potential ergogenic aid. In 2013, FDA declared products containing this ingredient to be illegal after it received 86 reports of deaths and illnesses associated with dietary supplements containing DMAA. These reports described heart problems as well as nervous system and psychiatric disorders. Furthermore, FDA had never approved DMAA as a new dietary ingredient that would reasonably be expected to be safe. Although products marketed as dietary supplements containing DMAA are illegal in the United States, discontinued, reformulated, or even new products containing DMAA might still be found in the U.S. marketplace. The Department of Defense's Human Performance Resource Center maintains a list of currently available products that contain DMAA or are labeled as containing DMAA, 1-3-dimethylamylamine, or an equivalent chemical or marketing name (e.g., methylhexaneamine or geranium extract).

The FDA also determined that dietary supplements containing 1,3-dimethybutylamine (DMBA), a stimulant chemically related to DMAA, are adulterated. As with DMAA, FDA had never approved this stimulant as a new dietary ingredient. The agency contended that there is no history of use or data offering sufficient assurance that this compound is not associated with "a significant or unreasonable risk of illness or injury".

Ephedra

Ephedra (also known as ma huang), a plant native to China, contains ephedrine alkaloids, which are stimulant compounds; the primary alkaloid is ephedrine. In the 1990s, ephedra—frequently combined with caffeine—was a popular ingredient in dietary supplements sold to enhance exercise and athletic performance and to promote weight loss.

No studies have evaluated the use of ephedra dietary supplements, with or without caffeine, as ergogenic aids. Instead, available studies have used the related synthetic compound ephedrine together with caffeine and typically measured the effects 1–2 hours after a single dose. These studies showed that the ephedrine–caffeine combination produced a 20–30% increase in power and endurance, but ephedrine alone had no significant effects on exercise-performance parameters, such as oxygen consumption or time to exhaustion. No data show any sustained improvement in athletic performance over time with continued dosing of ephedrine with caffeine.

Ephedra use has been associated with death and serious adverse effects, including nausea, vomiting, psychiatric symptoms (such as anxiety and mood change), hypertension, palpitations, stroke, seizures, and heart attack. In 2004, FDA banned the sale of dietary supplements containing ephedrine alkaloids in the United States because they are associated with "an unreasonable risk of illness or injury". The World Anti-Doping Agency prohibits the use of ephedrine in amounts that lead to urine concentrations of ephedrine (or the related methylephedrine) exceeding 10 mcg/ml.

Regulation of Dietary Supplements to Enhance Exercise and Athletic Performance

The FDA regulates dietary supplements for exercise and athletic performance in accordance with the Dietary Supplement Health and Education Act of 1994. Like other dietary supplements, exercise- and athletic-performance supplements differ from over-the-counter or prescription medications in that they do not require premarket review or approval by FDA. Supplement manufacturers are responsible for determining that their products are safe and their label claims are truthful and not misleading, although they are not required to provide this evidence to FDA before marketing their products. If FDA finds a supplement to be unsafe, it may remove the product from the market or ask the manufacturer to voluntarily recall the product. The FDA and Federal Trade

Commission (FTC) may also take regulatory actions against manufacturers that make unsubstantiated physical-performance or other claims about their products.

The FDA permits dietary supplements to contain only "dietary ingredients," such as vitamins, minerals, amino acids, herbs, and other botanicals. It does not permit these products to contain pharmaceutical ingredients, and manufacturers may not promote them to diagnose, treat, cure, or prevent any disease.

Safety Considerations

Like all dietary supplements, supplements used to enhance exercise and athletic performance can have side effects and might interact with prescription and over-the-counter medications. In some cases, the active constituents of botanical or other ingredients promoted as ergogenic aids are unknown or uncharacterized. Furthermore, many such products contain multiple ingredients that have not been adequately tested in combination with one another. People interested in taking dietary supplements to enhance their exercise and athletic performance should talk with their healthcare providers about the use of these products.

The Uniformed Services University of the Health Sciences and the U.S. Anti-Doping Agency maintain a list of products marketed as dietary supplements that contain stimulants, steroids, hormone- like ingredients, controlled substances, or unapproved drugs and that can have health risks for warfighters and others who take them for bodybuilding or other forms of physical performance.

Fraudulent and Adulterated Products

The FDA requires the manufacture of dietary supplements to comply with quality standards that ensure that these products contain only the labeled ingredients and amounts and are free of undeclared substances and unsafe levels of contaminants. However, FDA notes that products marketed as dietary supplements for bodybuilding are among those most often adulterated with undeclared or deceptively labeled ingredients, such as synthetic anabolic steroids or prescription medications. As one example, some products sold for bodybuilding are adulterated with selective androgen receptor modulators (SARMs); these synthetic drugs are designed to mimic the effects of testosterone. Using such tainted products can cause health problems and lead to disqualification of athletes from competition if a drug test shows that they have consumed prohibited substances, even if they have done so unknowingly. FDA has warned against the use of any body- building products that claim to contain steroids or steroid-like substances. It recommends that a user contact their healthcare provider if they experience symptoms possibly related to these products, especially nausea, weakness, fatigue, fever, abdominal pain, chest pain, shortness of breath, jaundice (yellowing of skin or whites of eyes), or brown or discolored urine.

Some dietary-supplement firms have hired third-party certification companies to verify the identity and content of their supplements to enhance exercise and athletic performance, thus providing some extra, independent assurance that the products contain the labeled amounts of ingredients and are free of many banned substances and drugs. The major companies providing this certification service are NSF (nsf.org) through its Certified for Sport program, Informed-Choice (informed-choice.org), and the Banned Substances Control Group (bscg.org). The products that meet the requirements of these companies may carry the certifier's official logo and are listed on the certifier's website.

Interactions with Medications

Some ingredients in dietary supplements used to enhance exercise and athletic performance can interact with certain medications. For example, intakes of large doses of antioxidant supplements, such as vitamins C and E, during cancer chemotherapy or radiotherapy could reduce the effectiveness of these therapies by inhibiting cellular oxidative damage in cancerous cells. Ginseng can reduce the anticoagulant effects of the blood thinner warfarin (Coumadin or Jantoven). Iron supplements can reduce the bioavailability of levodopa (used to treat Parkinson's disease) and levothyroxine (Levothyroid, Levoxyl, Synthroid, and others, for hypothyroidism and goiter), so users should take iron supplements at a different time of the day than these two drugs. Cimetidine (Tagamet HB, used to treat duodenal ulcers) can slow the rate of caffeine clearance from the body and thereby increase the risk of adverse effects from caffeine consumption.

Individuals taking dietary supplements and medications on a regular basis should discuss the use of these products with their healthcare providers.

Performance-enhancing Supplements

Performance-enhancing substances (PESs) are used commonly by children and adolescents in attempts to improve athletic performance.

Studies looking at the purity of supplements find high rates of contamination with possibly harmful substances. Also, many products do not contain the ingredients listed on the label.

Protein and Creatine

Young athletes sometimes take protein supplements or nucleic acid supplements *(creatine)* to help their sports performance. However, studies have not shown these supplements help improve sports performance in younger athletes.

During puberty athletes grow and become stronger and their performance often improves very quickly. Creatine does not appear to offer any additional benefit in this age group. Most young athletes who eat a healthy, well-balanced diet do not need and would not benefit from protein supplements. However, vegetarians may be at risk of not eating enough protein and may benefit from meal planning with a registered dietitian.

Energy Drinks and Stimulants

Caffeine is found in a variety of foods and drinks. About 3 out of 4 children consume caffeine on any given day.

The FDA regulates the amount of caffeine in items sold as foods and drinks; however, it does not have control over items sold as supplements, such as energy drinks. It is very difficult to know how much caffeine is in many of these products. Consuming too much caffeine, such as that found in powders, pills, and multiple energy drinks, can be dangerous.

Although caffeine appears to improve some parts of sports performance in adults, the effects vary a lot. The effects of caffeine are not as well studied in children.

Young athletes who take medicine for attention-deficit/hyperactivity disorder need to be very careful when using energy drinks that contain stimulants. They also need to keep track of their fluid intake and how they respond to severe heat and humid conditions when exercising or competing.

Vitamins and Minerals

Athletes do not need vitamins and mineral supplements if they are eating healthy, well-balanced meals. Low iron levels are associated with decreases in athletic performance, but high doses of iron, or of any other vitamin or mineral, have not been shown to improve sports performance in otherwise healthy athletes.

Anabolic Steroids

Anabolic steroids are drugs that are illegal without a doctor's prescription. Athletes sometimes use anabolic steroids to enhance muscle strength and size. Nonathletes may use anabolic steroids because they want to look more muscular. However, there are side effects. Anabolic steroids stop growth in children and teens who are still gaining height. They may also cause long-term problems with the heart, skin, and other organs that can be severe and may be irreversible.

Anti-inflammatory steroids, such as prednisone, that are used for asthma and other conditions are safe and often needed for young athletes when prescribed by a doctor.

Energy Bars

Energy bars are supplemental bars containing cereals and other high energy foods targeted at people that require quick energy but do not have time for a meal. They are different from energy drinks, which contain caffeine, whereas bars provide food energy.

Energy bars (also called nutrition or sports bars) vary in how much protein, fat and carbohydrates they contain, as well as in the vitamins, minerals and other compounds that are added. They may be marketed as "low-carb," "high-carb," "low-glycemic-index" or "high-protein" (all the diet fads are covered). A few boast organic ingredients or provide extras like herbs and omega-3 fats.

But they won't make you more energetic, stronger or faster than other foods. Nor will they improve brain function or do any of the other things that may be implied by the bar's name or promoters. Many, in fact, are just souped-up candy bars, loaded with sugar and fat and thus extra calories. But some can be good occasional snacks.

Raising the Bar

- Not all bars are created equal, so read the nutrition information and ingredients. Look for whole grains like rolled oats, nuts, peanut butter or fruit at or near the top of the ingredient list (not high-fructose corn syrup, brown rice syrup or maltitol—all sweeteners).
- Choose bars with more fibre. Fibre typically ranges from two to five grams.
- Calories usually range from 170 to 300. Lower-calorie bars simply tend to be smaller. Some bars have as many calories as a small meal.
- Look for low saturated fat. Most bars have two to five grams; Atkins bars have more.
- A high-protein bar or other high-protein snack after strenuous exercise may help older people build a little more muscle, but most people don't need extra protein.
- Don't judge a bar by how many added vitamins and minerals it has. You're better off getting these from natural food sources or a multivitamin/mineral supplements that provides 100 percent of the daily values.

Sports Drinks

Sports drinks are beverages that are specially formulated to help people rehydrate during or after exercise. They are usually rich in carbohydrates the most efficient source of energy.

As well as carbs, which are important in maintaining exercise and sport performance, sports drinks usually contain sweeteners and preservatives.

Sports drinks also contain electrolytes (minerals such as chloride, calcium, magnesium, sodium and potassium), which, along with body fluid, diminish as you exercise and sweat.

Replacing the electrolytes lost during training promotes proper rehydratio, which is important in delaying the onset of fatigue during exercise.

Keeping rehyrdated is particularly important for people with diabetes who have an increased risk of dehydration due to high levels of blood glucose.

Types of Sport Drinks

There are three main types of sports drinks available, all of which contain various levels of fluid, electrolytes and carbohydrate.

Isotonic

Isotonic drinks contain similar concentrations of salt and sugar as in the human body:

- Quickly replaces fluids lost through sweating and supplies a boost of carbohydrate.
- The preferred choice for most athletes, including middle and long-distance running or those involved in team sports.

Hypertonic

Hypertonic drinks contain a higher concentration of salt and sugar than the human body:

- Normally consumed post-workout to supplement daily carbohydrate intake and top-up muscle glycogen stores.
- Can be taken during ultra-distance events to meet the high energy demands, but must be used in conjunction with isotonic drinks to replace lost fluids.

Hypotonic

Hypotonic drinks contain a lower concentration of salt and sugar than the human body:

- Quickly replaces fluids lost by sweating.
- Suitable for athletes who require fluid without a carbohydrate boost, e.g. gymnasts.

Most sports drinks are moderately isotonic, containing between 4 and 5 heaped teaspoons of sugar per five ounce (13 and 19 grams per 250ml) serving.

Risk of Water Intoxication

While water is the best option for rehydrating your body, drinking excessive amounts can cause an imbalance of electrolytes in the body. This condition is known as water intoxication and although it is very rare, it can be fatal.

It occurs when large quantities of plain water are consumed to replace the fluid and electrolytes lost through heavy sweating caused by either hot weather or exercise, or a combination of the two.

The resulting low concentration of electrolytes can cause over hydratio, which disrupts nerve cell function. Severe over hydration can lead to disoriented behaviour, convulsions, coma, and even death.

To reduce the risk of water intoxicatio, most sports drinks comprise of ingredients that replenish fluids and electrolytes in a similar ratio to that usually found in the human body. However, some products contain low concentrations of electrolytes, so excess consumption of them could still cause an imbalance of these minerals.

Controversy Surrounding Sports Drinks

In July 2012, research published by the Guardian questioned the alleged benefits of sports drinks, such as enhanced performance and recovery, with experts from the University of Oxford claiming there is not enough evidence to support the claims from manufacturers and advertisers.

The research, which was published in the peer-reviewed medical journal BMJ Ope, involved a systematic assessment of magazine and website-based claims for improved sports performance and recovery made by advertisers for sports-related products, including drinks and supplements.

The researchers said they found a significant lack of evidence to support the beneficial effect claims made by the vast majority of products.

Of the websites and magazines that did provide evidence to back their claims, half of the evidence was deemed to be unreliable.

Based on their findings, they concluded that it is practically impossible for people to make informed choices about the pros and cons of advertised sports drinks and other sports-related products.

References

- Fitness-sports-nutrition-4157142: verywellfit.com, Retrieved 06 July, 2019
- Supplements-4014137: verywellfit.com, Retrieved 08 March, 2019
- ExerciseAndAthleticPerformance-HealthProfessional: ods.od.nih.gov, Retrieved 11 January, 2019
- Performance-Enhancing-Substances: healthychildren.org, Retrieved 19 August, 2019
- What-makes-good-energy-bar, healthy-eating: berkeleywellness.com, Retrieved 22 March, 2019
- Sports-drinks: diabetes.co.uk, Retrieved 25 August, 2019

Permissions

All chapters in this book are published with permission under the Creative Commons Attribution Share Alike License or equivalent. Every chapter published in this book has been scrutinized by our experts. Their significance has been extensively debated. The topics covered herein carry significant information for a comprehensive understanding. They may even be implemented as practical applications or may be referred to as a beginning point for further studies.

We would like to thank the editorial team for lending their expertise to make the book truly unique. They have played a crucial role in the development of this book. Without their invaluable contributions this book wouldn't have been possible. They have made vital efforts to compile up to date information on the varied aspects of this subject to make this book a valuable addition to the collection of many professionals and students.

This book was conceptualized with the vision of imparting up-to-date and integrated information in this field. To ensure the same, a matchless editorial board was set up. Every individual on the board went through rigorous rounds of assessment to prove their worth. After which they invested a large part of their time researching and compiling the most relevant data for our readers.

The editorial board has been involved in producing this book since its inception. They have spent rigorous hours researching and exploring the diverse topics which have resulted in the successful publishing of this book. They have passed on their knowledge of decades through this book. To expedite this challenging task, the publisher supported the team at every step. A small team of assistant editors was also appointed to further simplify the editing procedure and attain best results for the readers.

Apart from the editorial board, the designing team has also invested a significant amount of their time in understanding the subject and creating the most relevant covers. They scrutinized every image to scout for the most suitable representation of the subject and create an appropriate cover for the book.

The publishing team has been an ardent support to the editorial, designing and production team. Their endless efforts to recruit the best for this project, has resulted in the accomplishment of this book. They are a veteran in the field of academics and their pool of knowledge is as vast as their experience in printing. Their expertise and guidance has proved useful at every step. Their uncompromising quality standards have made this book an exceptional effort. Their encouragement from time to time has been an inspiration for everyone.

The publisher and the editorial board hope that this book will prove to be a valuable piece of knowledge for students, practitioners and scholars across the globe.

Index

A
Achilles Tendonitis, 156, 158, 202
Adductor Strain, 117-119
Ankle Arthroscopy, 35, 41-42
Ankle Sprain, 35, 38, 42-43, 73, 150, 155, 158, 160
Anterior Cruciate Ligament, 33, 57, 69, 89-90, 112-113, 150-151, 153, 155, 157, 160
Articular Cartilage, 11, 33, 51-53, 58, 72, 78, 81, 98-106, 112-113
Athletic Pubalgia, 116-118, 121-122
Atopic Dermatitis, 170

B
Bankart Lesion, 37
Bone Spurs, 10, 47

C
Cavus Foot Reconstruction, 48-49
Chevron Osteotomy, 40
Chiropractic Care, 4-6
Collagen Fibrils, 80, 83, 86
Compartment Syndrome, 24-25, 42, 72, 74, 78, 136
Computed Tomography, 9, 11, 29, 57, 121, 136
Coronal Image, 18
Cryotherapy, 35, 163, 167-171, 203

E
Edema, 13, 17-18, 23-26, 28, 47-48, 60, 94, 97, 121, 230
Endurance Exercise, 2, 195, 221, 226-227
Epimysium, 14, 27, 137
Extra Cellular Matrix, 80

F
Flatfoot, 44, 49-50
Foot Fusion, 50-51

G
Glenohumeral Internal Rotation, 36, 135
Glenoid Socket, 129-131, 133

H
Hematoma, 13, 15-17, 20-21, 25, 27-28, 97-98, 102, 138
Hip Tendonitis, 71, 115-116
Hyaluronic Acid, 56, 101
Hydrotherapy, 163, 171-173, 195-197, 204
Hypertension, 2, 172, 240

I
Isotope Bone, 10-11

K
Kinesiology Taping, 60
Knee Stability, 33-34, 54, 160

L
Labral Tears, 34, 58
Lateral Epicondylitis, 140-143, 146-147, 159
Lumbar Lordosis, 68

M
Magnetic Resonance Imaging, 9, 11, 57, 117, 124, 136, 146
Medial Collateral Ligament, 33, 89, 112, 157, 159
Meniscal Tear, 52, 104, 155
Meniscus, 32, 52-55, 112-114, 148, 150, 155
Migraine, 169-170
Muscle Contraction, 27, 93, 208
Muscle Hernias, 14, 28
Muscle Lesion, 14
Muscular Strength, 2, 230, 239
Musculoskeletal Injuries, 4, 92, 182, 201, 203
Myofibril, 26, 136
Myotendinous Junction, 12

N
Nonsteroidal Anti-inflammatory Drugs, 57, 118, 175

O
Orthopaedic Rehabilitation, 56
Orthopedic Physical Therapy, 60-65, 67-69
Orthopedic Sports Medicine, 32
Osteoarthritis, 34, 50, 56, 59-60, 72, 78, 100, 102, 144, 172, 176, 181
Osteochondritis Dissecans, 45-46, 48, 145
Osteonecrosis, 11, 45-47
Oswestry Disability Index, 57

P
Palpable Gap, 13, 16-17
Palpation, 62, 64, 117, 143
Partial Meniscectomy, 53-54
Patella Tendons, 85
Perifascial Fluid, 16-17, 21, 23-24

Perimysium, 14-15, 92, 137
Positive Performance, 8, 200
Posterior Cruciate Ligament, 33, 112-114

Q
Quadriceps Tendon, 33, 87, 112
Quality Metrics, 54

R
Rectus Femoris Muscle, 29
Reflect Lipomatous, 29
Rotator Cuff Tears, 9, 37, 58, 77, 133, 135-136

S
Scarf Osteotomy, 40
Sciatic Nerve, 15, 177

Shear Stiffness Values, 23
Sheathed Tendons, 81, 90
Shin Splints, 71, 124-127, 149, 152, 156
Spondylolisthesis, 174, 178-179
Sport Psychology, 1, 6-8
Sports Hernia, 122-124, 193
Sports Nutrition, 1, 205-213, 216, 222
Sports Vision, 1, 211
Stress Fractures, 45, 47, 125, 127, 174, 180
Stress Relaxation, 84-85

T
Tendon Transfer, 34, 43-45, 49
Tenoperiosteum, 125-126

CPSIA information can be obtained
at www.ICGtesting.com
Printed in the USA
BVHW051703180820
586707BV00003B/73